THE IMMUNE SYSTEM

GENES, RECEPTORS, SIGNALS

ACADEMIC PRESS RAPID MANUSCRIPT REPRODUCTION

The Proceedings of a Conference
Held at Squaw Valley, California
March 1974

THE IMMUNE SYSTEM

GENES, RECEPTORS, SIGNALS

edited by

ELI E. SERCARZ

Department of Bacteriology
University of California
Los Angeles, California

ALAN R. WILLIAMSON

Department of Biochemistry
National Institute of Medical Research
London, England

C. FRED FOX

Department of Bacteriology
University of California
Los Angeles, California

ACADEMIC PRESS New York and London 1974
A Subsidiary of Harcourt Brace Jovanovich, Publishers

ACADEMIC PRESS, INC.
111 Fifth Avenue, New York, New York 10003

United Kingdom Edition published by
ACADEMIC PRESS, INC. (LONDON) LTD.
24/28 Oval Road, London NW1

LIBRARY OF CONGRESS CATALOG CARD NUMBER: 74-11114

PRINTED IN THE UNITED STATES OF AMERICA

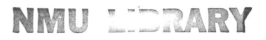

CONTENTS

I. V REGION: STRUCTURE AND GENETICS—
MOLECULAR BASIS OF ANTIBODY SPECIFICITY

II. V REGION: STRUCTURE AND GENETICS—
GENETIC CONTROL OF VARIABLE REGION STRUCTURE

v

VI. B-CELL ACTIVITIES–
DEVELOPMENT AND PROPAGATION OF CLONES

VII. T CELL EFFECTS ON OTHER CELLS–
SUPPRESSOR T CELLS

VIII. T CELL EFFECTS ON OTHER CELLS— MEDIATORS AND MATRICES

IX. ON-OFF SIGNALS: CELLULAR DISCRIMINATION AND GENETIC CONTROL

LIST OF CONTRIBUTORS

Diana F. Amsbaugh, Laboratory of Microbial Immunity and the Laboratory of Microbiology, National Institute of Allergy and Infectious Diseases, Bethesda, Maryland 20014

L. M. Amzel, Johns Hopkins University School of Medicine, Baltimore, Maryland 21205

Phillip J. Baker, Laboratory of Microbial Immunity and the Laboratory of Microbiology, National Institute of Allergy and Infectious Diseases, Bethesda, Maryland 20014

P. Barstad, Division of Biology, California Institute of Technology, Pasadena, California 91109

Kathleen B. Bechtol, Division of Immunology, Department of Medicine, Stanford University School of Medicine, Stanford, California 94305

Baruj Benacerraf, Department of Pathology, Harvard Medical School, Boston, Massachusetts 02115

S. Z. Ben-Sasson, National Institute of Allergy and Infectious Diseases, Bethesda, Maryland 20014

Hans Binz, Department of Medical Microbiology, University of Zurich, Zurich, Switzerland

Barbara K. Birshtein, Department of Cell Biology, Albert Einstein College of Medicine, Bronx, New York 10461

Bonnie Blomberg, The Salk Institute, P. O. Box 1809, San Diego, California 92112

Jacques M. Chiller, Department of Experimental Pathology, Scripps Clinic and Research Foundation, La Jolla, California 92037

G. H. Cohen, Laboratory of Molecular Biology, National Institute of Arthritis, Metabolism and Digestive Diseases, Bethesda, Maryland 20014

Melvin Cohn, The Salk Institute, P.O. Box 1809, San Diego, California 92112

Robert E. Cone, Basel Institute for Immunology, 487 Grenzacherstrasse, CH-4058 Basel, Switzerland

Richard G. H. Cotton, MRC Laboratory of Molecular Biology, Hills Road, Cambridge, CB2 2QH, England

Nicholas J. Cowan, MRC Laboratory of Molecular Biology, Hills Road, Cambridge, CB2 2QH, England

Susan E. Cullen, Department of Cell Biology, Albert Einstein College of Medicine, Bronx, New York 10461

A. J. Cunningham, Department of Microbiology, The John Curtin School of Medical Research, Canberra, Australia

D. R. Davies, Laboratory of Molecular Biology, National Institute of Arthritis, Metabolism and Digestive Diseases, Bethesda, Maryland 20014

Terry L. Delovitch, Division of Immunology, Department of Medicine, Stanford University School of Medicine, Stanford, California 94305

A. Faye Dewey, Department of Pathology, University of Pennsylvania Medical School, Philadelphia, Pennsylvania 19174

Michael Doenhoff, The Chester Beatty Institute, London, England

Wulf Droege, Basel Institute for Immunology, 487 Grenzacherstrasse, CH-4058 Basel, Switzerland

Richard W. Dutton, Department of Biology, University of California, San Diego, La Jolla, California 92037

Marc Feldmann, ICRF Tumour Immunology Unit, University College, London, England

F. Finkelman, National Institute of Allergy and Infectious Diseases, Bethesda, Maryland 20014

William Geckeler, The Salk Institute, P.O. Box 1809, San Diego, California 92112

Richard K. Gershon, Department of Pathology, Yale University School of Medicine, New Haven, Connecticut 06510

Melvyn Greaves, ICRF Tumour Immunology Unit, University College, London, England

LIST OF CONTRIBUTORS

I. Green, National Institute of Allergy and Infectious Diseases, Bethesda, Maryland 20014

Günter J. Hämmerling, Division of Immunology, Department of Medicine, Stanford University School of Medicine, Stanford, California 94305

Leonore A. Herzenberg, Department of Genetics, Stanford University School of Medicine, Stanford, California 94305

T. Honjo, Laboratory of Molecular Genetics, National Institute of Child Health and Human Development, Bethesda, Maryland 20014

L. Hood, Division of Biology, California Institute of Technology, Pasadena, California 91109

John K. Inman, National Institute of Allergy and Infectious Diseases, Bethesda, Maryland 20014

George Janossy, Department of Immunology, Clinical Research Centre, Harrow, Middlesex, England

David H. Katz, Department of Pathology, Harvard Medical School, Boston, Massachusetts 02115

T. J. Kindt, The Rockefeller University, New York, New York 10021

D. G. Klapper, The Rockefeller University, New York, New York 10021

Norman R. Klinman, Department of Pathology, University of Pennsylvania Medical School, Philadelphia, Pennsylvania 19174

E. Kölsch, Heinrich-Pette-Institut für experimentelle Virologie und Immunologie, an der Universität Hamburg, 2 Hamburg 20, Martinistrasse 52, Germany

W. H. Konigsberg, Yale University School of Medicine, New Haven, Connecticut 06510

Nitza Lahat, Rogoff-Wellcome Medical Research Institute and Tel-Aviv University Medical School, Beilinson Hospital, Petah Tikva, Israel

P. Leder, Laboratory of Molecular Genetics, National Institute of Child Health and Human Development, Bethesda, Maryland 20014

Jean Lindenmann, Department of Medical Microbiology, University of Zurich, Zurich, Switzerland

E. Loh, Division of Biology, California Institute of Technology, Pasadena, California 91109

Peter Lonai, Division of Immunology, Department of Medicine, Stanford University School of Medicine, Stanford, California 94305

Francis Loor, Basel Institute for Immunology, 487 Grenzacherstrasse, CH-4058 Basel, Switzerland

Jacques A. Louis, Department of Experimental Pathology, Scripps Clinic and Research Foundation, La Jolla, California 92037

B. N. Manjula, Yale University School of Medicine, New Haven, Connecticut 06510

John J. Marchalonis, Walter & Eliza Hall Institute of Medical Research, Royal Melbourne Hospital, Melbourne, Victoria, Australia

Hugh O. McDevitt, Division of Immunology, Department of Medicine, Stanford University School of Medicine, Stanford, California 94305

A. J. McMichael, National Institute of Medical Research, Mill Hill, London HW7 1AA, England

R. Mengersen, Heinrich-Pette-Institut für experimentelle Virologie und Immunologie, an der Universität Hamburg, 2 Hamburg 20, Martinistrasse 52, Germany

Henry Metzger, National Institute of Arthritis, Metabolism and Digestive Diseases, Bethesda, Maryland 20014

Charles M. Metzler, Department of Genetics, Stanford University School of Medicine, Stanford, California 94305

Cesar Milstein, MRC Laboratory of Molecular Biology, Hills Road, Cambridge, CB2 2QH, England

Chaya Moroz, Rogoff-Wellcome Medical Research Institute and Tel-Aviv University Medical School, Beilinson Hospital, Petah Tikva, Israel

M. Mudgett, The Rockefeller University, New York, New York 10021

Stanley G. Nathenson, Department of Microbiology and Immunology, Albert Einstein College of Medicine, Bronx, New York 10461

M. Nau, Laboratory of Molecular Genetics, National Institute of Child Health and Human Development, Bethesda, Maryland 20014

B. Norman, Laboratory of Molecular Genetics, National Institute of Child Health and Human Development, Bethesda, Maryland 20014

C. Nottenburg, Division of Biology, California Institute of Technology, Pasadena, California 91109

S. Packman, Laboratory of Molecular Genetics, National Institute of Child Health and Human Development, Bethesda, Maryland 20014

E. A. Padlan, Laboratory of Molecular Biology, National Institute of Arthritis, Metabolism and Digestive Diseases, Bethesda, Maryland 20014

W. Paul, National Institute of Allergy and Infectious Diseases, Bethesda, Maryland 20014

Israel Pecht, Weizmann Institute of Science, Rehovot, Israel

Stefanello de Petris, Basel Institute for Immunology, 487 Grenzacherstrasse, CH-4058 Basel, Switzerland

Linda M. Pilarski, Department of Microbiology, The John Curtin School of Medical Research, Canberra, Australia

R. J. Poljak, Johns Hopkins University School of Medicine, Baltimore, Maryland 21205

M. Potter, Laboratory of Cell Biology, National Cancer Institute, Bethesda, Maryland 20014

Benjamin Prescott, Laboratory of Microbial Immunity and the Laboratory of Microbiology, National Institute of Allergy and Infectious Diseases, Bethesda, Maryland 20014

Joan L. Press, Department of Pathology, University of Pennsylvania Medical School, Philadelphia, Pennsylvania 19174

Jean-Louis Preud'homme, Laboratoire d'Immunochimie, Université de Paris, Faculté de Medecine, Institut de Recherches sur les Malades du Sang, Hôpital Saine-Louis, 2, Place du Docteur-Fournier, Paris-Xe, France

Martin C. Raff, MRC Neuroimmunology Project, Department of Zoology, University College, London WC1E 6BT, England

William C. Raschke, The Salk Institute, P.O. Box 1809, San Diego, California 92112

Roy Riblet, The Salk Institute, P.O. Box 1809, San Diego, California 92112

Frank F. Richards, Yale University School of Medicine, New Haven, Connecticut 06510

Georges E. Roelants, Basel Institute for Immunology, 487 Grenzacherstrasse, CH-4058 Basel, Switzerland

R. W. Rosenstein, Yale University School of Medicine, New Haven, Connecticut 06510

S. Rudikoff, Laboratory of Cell Biology, National Cancer Institute, Bethesda, Maryland 20014

F. Saul, Johns Hopkins University School of Medicine, Baltimore, Maryland 21205

Matthew D. Scharff, Department of Cell Biology, Albert Einstein College of Medicine, Bronx, New York 10461

David S. Secher, MRC Laboratory of Molecular Biology, Hills Road, Cambridge, CB2 2AH, England

D. M. Segal, Laboratory of Molecular Biology, National Institute of Arthritis, Metabolism and Digestive Diseases, Bethesda, Maryland 20014

E. M. Shevach, National Institute of Allergy and Infectious Diseases, Bethesda, Maryland 20014

Barry J. Skidmore, Department of Experimental Pathology, Scripps Clinic and Research Foundation, La Jolla, California 92037

Philip W. Stashak, Laboratory of Microbial Immunity and the Laboratory of Microbiology, National Institute of Allergy and Infectious Diseases, Bethesda, Maryland 20014

Ronald H. Stevens, National Institute of Medical Research, Mill Hill, London NW7 1AA, England

D. Swan, Laboratory of Molecular Genetics, National Institute of Child Health and Human Development, Bethesda, Maryland 20014

A. L. Thunberg, The Rockefeller University, New York, New York 10021

Janos M. Varga, Yale University School of Medicine, New Haven, Connecticut 06510

James Watson, The Salk Institute, P.O. Box 1809, San Diego, California 92112

G. Weber, Heinrich-Pette-Institut für experimentelle Virologie und Immunologie, an der Universität Hamburg, 2 Hamburg 20, Martinistrasse 52, Germany

Martin Weigert, Institute for Cancer Research, Philadelphia, Pennsylvania 19111

William O. Weigle, Department of Experimental Pathology, Scripps Clinic and Research Foundation, La Jolla, California 92037

Hans Wigzell, Department of Immunology, University of Uppsala, Uppsala, Sweden

A. R. Williamson, Department of Biochemistry, The University of Glasgow G12 8QQ, England

Leon Wofsy, Department of Bacteriology and Immunology, University of California, Berkeley, California 94720

Robert T. Woodland, Department of Pathology, University of Pennsylvania Medical School, Philadelphia, Pennsylvania 19174

I. M. Zitron, Building 30, Room 327, National Institutes of Health, Bethesda, Maryland 20014

PREFACE

We came together in Squaw Valley on March 17, 1974 hoping for clarification of some problems and, perhaps, answers to certain questions. We left exhilarated by the interchange of much exciting information. In many cases the answers which were offered only served to raise more questions, indicating the complexity of immune mechanisms. It seemed that a molecular approach to their understanding was pervasive.

The papers presented in this volume illustrate the high standard of the meeting. The free-flowing, informal workshops held each afternoon on the session material and related topics were at least as valuable as the formal sessions, the main criticism being that the workshops were too short! This introduction attempts to convey the flavor of the meeting and some of the interesting findings which were reported at the workshops. We have made no attempt at being comprehensive and only hope that we are accurate in the comments we have chosen to make.

The genetic level seems the most appropriate place to start. Further information emerged to support the idea that multi gene systems encode antibody structure. Papers describing the Ir (immune response) genes and products point to yet another multigene system controlling immune responsiveness, independent of antibody structure. As more amino acid sequences of V-regions are obtained, the existence of multiple V_H and V_L genes has become more widely accepted, even by reluctant theorists such as Mel Cohn. The reality of multiple V-genes leaves us unclear as to the role which a somatic generator of diversity might play.

RNA/DNA hybridization studies are as yet incomplete. Leder's paper points to the existence of a unique C-gene and multiple V-genes. Although the number of V-genes varies dramatically in other reports, the unique C-gene and separate V-gene pool are generally agreed upon. Tonegawa introduced a radical piece of data at this meeting which awaits confirmation. He finds a reiterated sequence, of about 70–80 nucleotides in length, common to κ, λ, and γ chain mRNA molecules.

The number of known V-genes is growing and this meeting saw the beginnings of a simple V-gene map. Five loci can be identified with confidence: $\alpha 1{:}3$ dextran; phosphoryl choline (T15); p-azophenylarsonate (ARS); streptococcal A variant carbohydrate (A5A); and nitrohydroxyphenyl(NP)/nitroiodohydroxyphenyl (NIP).

Most of these results will be presented in a mid-'74 issue of the journal, *Immunogenetics*. This tentative map is based on (a) study of idiotype inheritance pattern of responsiveness, with anti-idiotype antibodies (Lieberman; Davie; Capra) (b) analysis of rare recombinants to give map distances relative to known Ig map positions (Riblet; Eichmann) (c) study of the inheritance of unusual specificities. Mäkelä and Imanishi followed the ability of mice to make antibody against NP which in fact binds NIP with much higher affinity (heteroclitic antibody); this marker was found to be controlled by a single gene linked to the Iglb allotype. McMichael and Williamson added to this data the identification of the major monoclonal heteroclitic antibody by its isoelectric spectrum. Inheritance of this clonal antibody was apparently controlled only by a single gene, linked to Iglb; light chain genes were thus indicated to be common to the strains studied.

Birshtein's fascinating paper on mutations affecting Ig production heralds in a new area of somatic cell genetics which should lead to exciting information on the arrangement and rearrangement of genes coding for Ig. Secher added a short description of the MRC-Cambridge group's work on two spontaneous, non selected myeloma cell variants. Both of these variants involve deletion of a portion of the H chain approximating a complete domain. This fact could be considered along with the results of Kuehl and Honjo which were described in a workshop. Kuehl and Scharff have shown the production of a light chain fragment which appears to correspond to the constant region by a variant MPC11 clone. Honjo and Leder have shown that the mRNA coding for this fragment is about half the size of complete L chain mRNA. Linking these mutant phenotypes with H-chain disease and L-chain fragments found associated with Bence-Jones proteins led to fresh speculation on the joining of V regions and C regions (or even separate C domains) at the polypeptide level or the mRNA level. (The weight of contrary evidence is against such speculation.) Provocative findings such as those in Kindt's paper do lend themselves to unorthodox explanations at a level of somatic gene rearrangement. Pappenheimer presented an intriguing story of a rabbit expressing a series of clones of anti-pneumococcal-type III – polysaccharide of increasing affinity but all showing cross reaction with type VIII polysaccharide.

Even if we were to know the number and arrangement of genes coded for, there are still going to be plenty of questions to ask about control of gene expression. Stevens is approaching the question of control at a molecular level, and in his paper he documents a very specific interaction between Ig and H-chain mRNA of a similar sort to the repressor-DNA interaction. Although this binding has been shown to effect a translational control under certain conditions, it is possible that such a high affinity interaction has some other role during an immune response.

Other questions of control were raised by the report from Liacopoulos on a human double myeloma with the products of each cell being a $(\kappa\gamma_1)_2$ and a $(\lambda\gamma_1)_2$. By idiotype the $\gamma1$ chains of the two molecules were indistinguishable and no molecules were found with mixed L chains.

A revolutionary model was proposed by Cunningham to explain the results presented in his paper. He and Pilarski have performed some challenging experiments which taken at face value point to rapid changes of phenotype occurring within an expanding clone of antibody forming cells. Their results depend heavily on the absolute reliability of plaque morphology as a stable phenotypic marker. Concern was voiced in discussion over the cause of changes in plaque morphology (affinity?, rate or amount of production?) or that the apparent change in specificity was owing to a multispecific parent cell producing monospecific daughter cells. Further clarification will be awaited eagerly.

Other changes during clonal expansion, e.g. M→ G, were raised. B. Andersson presented column fractionation evidence to show that IgM-receptor bearing cells do not give rise directly to G secreting cells. Herzenberg presented evidence from the cell-sorting machine which favored an M→ G switch. In a workshop on biosynthesis, Kaji presented evidence that myeloma cells making IgG also synthesize J chain. Kaji and Parkhouse speculate that this may be molecular evidence of M synthesis at an earlier stage in the expansion of that clone.

Liacopoulos pointed to a transient stage early in the antigen driven maturation of B cells during which antibodies of two specificities can be secreted by the same cell.

Discussion over the need for two signals as opposed to a single signal for induction of clonal expansion and antibody formation (or effector function) took place as expected. Two-signal model (AG = signal one, non specific mediator = signal two) is versatile in providing phenomenological explanations. However, G. Möller and Coutinho pointed to the difficulty of finding an antigen lacking intrinsic mitogenicity. The central questions at issue are whether immunogens and mitogens each act on *different* cell-surface sites to trigger similar initiative signals, or whether they might act on the *same* sites. The nature of the two signals was hotly debated as may be judged in part from the papers of Greaves and Watson. The area of combat was the meaning of "activation." The point was made that this could be subdivided into a triggering phase and a subsequent potentiation phrase allowing full expression of the initiated clonal development. Thus, Greaves was willing to grant some potentiating role to cAMP and cGMP, but not a primary role. Greaves underlined the heterogeneity of the target cells, suggesting that certain B cells (IgM precursors) might require much less "second signal" involvement than IgG precursor B cells. Watson saw the ratio of levels of cAMP and cGMP as the determinant of immune or tolerance pathways. Chiller was able to use lipopolysaccharide (LPS) to prevent tolerance induction, but only when the LPS was mitogenic in the particular strain of mouse.

Williamson in describing the generation of memory in B-cell clones, appropriated "signal 2" effectors in driving clones towards antibody formation, and a high signal 1/signal 2 ratio as a driving force towards memory cell expansion. Miller and Cudkowicz reported memory in the absence of T-cell help, as did Kölsch.

That B-cell division could occur in the presence of AG and the absence of "signal 2" was shown by Dutton. In his nude spleen cell *in vitro* system, B-cell expansion is AG dependent and stimulation by allogeneic culture supernates could be withheld for 48 hours without any effect on final clonal burst size. Thus, the *initiation* of B-cell division does not seem to require signal 2.

The Great Debate over the chemical nature of the T-cell receptor still is unresolved! An impressive amount of support was presented for the view that the binding of, and reactivity to Ag by T-cells could be attributed to a membrane bound, 8S-IgM-like immunoglobulin (IgT). (Two of the most startling data at the meeting were presented by Chaya Moroz, showing α rather than μ chains on Balb/c thymocytes and non associated heavy and light chains at that.) Subsequently, Ag-IgT complexes can be found attached to macrophages, ready for delivery to B cells. Cone reported evidence that this T-related Ig could not bind to T-cells or B-cells but rather only to macrophages: the undercurrent of doubt was whether the complexes would not also bind to activated T-cells. Disbelievers in the T-cell origin of the Ig welcomed experiments demonstrating biosynthesis by normal T cells (which have been performed by F. Loor and D. DeLuca with their respective colleagues).

Jan Decker's finding of antigen-binding cells in fetal 14-day mouse thymus for five diverse antigens was also difficult to attribute to passively acquired AB.

The persistent puzzle was why there are some groups which cannot find the T-cell related Ig, whatever its origin. There was a rousing ovation at the T-cell receptor workshop when Bob Cone and Mike Parkhouse offered to be "locked" in a room until a definitive statement could be made on the effectiveness of the difficult techniques used in this field.

It is the era of suppression! This meeting saw a common acceptance of a new paradigm that the outcome of immune cellular interactions was due to competition between synergistic and suppressive T-cells. Whether it be suppression of allotypes in the newborn, genetic inability to respond to a particular antigen, or low-zone tolerance phenomena, it is clear that future experiments will have to consider whether a dominant, actively responding T-cell suppressive subpopulation is exerting its influence. Gershon pointed especially to experiments showing the homeostatic role of opposing regulatory T-cell effects. This was cleverly illustrated in Figs. 1 and 2 showing the T_2 cell as the key figure in immunocyte regulation.

An implicit corollary of the T-B cell paradigm has been rapidly crumbling— that distinct, non overlapping T and B-subpopulations are necessary and sufficient for immune responsiveness. There was a consensus of awareness that we are in the midst of a complexity explosion concerning the nature of cellular participants in the immune system and the markers displayed on their surfaces. Francis Loor reported that nude mouse spleen contains 34% cells staining with an anti-mouse brain specific for T-cells, casting doubt on conclusions made from this widely used animal model. Fully one-third of these T cells also bore obvious Ig on their surface, a much larger proportion than was found in normal spleen, suggesting an interesting regulatory system.

Basch reminded us that bone marrow cells were just 2 hours away from expressing θ and TL after transformation with thymin.

In a similar vein, Droege described experiments characterizing a bursal-dependent T-cell, a "heavy" cell type, absent from bursectomized chickens, as a prime candidate for the suppressor cell, especially in the younger chicken. Mosier also described a prevalent suppressor population in the neonatal mouse spleen.

The nylon wool method of separating out T lymphocytes won the award for the most-used, novel method of the year. Elizabeth Simpson could separate T-subpopulations with the laser activated cell sorter at low or high concentrations of θ, representing different maturational T-cell stages.

On the B-cell side, Sam Strober discussed the development of B cells from a pre-B cell in the marrow through a generator B cell in the spleen which continually provides virgin precursors that are saved from rapid extinction by antigen, driving them into the memory state. As for the very beginnings, Max Cooper's findings were that fetal liver rather than gut-associated lymphoid tissue seemed to be the site of origin of B-cells.

We may finish with mention of the role of Ir genes in triggering the B-cell response. Although immune response genes appear to affect carrier recognition function, a variety of reports indicated more Ir product on the B-cell, or its easier availability as antigen. The Ia antigens (I-region associated antigens) are different chemically and in tissue distribution from histocompatibility antigens.

It soon will be known by Katz and colleagues whether the Ir genes as well as the H-2 K or D ends of the major histocompatibility region must be identical before T and B-cells can interact effectively. The structural relationship of the Ir gene products to antigen receptors and the cell membrane in general, promises to be a major focus for several years.

We left Squaw Valley after a week of exotic spring weather and exciting progress. One could think backwards to the Cold Spring Harbor meeting in 1967 as a time of innocent simplicity. Confidence was rampant that the vigor of the current fundamental and molecular explorations would continue to yield many new insights into the controlling elements in immune responsiveness.

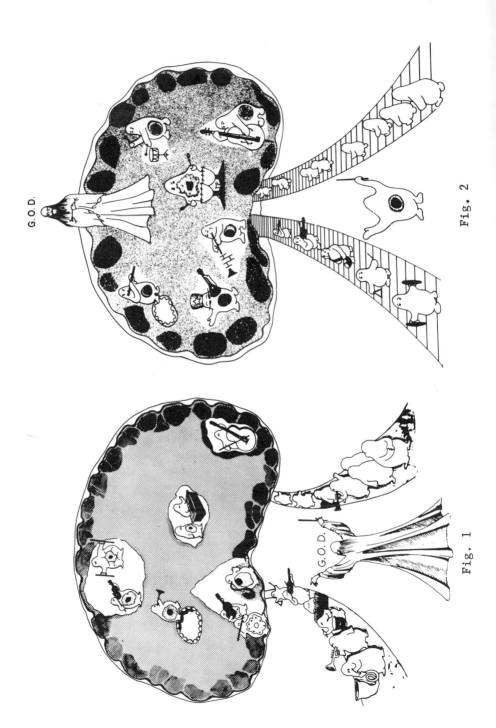

G.O.D.

Fig. 2

G.O.D.

Fig. 1

THE CONDUCTOR OF THE IMMUNOLOGICAL ORCHESTRA

In 1968, shortly after his discovery that thymus derived lymphocytes did not make antibody but rather assisted bone marrow derived lymphocytes to do so, Tony Davis suggested that immunologists might do well to adopt an idea from endocrinologists (Lancet 1:185, 1968). They spoke of an endocrine orchestra, implying an interaction between various components of the system which determines overall endocrine function. Thus, the notion of an immunological orchestra was conceived. How that orchestra might have looked circa 1968 is depicted in Figure 1. At that time a great deal of attention was being focused on the generator of diversity (G.O.D.). T cells and B cells and macrophages were the players. Since that time the orchestra has expanded to include sub-populations of the above cells and also eosinophils and basophils have been added as members. In addition, it has been shown that T cells act not only to amplify immune responses but also to suppress them, suggesting that some T cells should be thought of as regulatory cells. This new concept is depicted in Figure 2 which suggests that in 1974 the T-cell (probably T_2) may be considered to be the conductor of the immunological orchestra.

(by R. K. Gershon)

ACKNOWLEDGMENTS

This conference is the third in an interdisciplinary series sponsored by ICN Pharmaceuticals, Inc. and organized through the Molecular Biology Institute of the University of California, Los Angeles. We are grateful to Gerald Camiener and Tom Fulton of the Life Sciences Division of ICN Pharmaceuticals, Inc. for their continued efforts in support of these conferences. We also express gratitude to Hans Neurath, editor of *Biochemistry* and to the editorial boards of *European Journal of Immunology, Journal of Immunology,* and *Cellular Immunology* for arranging to publish announcements of this conference in their respective journals. We thank Steven Kallestad of Kallestad Laboratories for a gift to support social activities at the conference; Bettye Knutsen and George Sullivan of United Air Lines, Los Angeles for coordination of travel arrangements for all conferees, and William Parson and Olive Nielson of the Olympic Village Hotel and Squaw Valley Convention Bureau for their untiring efforts prior to and during the conference. Finally we thank Charlotte Miller and Fran Stusser of the ICN-UCLA conference staff for creating the illusion that the organizers of the conference were organized.

ANTIBODY STRUCTURE AND THE IMMUNE RESPONSE

Henry Metzger

National Institute of Arthritis, Metabolism
and Digestive Diseases
National Institutes of Health
Bethesda, Maryland 20014

It is customary in a conference such as this one to
begin with a symposium on antibody structure. I suspect
that especially in recent years, with the extraordinary
flourishing of cellular immunology, this custom has been
largely maintained in deference to tradition rather than
for compelling scientific reasons on the part of the
organizers. In this introduction I want to summarize why
I think this custom has not outgrown its usefulness; why
the details of antibody structure continue to be of para-
mount importance to an understanding of the regulation of
the immune reactions in which we here are all interested.

Role of antibodies in immune reactions. The immune
reactions of vertebrates have two fundamental components:
recognition and response. The first is the sin qua non.
It is of course required for all positive responses and
contemporary concepts suggest that it also is required in
various refractory states (i.e. that tolerance is not
simply the lack of recognition). Recognition in the
immune system occurs in a variety of situations (Table 1).
In almost all of these immunoglobulin is the molecular
basis of the recognition. Only with respect to the thymus
processed cells (T-cells) do we have experimental data
which implicate a different type of recognition system;
the question of whether immunoglobulins are also involved
remains moot.
    The immune system responds in two ways: There is a
proliferation of recognition units and a stimulation of
reactions which can be broadly characterized as directed
to antigen elimination. Proliferation of recognition
units occurs both by multiplication of immunocompetent
cells and by differentiation e.g. into antibody secreting
cells. The role of immunoglobulins in these reactions is
uncertain. While it may well be true that antigens trigger
cells by interacting with surface-bound antibody, alternative mechanisms cannot be ruled out and may at the very
least contribute. Thus antigens may form a link between
antibody bound to macrophages and B-cells, macrophages and

1

Table 1

DISTRIBUTION OF RECOGNITION UNITS IN IMMUNE SYSTEM

Class	Function	Molecular Basis of Specific Recognition
	CELLULAR	
B	1. Precursor of antibody forming cell 2. Memory cell	Immunoglobulin
T	1. 'Helper' cell 2. Mediator of cellular reactions 3. Memory cell	?Immunoglobulin ?Ir gene product
Misc.	1. Antigen presentation e.g. macrophage 2. Antigen elimination e.g. macrophage 3. Mediator release e.g. mast cells	?Immunoglobulin Immunoglobulin Immunoglobulin
	NON-CELLULAR	
Serum, secretions, other extra-cellular fluids	1. Antigen elimination 2. ?Antigen presentation	Immunoglobulin

T-cells, T-cells and B-cells. It is these cellular interactions which may provide the critical signal, the antibody
simply serving to set limits on the number of cells which
will respond. To the extent that this is not the case, i.e.
that a critical signal is mediated via the antibody it is
pertinent to ask how the structure of the immunoglobulins,
their surface distribution, and their density affect the
generation of the signal.

With regard to some of the complex reactions involved in
antigen elimination (opsonization, complement fixation,
mediator release from mast cells, etc.) there is no question
that antibodies are directly involved. In other instances
(lymphocyte cytotoxic reactions) we are uncertain of the
importance of antibodies.

Thus in the two fundamental phenomena of what we call an
immune reaction, recognition and response, antibodies are
suspected or known to play a major role.

Antibody structure in relation to recognition function.
How do antibodies perform their functions? What is the
structural basis of recognition and for the signal that will
lead to a response?

The first part of the latter question can now be responded to with considerable sophistication. The 'answer'
has been contributed to by a variety of approaches. Protein-
chemical and electronmicroscopic investigations defined where
on the immunoglobulin molecule recognition occurred. Affinity labeling data pin-pointed the relevant stretches of the
hyper-variable segments and sequence analyses provided a completely independent, albeit indirect, confirmation. In 1973
and 1974 we will be provided with several detailed X-ray
diffraction views of antibody combining sites. It is likely
that these results will point the direction but not mark the
end of the road to a complete understanding of these sites.
Many questions remain: Are there generic features which
distinguish antibody combining sites from binding sites on
other biopolymers? If so, how do these features differ among
antibodies of different species? Is there a recognizable
evolutionary trend? Are the 3-dimensional structures of the
variable regions which form the sites influenced at all by
the type of class-specific constant regions to which they are
covalently linked? What is the true functional multiplicity
of combining sites and how does it relate to structural diversity? If there are subsites within the general area we
call the antibody combining site does the homologous antigen
(the immunogen) always occupy one of these? The work of the
speakers in this first symposium is providing us with some of

3

the answers to these questions.

Antibody structure in relation to response function.

I have elsewhere reviewed the available data on how antigen
affects the structure of antibody (1). On the basis of information on the structure of antibodies, on the structure
of antigen-antibody complexes, and on the characteristics of
antibody mediated responses I concluded that 1) it was unlikely that antigen induced significant conformational changes in
the relevant regions (i.e. the Fc regions) of antibodies and
2) that aggregation of immunoglobulin could explain most and
perhaps all antibody-mediated phenomena. Others find such a
formulation inadequate (2) and the recent experiments of
Watson et al. (3) provide a challenge to the "associative"
theory of antigen action. Rather than re-review the data I
would like to briefly describe the approach my own laboratory
is taking towards collecting more helpful information.

The IgE System: A model system for antibody mediated responses.

We have chosen the IgE mediated degranulation
of mast cells and basophils as a useful system to explore.
IgE like other immunoglobulins are secreted by plasma cells.
Because of their unique Fc region they become attached to
the surface membrane of mast cells and basophils. If such
cells are reacted with an antigen with which the membrane-
bound IgE can combine, rapid degranulation (a non-cytotoxic
reaction) occurs. Degranulation can also be induced by reacting the surface IgE with anti-immunoglobulin. The system
is relatively simple in so far as no additional extrinsic
factors other than Ca^{++} and Mg^{++} are required. There
appears to be no helper cell necessary nor any high molecular
weight soluble factors. The available data clearly indicate
that the IgE must be cross-linked (by antigen or anti-Ig) in
order to obtain a response. The few experiments which suggest otherwise (i.e. appear to demonstrate hapten evoked responses) (4) may be explainable simply by assuming that the
monofunctional ligands become bound to other cells and then
present themselves as multifunctional antigens to the mast
cell (5). It is not easy to "prove" such an explanation.

When B-lymphocytes are reacted with bivalent anti-
immunoglobulins or antigens two phenomena are observed:
Rapid redistribution of surface immunoglobulin (patching,
capping) and blast transformation. Since in many experiments
cross-linking of immunoglobulins appears to be a requirement
for both reactions it is reasonable to ask whether the former
phenomenon is in fact a requirement for the latter. Early

biochemical correlates of blast transformation have not yet
been sufficiently characterized so this question is not
easily answered in the lymphocyte system. In the IgE-basophil system we were however able to obtain a definite answer
(6). IgE on basophils can also be redistributed and like
anti-Ig induced histamine release requires the presence of
bivalent (cross-linking) antibody. We showed unambiguously
that gross redistribution of the surface IgE was not required
for histamine release (Fig. 1). Indeed it was interesting
that doses of anti-Ig so high that capping occurred rapidly
- within the time period when histamine release would be
expected - in fact suppressed degranulation completely.
Doses which were adequate to cause capping but only after a
more prolonged lag period did not interfere with optimal
histamine release. These results indicate that the topological arrangement of the immunoglobulin during a critical
period in the triggering reaction may markedly affect the
cell's response. There are a few published experiments
which suggest lymphocytes may behave similarly (7).

To understand the biochemical sequelae of antibody-
mediated antigen-induced phenomena we need to characterize
the 'next-step' down the line i.e. the molecules which
interact with the immunoglobulin. We are attempting this
in the IgE-basophil system. We have recently successfully
adapted a rat basophil leukemia (8) to cell culture. These
cells appear highly differentiated morphologically and bind
monomeric IgE with high specificity (9). We have determined
that the IgE binds with the expected bimolecular kinetics
with a K_A of approximately 10^{10} M^{-1} (10). Depending on the
conditions of growth the receptor number per cell can vary
widely (0.25 to 1.5 x 10^6/cell) though its binding properties
appear unchanged (11). We are attempting to isolate this
receptor and study its interaction with IgE in detail.
In this way we hope ultimately to increase our understanding
of how antibodies mediate antigen-induced phenomena at
least in this system.

As an introduction to a symposium on antibody structure
it may seem that I have wandered far afield. Yet I think
these are the directions we wish ultimately to take.

Those who study how the immune system functions can try
to estimate what is required of antibodies; those who investigate the structure of immunoglobulins can suggest what
antibodies can potentially do; cooperatively we can find out
what actually happens.

Now let us return to the combining site where the
action begins.

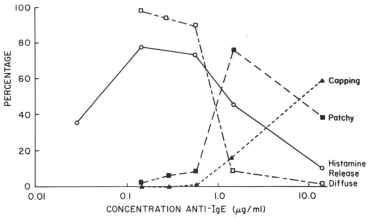

EFFECT OF CONCENTRATION OF ANTI-IgE ON
HISTAMINE RELEASE AND CELL SURFACE IgE

Figure 1. Relationship between anti-IgE induced redistribution of membrane bound IgE and histamine release. Concentrations of antibody which lead to gross redistribution (patching and capping) inhibit the release of histamine. Other studies indicated, however, that cross-linking of the membrane bound IgE was a prerequisite for histamine release. Reprinted from (6) by permission of the Journal of Experimental Medicine

REFERENCES

1. H. Metzger, Adv. Immunol. 18, 169 (1974).
2. M. Cohn, Ann. N. Y. Acad. Sci. 190, 529 (1971).
3. J. Watson, E. Trenkner and M. Cohn, J. Exp. Med. 138, 699 (1973).
4. L.T. Rosenberg, A.A. Amkraut, R.S. Corp and S. Raffel, J. Immunol. 107, 1175 (1971).
5. A.L. de Weck, C.H. Schneider, H. Spengler, O. Taffler and S. Lazary, Mechanisms in Allergy: Reagin-mediated Hypersensitivity, L. Goodfriend, A.H. Sehon and R.P. Orange (Eds.) Marcel Dekker, Inc., New York, 1973, p. 323.
6. K. Becker, T. Ishizaka, H. Metzger and K. Ishizaka, J. Exp. Med. 138, 394 (1973).
7. C.J. Elson, J. Singh and R.B. Taylor, Scand. J. Immunol. 2, 143 (1973).
8. E. Eccleston, B.J. Leonard, J.S. Lowe and H. J. Welford, Nature New Biol. 244, 73 (1973).
9. A. Kulczycki, Jr., C. Isersky and H. Metzger, J. Exp. Med. 139, 600 (1974).
10. A. Kulczycki, Jr. and H. Metzger, in preparation (1974).
11. C. Isersky, H. Metzger and D. Buell, in preparation (1974).

THE THREE-DIMENSIONAL STRUCTURE OF THE ANTIGEN BINDING SITE OF McPC 603 PROTEIN

E. A. Padlan, D. M. Segal, G. H. Cohen, D. R. Davies

Laboratory of Molecular Biology
National Institute of Arthritis,
Metabolism and Digestive Diseases
and
S. Rudikoff and M. Potter
Laboratory of Cell Biology
National Cancer Institute
National Institutes of Health
Bethesda, Maryland 20014

ABSTRACT. The structure of the Fab fragment of McPC 603 protein has been determined by crystallographic analysis to 3.1 Å resolution. The site of phosphorylcholine binding was located in a cleft formed by the three heavy chain hypervariable loops and the first and third hypervariable regions of the light chain. There are strong interactions between the phosphate group of the hapten and the side groups of Tyr 33 and Arg 52 both of the heavy chain. Acidic side groups from both light and heavy chains are in the immediate vicinity of the positively charged choline group. The hapten is in van der Waals contact with various portions of the hypervariable loops. Phosphorylcholine occupies only a small portion of the cleft between the variable domains.

INTRODUCTION

Antigen binding activity has been demonstrated for many mouse myeloma proteins (1). We are attempting to crystallize a number of these proteins for the purpose of making a comparative study of antigen-binding sites. We have obtained crystals of Fab fragments of two of these, McPC 603 and J 539 (2), and in this paper we report the preliminary results of a crystallographic study of the Fab of McPC 603 protein at 3.1 Å resolution.

McPC 603, an IgA(K) protein, binds to natural antigens from a variety of organisms, including *Pneumococcus, Lactobacillus, Trichoderma, Aspergillus, Proteus morganii* and *Ascaris* (3). Phosphorylcholine is an immunodominant group in these antigens for the mouse and McPC 603 protein has been demonstrated to bind phosphorylcholine (3). The Fab fragment binds phosphorylcholine in solution (K_A = 1.7 x $10^{-5}$$M^{-1}$) and in the crystal($K_A$ = 3.9 x $10^{-3}M^{-1}$)

7

(2).

We have previously reported a low resolution structure for McPC 603 Fab (4) in which it was apparent that the molecule is made up of four distinct structural units corresponding to the four domains. This structure closely resembled the structure reported for a human myeloma protein Fab fragment (5). We have also reported the location of the hapten binding site at one end of the molecule in a cleft between two domains in what we identified as the variable region of the fragment. By difference Fourier techniques we examined the binding of phosphorylcholine and of a mercury thiophene derivative of phosphorylcholine. Our results clearly showed that the choline moiety is bound towards the interior of the cleft while the phosphate group is more towards the exterior. In the unsubstituted protein crystals a sulfate ion binds in the phosphate position, presumably the result of the high concentration of ammonium sulfate from which the crystals are grown.

The binding of phosphorylcholine to McPC 603 Fab in the crystal does not produce gross conformational changes in the structure. This implies that hapten binding in solution will leave the overall configuration of the fragment unchanged in agreement with low-angle X-ray scattering observations (6). However, we cannot rule out the possibility that the presence of a sulfate ion in the hapten binding site may have already frozen the structure in the "liganded" conformation.

RESULTS

Whereas the low resolution electron density map could not reveal the atomic details of the molecule, our present 3.1 Å map has enabled us to trace clearly the course of the polypeptide chains. In addition, we can correlate peaks in the map with the corresponding amino acid residues that are known from the sequence (7).

A molecular model has been constructed of the variable region. The overall tertiary structure of the McPC 603 V_L and V_H domains is very similar to those of the V_λ and V_K domains from two human Bence-Jones proteins (8,9) and the V_L and V_H domains of a human Fab (New) (10). Moreover, the way in which the V_L and V_H domains are combined in the McPC 603 protein, involving as they do an approximate two-fold axis, is very similar to the combination of the V_L and V_H domains in the New protein and the combination of the V_λ and V_K domains in the two Bence-Jones dimers.

One end of the McPC 603 Fab consists almost entirely of the hypervariable regions (11) in the form of loops. There is a wedge-shaped cleft in this region, the walls of which are formed by 5 of the 6 hypervariable loops. This cleft is approximately 15 Å wide at the mouth, 12 Å deep and 20 Å long. The conformation in this region is quite different from that reported for the human Fab (10). In the latter this part of the molecule is described as being relatively flat with the exception of a shallow groove, 15 Å x 6 Å x 6Å.

In McPC 603 the phosphorylcholine binding site is observed to be located at this end of the molecule roughly in the middle of the cleft. The relation between the hapten and the hypervariable loops is shown schematically in Fig. 1. It is clear that the phosphorylcholine is situated closer to the heavy chain than to the light chain hypervariable regions. In fact, the second hypervariable region of the light chain is quite removed from the binding site and is screened from it by the first light chain hypervariable loop.

Side groups from several residues in the other five hypervariable loops project into the cleft and interact with the hapten. The two residues that are closest to the hapten are Tyr 33 and Arg 52, both from the heavy chain (Fig. 2). The hydroxyl group of Tyr 33 is apparently hydrogen-bonded to one of the oxygens of the phosphate as is one of the NH_2 groups of the arginine side chain. Moreover, the close proximity of the positively charged guanidinium group of Arg 52 to the negatively charged phosphate should produce a large favorable electrostatic interaction. There is also in the immediate vicinity of the phosphate another positive group, that of Lys 54, also of the heavy chain, which could help neutralize the negative charge of this portion of the hapten.

Whereas the phosphate interacts only with the heavy chain, the choline group interacts with both light and heavy chains. There are possible electrostatic interactions with acidic side groups which are in close proximity to the positively charged choline group. In addition, there are van der Waals interactions between the choline and main chain atoms of residues 102-103 of the heavy chain and residues 91-94 of the light chain. The entire hapten is in close van der Waals contact with the ring atoms of Tyr 33 of the heavy chain.

Phosphorylcholine does not fill the entire cleft outlined by the hypervariable loops (Fig. 3). Thus, there appears to be room for a much larger ligand.

The complete description of the protein-hapten interactions, especially those involving the choline group, must await the complete sequence of residues in the third hypervariable region of the light chain.

9

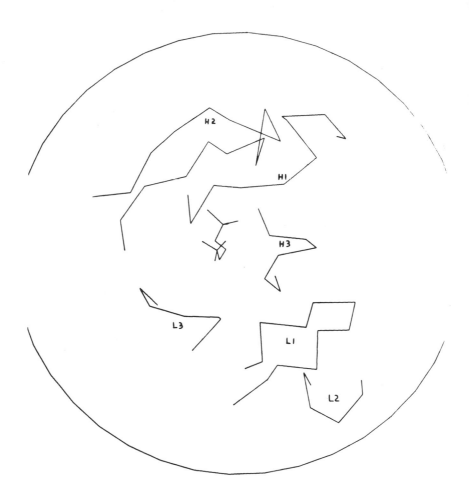

Fig. 1. Schematic drawing of the hypervariable loops of
McPC 603 protein in relation to the phosphorylcholine hapten.
L1, L2 and L3 are the first, second and third light chain
hypervariable regions, respectively, and H1, H2 and H3 are
the corresponding heavy chain regions.

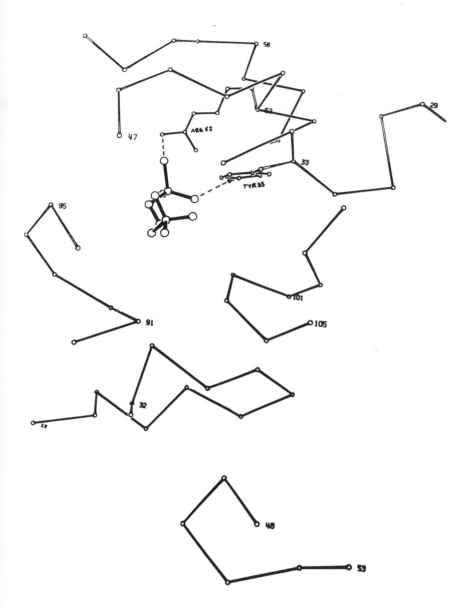

Fig. 2. Schematic drawing of the hypervariable loops including the side groups of Tyr 33 and Arg 52. Hydrogen-bonds (- - - -) could be formed between these side chains and oxygen atoms of the phosphate group of phosphorylcholine.

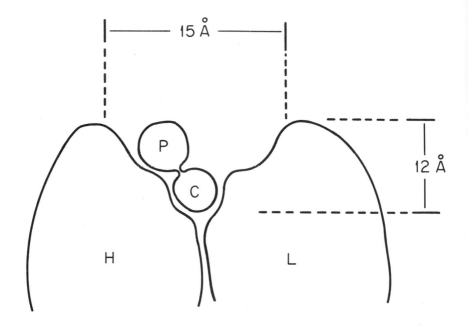

Fig. 3. Schematic drawing of the binding of phosphorylcholine (PC) in the cleft formed by the hypervariable loops of the heavy (H) and light (L) chains of McPC 603 protein.

DISCUSSION

The close similarity between this mouse IgA(K) Fab and the human IgG (λ) Fab (10) in both their tertiary and quaternary structures, coupled with the similar structures observed for human Bence-Jones dimers (8,9), strongly implies the invariance of these structural features in the architecture of antibodies. However, the considerable differences in the overall shape, size and general chemical nature of the antigen-binding sites provides a structural basis for antibody variability.

In McPC 603 the light and heavy variable domains are in general related to each other by a dyad axis, except in the combining site region where the two chains are quite different. This is illustrated by the asymmetry of phosphorylcholine binding. The hypervariable surface of $V_L.V_L$ or $V_H.V_H$ dimers of McPC 603 would be much more symmetric and would be expected to have quite different binding properties.

It is interesting to note that the amino acid sequences of the heavy chains of five phosphorylcholine-binding mouse myeloma proteins are identical through the first hypervariable region (12). The light chain sequences of those not exhibiting idiotypic identity are quite different. This correlates well with our observation of strong specific interactions between the hapten and the heavy chain.

Phosphorylcholine, being a small molecule, interacts with relatively few amino acid residues in the binding site. It is well known that antigenic determinants can be much larger than phosphorylcholine and further that phosphorylcholine itself may be only a part of the natural antigenic determinant. In this respect it is pertinent to observe that the hypervariable loops of McPC 603 are gathered together to form a continuous hypervariable surface that is much more extensive than that which is involved simply in phosphorylcholine binding.

REFERENCES

1. M. Potter, *Physiol. Rev. 52*, 631 (1972).
2. S. Rudikoff, M. Potter, D. M. Segal, E. A. Padlan and D. R. Davies, *Proc. Nat. Acad. Sci. U.S. 69*, 3689 (1972).
3. M. Potter, *Ann. N. Y. Acad. Sci. 190*, 306 (1971).
4. E. A. Padlan, D. M. Segal, T. F. Spande, D. R. Davies, S. Rudikoff and M. Potter, *Nature New Biology 245*, 165 (1973).
5. R. J. Poljak, L. M. Amzel, H. P. Avey, L. N. Becka and A. Nisonoff, *Nature New Biology 235*, 137 (1972).

6. I. Pilz, O. Kratky, A. Licht and M. Sela, *Biochemistry* *12*, 4998 (1973).

7. S. Rudikoff and M. Potter, manuscript in preparation.

8. M. Schiffer, R. L. Girling, K. R. Ely and A. B. Edmundson, *Biochemistry* *12*, 4620 (1973).

9. O. Epp, P. Colman, H. Fehlhammer, W. Bode, M. Schiffer and R. Huber, *Eur. J. Biochem.* in press.

10. R. J. Poljak, L. M. Amzel, H. P. Avey, B. L. Chen, R. P. Phizackerley and F. Saul, *Proc. Nat. Acad. Sci. U.S.* *70*, 3305 (1973).

11. T. T. Wu and E. A. Kabat, *J. Exp. Med.* *132*, 211 (1970).

12. P. Barstad, S. Rudikoff, M. Potter, M. Cohn, W. Konigsberg and L. Hood, *Science* *183*, 962 (1974).

KINETIC MAPPING OF ANTIBODY BINDING SITES

Israel Pecht
Department of Chemical Immunology
The Weizmann Institute of Science
Rehovot, Israel

ABSTRACT. The specificity and affinity exhibited by the binding sites of antibodies is a result of the interactions of a particular spatial combination of certain residues within the site with the complementary counterpart groups of the hapten. The dynamic equilibrium between hapten and antibody has been shown to involve a single step: $Ab + H \underset{k_{21}}{\overset{k_{12}}{\rightleftharpoons}} AbH$

In order to probe the dimensions of the antibody combining site and to determine the nature and localization of the attracting forces, a correlation between structure of a series of systematically varied ligands and their specific rates of binding (k_{12}) and dissociation (k_{21}) to a certain binding site is carried out using the chemical relaxation T-jump method to determine these rates.

The combining site of the homogeneous murine IgA protein 315 which has affinity to polynitrophenyl derivatives has been probed using over 40 different ligands. The results enabled the construction of a proposed model for the site; four subsites of interaction are observed: (a) The polynitrophenyl binding subsite, (b) two hydrophobic subsites, and (c) an electrostatic (positive) subsite. The overall minimal dimensions of this site are 12 x 6Å.

Another homogeneous site which is at present being studied is that of the phosphoryl choline binding protein HOPC 8.

Normally induced, heterogeneous antibodies binding oligoalanine peptides have also been investigated by this kinetic method. Specific rates were determined for the interaction of haptens of different lengths with different eluates of the antibody population. Using fluorescent probes, covalently attached to the hapten (oligoalanines or DNP) the depth of the combining site has been examined. This has been accomplished by measurements of the circular and linear polarized components of the bound ligands carrying the fluorophores.

INTRODUCTION

The three-dimensional structure of immunoglobulins and particularly the combining sites for antigen at their variable regions are now becoming resolved at an increasingly higher resolution by X-ray crystallography (1,2,3). In solution the antibody-antigen (or hapten) complex exists in a dynamic binding equilibrium and the rather fast elementary steps by virtue of which this complex is formed and dissociates have been followed by fast kinetic methods, mainly the chemical relaxation-temperature jump technique (4-8). In all cases hitherto examined the interaction mechanism between haptens and their respective antibodies was found to be a single step process involving a bimolecular binding and a monomolecular dissociation reaction. This is expressed in the experimental observation that the chemical relaxation times of the perturbed equilibrium of the antibody hapten are reciprocally dependent on the free concentrations of the reactants (figure 1). The mechanistic implication of this behaviour is as stated above the following single step equilibrium: $Ab + H \underset{k_{21}}{\overset{k_{12}}{\rightleftarrows}} AbH$. This is in contrast to the

mechanism resolved or the interactions between enzymes and their respective ligands (substrates, substrate analogs or inhibitors) where even for small, single polypeptide chain enzymes, the common feature of the binding process is a two step mechanism: a rapid bimolecular step between the enzyme and the ligand followed by a relatively slow monomolecular step This is illustrated in the upper part of figure 1 where the reciprocal relaxation times of the T-jump perturbed equilibrium of the complex of lysozyme and a substrate analog are plotted as function of free enzyme and substrate analog concentrations. The type of non linear dependence has been found for a variety of similar systems (9) and was shown to fit the following two steps mechanism: $E + L \underset{k_{21}}{\overset{k_{12}}{\rightleftarrows}} EL^* \underset{k_{32}}{\overset{k_{23}}{\rightleftarrows}} EL$

where E and L are the enzyme and ligand and EL* and EL are two conformers of the complex formed between them.

For the single step equilibrium between antibody and hapten, the equilibrium constant is given by $K = k_{12}/k_{21}$. It is evident that variation in K may result from changes in either k_{12} or k_{21} or in both. Thus, a correlation between the structural features of a series of systematically varied

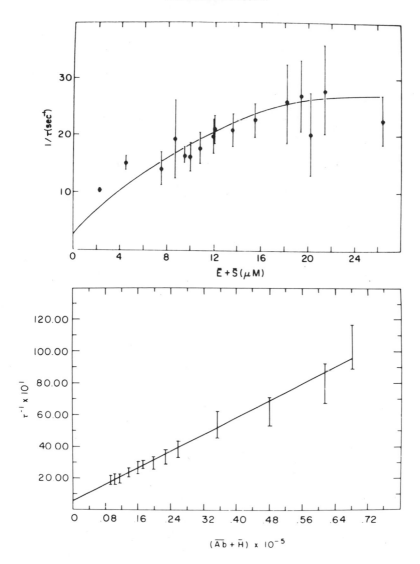

Figure 1. The dependence of the reciprocal of the observed relaxation times and the sum of free equilibrium concentrations of: (Upper part) iodine modified lysozyme + te-
tra N- acetyl glucoseamine (Lower part) MOPC 315 + ε-N-DNP
lysine.

ligands and their specific rates of interaction with the
antibody combining site may lead to the resolution and mapping of the different elementary interacting forces in a
homogeneous combining site (10). This is mainly so because
the specific rate of binding (k_{12}) varies only over a limited range and that k_{21} the specific rate of dissociation
being a measure of the residence time of the hapten in the
site reflects their interaction forces and complementarity
The first and most extensively investigated site by this
method is that of the murine protein 315. This protein,
possessing affinity towards polynitrophenyl ligands has
been studied (8,10,11) by measuring the specific rates of
binding (k_{12}) and dissociation (k_{21}) of more than 50 different derivatives which belonged to 5 structurally different
series: (a) nitrophenyl derivatives differing in the number
and position of the nitro group or in the nature of the
substituent on the ring; (b) 2,4-dinitroaniline derivatives,
mono-substituted at the amino group by branched and straight
alkyl chains including alkyl carboxylates and ammonium
groups; (c) 2,4-dinitroaniline di-substituted by alkyl
groups at the amino group, (d) $\overline{\alpha}$-N-DNP derivatives of glycine
and alanine and their dipeptides, including the different
diastereoisomers of alanine and alanyl alanine, (e) ε-N-DNP
lysyl (lysine)$_n$ derivatives where n = 0 to 8.

Four types of elementary interactions with the haptens
within the combining site were resolved in terms of their
chemical nature and localization relative to the nitrophenyl
binding subsite. On the basis of these data a model of the
site is delineated.

Another homogeneous combining site being investigated
is that of the phosphoryl choline binding murine myeloma
protein HOPC 8. For this protein again a single step interaction mechanism is found. The specific rates of binding
and dissociation vary in a range similar to that observed
for the respective rates of the MOPC 315.

Possible application of the kinetic mapping to combining sites of an heterogeneous population has been investigated on polyalanine antibodies which have been fractionated
by elution with oligo alanines of increasing length (13,17).
For this purpose alanine and dialanine derivatives carrying
a fluorescent side chain were synthesized (15) and their
kinetics of interaction with different eluates were studied.
Here also a single step reaction was found to fit the data.
Though the heterogeneity of the binding sites population

precludes a detailed and unambiguous mapping of the sites in the manner applicable to homogeneous systems, an interesting correlation between the specific combination of eluate and ligand and the kinetic parameters is observed. The architecture of the MOPC 315 binding site evolving from the kinetic mapping is extended by measuring the linear and circular fluorescence polarization of the complexes formed be tween the protein and a series of 2,4-dinitrophenyl(DNP) derivatives carrying, at an increasing distance a covalently linked fluorophore(16). Only those derivatives where the fluorophore is closer than 7Å to the center of the DNP ring exhibit induced circularly polarized fluorescence. This indicates the spatial boundaries of interaction posed by the combining site and is in accord with all the other data.

MATERIALS AND METHODS

MOPC 315 protein in its reduced and alkylated monomeric form was prepared as previously described (11). HOPC 8 was kindly supplied by Drs. M. Potter and S. Rudikoff, National Institutes of Health, USA. Antibodies to poly-D-alanine were prepared as described by Schechter et al. (13). The series of different 2,4-dinitroaniline derivatives were synthesized in our laboratory by procedures which have been described (8). The ε-N-DNP lysyl-oligolysine derivatives were prepared by Dr. A. Yaron and his collaborators (14). Oligoalanine derivatives carrying a 1-dansylethane diamine residue at the C-terminal were prepared by Mr. A. Licht in our laboratory (15). The DNP derivative of the general formula $DNP-\underset{H}{N}-(CH_2)_n-$(9-amino acridine) were synthesized (Miss U. Hartmann) in our laboratory (16).

Kinetic measurements were carried out by following the fluorescence changes. For the MOPC 315 and the HOPC 8 protein fluorescence intensity which is known to be quenched for the first (12) and enhanced (18) for the second upon ligand binding has been monitored. The binding of ligands to the anti-polyalanine antibodies was followed by measuring the fluorescence energy transfer to the dansyl covalently linked to the bound alanine hapten. The experimental procedure of measurements carried out on the temperature jump spectrofluorometer have been described earlier (7).

Fluorescence spectra were measured on either Turner model 210 or Hitachi Perkin Elmer MF3 spectro fluorometers. The circular polarization of fluorescence was measured on an apparatus constructed by Prof. I.Z. Steinberg and Drs. A. Gafni and J. Schlessinger of our Institute (19,20).

RESULTS AND DISCUSSION

In all antibody hapten systems hitherto examined only a single chemical relaxation was effected by the temperature jump perturbation. Moreover, in all cases the measured relaxation times depended reciprocally, over an extensive concentration range, on the free binding sites and haptens (4,6,10). It has already been explained in the introduction that this dependence of τ^{-1} is in agreement with a single step binding mechanism. The first series of ligands used for the kinetic mapping of the MOPC 315 site was that of nitrophenyl ligands where substitutions in the aromatic nucleus have been varied. Pronounced differences were observed in both specific rates of binding (k_{12}) and dissociation (k_{21}). However, in this group of derivatives both topological and electron density changes are caused by varying ring substitutions and it is difficult at the moment to clearly correlate the kinetic data with ligands structure. Thus, main effort was concentrated on varying the side chains attached to the DNP ring.

Dinitroaniline derivatives in which one or both amino group hydrogens were substituted by alkyl residues showed the following interesting trend: the changes in the specific rate of binding is decreasing by 50% from the unsubstituted (2,4-dinitroaniline-DNA) 4.8×10^8 mole $^{-1}$sec^{-1} to 2.1×10^8 mole $^{-1}$sec^{-1} for the N,N-diethyl dinitroaniline. The changes in k_{21} are much more pronounced, decreasing from 927 sec^{-1} to 373 sec^{-1} for N,N-dimethyl DNA and rising again to 555 sec^{-1} for the N,N-diethyl DNA. The data obtained with a more extensive series of normal and branched alkyl substituents on the amino nitrogen is summarized in Table 1. Again we find that both specific rates (k_{12} and k_{21}) vary, though to a different extent, as a function of the structure of the side chain. In the variation of the reciprocal lifetime (k_{21}) of the site-hapten complex, as a function of length and more pronounced on branching of the alkyl side chain, a well defined minimum is observed when a bulky, hydrophobic group is present adjacent to the 1 amine nitrogen of the aromatic ring (table 1 lines 9 and 10). It is remarkable to observe how sensitive k_{21} is to small structural changes. For example for isobutyl and tert butyl side

Table 1

Rate and equilibrium constants for the interaction between protein 315 and: 1) a homologous series of DNP alkylamines and 2) DNP derivatives containing branched, cyclic or aromatic side chains.

Hapten	$k_{12}^* \times 10^{-8}$ $M^{-1} Sec^{-1}$	k_{21}^* Sec^{-1}	$K=(k_{12}^*/k_{21}^*) \times 10^{-6}$ M^{-1}	$K_{st} \times 10^{-6}$ M^{-1}
1) $2ON$–⟨benzene, NO_2⟩–NH––CH_3	3.5 ± 0.24	373 ± 30	0.94	
2) –"– –CH_2–CH_3	2.8 ± 0.18	143 ± 24	1.95	2.04
3) –"– –CH_2–CH_2–CH_3	2.6 ± 0.18	94 ± 11	2.70	
4) –"– –CH_2–CH_2–CH_2–CH_3	2.5 ± 0.3	79 ± 10	3.20	3.40
5) –"– –CH_2–CH_2–CH_2–CH_2–CH_2–CH_3	1.2 ± 0.12	123 ± 18	1.00	1.10
6) –"– –CH⟨CH_3/CH_3	3.7 ± 0.22	108 ± 8.6	3.40	
7) –"– –CH⟨CH_2–CH_2/CH_2–CH_2⟩CH_2	2.55 ± 0.25	116 ± 10	2.20	
8) –"– –CH_2–CH⟨CH_3/CH_3	2.0 ± 0.14	83 ± 11	2.40	2.70
9) –"– –C⟨CH_3 CH_3/CH_3	3.6 ± 0.3	58 ± 6	6.10	
10) –"– –CH_2–⟨phenyl⟩	1.8 ± 0.15	47 ± 9	3.80	

chains a 30% difference is found in favour of stabilizing
the latter derivatives. If the side chain is not compact
and exceeds a certain degree of bulkiness it also is reflected immediately in k_{21} as found inter alia with the N,N di-
ethyl DNA (cf. above) or N-cyclohexyl DNA derivatives (table
1 - No. 7). The interesting feature evolving from these data
is the presence of a hydrophobic subsite available to interact with the appropriately located side group(s) of the DNP.
To estimate the dimension of this subsite the extended dimensions of the alkyl groups were used. Since both straight
chain and branched aliphatic side groups reduce k_{21} the
hydrophobic subsite may be quite extended up to 8Å length.
That this is indeed the case and that the straight aliphatic
chains are not bound in a folded form is corroborated by the
data obtained for the series of DNA with electrostatic char-
ges carried at increasing distance from the ring on aliphatic side chains. These data are shown diagramatically in
figure 2. The change in k_{21} as a function of the distance
of the negatively charged carboxylate from the DNA nucleus
is rather dramatic: while when it is close to the ring, k_{21}
is of the order of 10^3 sec^{-1}, it decreases sharply as it is
becoming more distant to a minimum value of 45 sec^{-1} at a
distance of ca. 8.5 Å from the ring's center. Significantly
no marked further change is found when the carboxylate is
further out from the ring (fig. 2). The identification of
the electrostatic subsite of interaction and its location
are further confirmed by the k_{21} values of a series of DNA
derivatives carrying a positively charged ammonium group at
varying distances from the ring (fig. 2). Thus, high k_{21}
values (8 x 10^2 sec^{-1}) are observed practically for the
three, positive charge carrying homologous ligands with
closer distance to the ring (fig. 2) and only when the charge is as far out as 6 methylene groups (~9 Å) this effect of
the charge repulsion diminishes and k_{21} drops to 120 sec^{-1}.
It is worthwhile noticing that both types of charged side
chains are causing repulsion (i.e. large values of k_{21}) when
close to the ring, possibly because of existence of the hydrophobic region (table 1). When their distance from the ring
increases, the specific preference of the negatively charged
ligand is expressed in the decrease of k_{21} values.

Further refinement of our mapping of the site is achieved by comparing specific rates of interactions of DNP
derivatives carrying stereoisomeric side chains. Data for

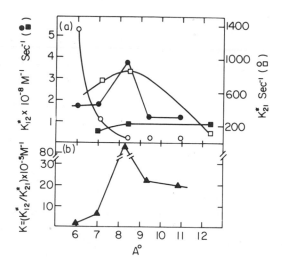

Figure 2.   The dependence of (a) k_{12} (-●- and -■-), k_{21} (-o- and -□-) and (b) K on the distance of the carboxylate or ammonium respectively group of the alkyl side chain from the DNP ring.   (Only extended chain length is shown).

α-N-DNP derivatives of glycine, D and L alanine and of their dipeptides (Gly_2, DD, LL, DL and LD Ala_2) were collected. Rather small variation in the k_{12} values were recorded. The k_{21} values did however span a larger range: both DNP gly and $DNP(gly)_2$ have relatively short residence time in the site (k_{21} = 1340 and 1058 respectively). For the alanine derivatives, the following sequence is found: $DNP-LD-Ala_2$ (880 sec^{-1}) > $DNP-LL-Ala_2$ (721 sec^{-1}) > DNP-L-Ala (664 sec^{-1}) > $DNP-DD-Ala_2$ (470 sec^{-1}) > $DNP-DL-Ala_2$ (330 sec^{-1}) > DNP-D-Ala (314 sec^{-1}).

In order to analyse the structural implication of these differences in k_{21} values in terms of the structure of the combining site, models of the different ligands were constructed and the relative distances from the ring of the various groups on the peptide side chains were measured for the different isomers. The large decrease in k_{21} upon changing the gly or gly_2 side chain to an ala derivate (i.e. substituting an α hydrogen by a methyl group) is another reflection of the presence of a hydrophobic subsite adjacent to the DNP binding subsite. The differences between the k_{21} values of the different combinations of ala isomers may be accounted for, in a fully self consistent manner, in terms of the proposed structure of the site (8) concluded from all above data: a) Though contribution to the binding of ligands to the site are mainly due to interactions with the polynitro-aromatic ring, there are available further contributions from other types of forces. b) Two types of interaction forces were identified and localized in terms of three subsites found in regions of increasing distance from the subsite of the polynitrophenyl ring. Two hydrophobic subsites of different dimensions and an positively charged electrostatic subsite (figure 3).

The measurements of specific rates of binding and dissociation of a series of derivatives where the structural parameter is changing in a different way is that of oligo-lysyl-ε-N-dinitrophenyl lysine ($(lysyl)_n$ ε-N-DNP lysine, n = 0 - 8). The data are shown in table 2 and clearly show that here, larger changes are observed in k_{12} than in k_{21} (11). This illustrates the case where no significant changes in the available interactions from the ligands with site contact residues occur beyond the dipeptide. Therefore, the k_{21} values remain practically constant for all longer derivatives. The k_{12} values however change over a range of 3 to

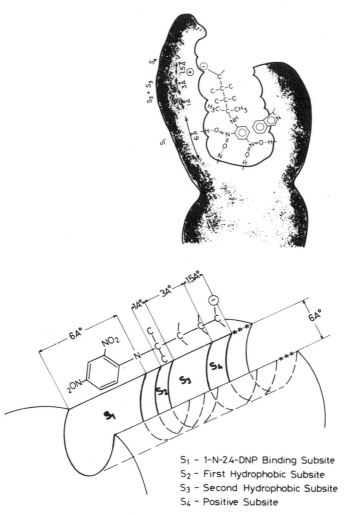

S₁ – 1-N-2,4-DNP Binding Subsite
S₂ – First Hydrophobic Subsite
S₃ – Second Hydrophobic Subsite
S₄ – Positive Subsite

Figure 3. Two hypothetic model views of the binding site of MOPC 315 indicating the different subsites of interaction.

Table 2

Rate and equilibrium constants for the interaction between protein 315 and oligolysyl ε-N-DNP lysine.

$(lys)_n$-εN-DNP-lysine	$k_{12}^* \times 10^{-7}$ $M^{-1} Sec^{-1}$	k_{21}^* Sec^{-1}	$K=(k_{12}^*/k_{21}^*) \times 10^{-6}$ M^{-1}
n=0	14.0 ± 1.4	53 ± 5	2.60
αN–Acetyl–εN– DNP–lysine	12.0 ± 1	51 ± 7	2.36
n=1	8.7 ± 0.78	35 ± 4	2.50
n=2	8.1 ± 0.64	27 ± 4	3.00
n=3	8.0 ± 0.6	32 ± 5.8	2.50
n=4	7.0 ± 0.7	31 ± 5.6	2.30
n=5	4.8 ± 0.85	29 ± 5.8	1.65
n=6	3.7 ± 0.55	29 ± 4.3	1.30
n=7	3.3 ± 0.4	31 ± 4.6	1.10
n=8	3.3 ± 0.2	32 ± 4.5	1.00

$14 \times 10^7 \text{ M}^{-1} \text{ sec}^{-1}$ which is relatively large and in our opinion (11) reflects the effect of non specific interactions between the highly charged oligolysyl chain and the negatively charged surface of MOPC 315. These data illustrates the importance of resolving the variations caused in the overall equilibrium constants (table 2) into their different causes as expressed in the changes in k_{21} and k_{12}. While in the first case the changes reflect variations in complementarity and forces of interaction, changes in the second are usually a result of the events occuring outside the site.

An independent criterion for the dimensions or more precisely range of interactions within the combining site (again relative to a certain reference point like the DNP subsite of binding) is obtained from measurements of the linear and circular polarization of the fluorescence (20) emitted by complexes formed between the MOPC 315 and a series of appropriately designed DNP derivatives. A fluorescent group, e.g. 9-amino acridine has been covalently linked to DNP derivatives to form the homologous series of the following structure: DNP-$\overset{\text{H}}{\text{N}}$-$(CH_2)_n$-$\overset{\text{H}}{\text{N}}$-Acridine where n = 2 to 6. The fluorescence emission spectrum of the complex formed between MOPC 315 and these ligands is shown in figure 4. Also included in this figure is the circularly polarized emission spectrum expressed in terms of g_{em} the emission anisotropy factor (20), which reflects the degree of a symmetry in the excited state of the emitter or it's environment.

Table 3 summarizes the data obtained from both linear and circular fluorescence polarization for complexes between MOPC 315 and three different ligands. It is interesting to note that while all three ligands show practically the same change in their linear polarized emission upon binding to the sites of MOPC 315, only the shorter derivative, i.e., the one where the fluorophore is only ca. 7.5 Å from the DNP ring center shows a significant component of circularly polarized emission. This indicates that the acridine part of this ligand is sensing part of the contact residues of the combining site. The relatively low value of g_{em} may imply that these interactions are quite on the external boundaries of the site and in order to check this ligand with shorter spacer are being investigated at present. The increase in linear polarization is due to the partial immobilization of the fluorophores in the complex where the DNP part of the ligand is anchored in the site.

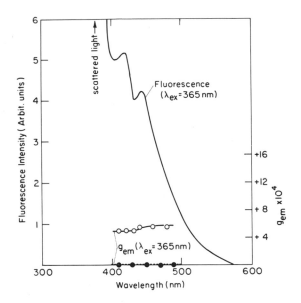

Figure 4. Spectra of the fluorescence and of the emission anisotropy factor of free and bound (2', 4' dinitro) anilino-2(9"amino)acridinylethane (-0-0-0-), complex with MOPC 315; (-●-●-●-) free hapten; (----) in presence of normal mice IgG. Hapten concentration - 10^{-4}M; protein concentration - 5.10^{-5}M. Excitation wavelength - 365nm.

Table 3

Linear and circular polarization measurements of the
complexes between MOPC 315 and DNP derivatives

λ_{Ex} nm	$\frac{I}{I}$	P	g_{em}	$\frac{I}{I}$	P	g_{em}
DNP-N-(CH$_2$)$_2$-9 amino acridine H				+ MOPC 315		
315	1,03	~0	~0	1,55	0,22	$+9 \cdot 10^4$
365	1,04	~0	~0	1,45	0,19	$+9 \cdot 10^4$
DNP-N-(CH$_2$)$_3$-9 amino acridine H				+ MOPC 315		
315	1,02	~0	~0	1,53	0,21	~0
365	1,02	~0	~0	1,48	1,9	~0
DNP-N-(CH$_2$)$_6$-9 amino acridine H				+ MOPC 315		
315	1,08	~0	~0	1,53	0,21	~0
365	1,05	~0	~0	1,44	1,8	~0

In figure 3 the model of the MOPC 315 binding site is presented in two concepts; a schematic groove like structure and a cross section of a deeper cleft structure which may be shalower and more groove like in other cross sections. The significant points are obviously the different subsites of interaction and their locations. The dimensions may be misleading to a certain extent since we were carrying out an analysis of a three dimentional site in two dimentional terms. It is however, gratifying that the position where we find the fluorophore to begin sensing the site are compatible with the model evolving from the kinetic mapping. The results of a different physical technique applied to probing antibody binding sites, namely the use of spin labelled haptens (21-23), are rather interesting in the context of our use of fluorophores labelled haptens. The immobilization of the spin label part of the compound DNP ligand is used as a criterion for its interaction with the site and recently complexes of two different DNP-spin label derivatives with MOPC 315 were studied (23). In these derivatives, the spin label is about 7 Å and less away from the center of the DNP ring and the electron spin resonance (ESR) spectra of the complexes show strong immobilization of the spin labels. These results are therefore in accord with the structural model proposed in this discussion.

The phosphoryl choline binding mouse myeloma proteins (24,25), offer an interesting possibility of extending our kinetic mapping to homogeneous binding site of distinctly different specificity. The measurements on HOPC-8 have already began following the proteins tryptophan fluorescence enhancement occurring upon ligand binding (26). With phosphoryl choline as ligand, again a single step interaction mechanism was found and the specific rates of binding $k_{12}=4.6 \times 10^7$ M^{-1} sec^{-1} and dissociation $k_{21} = 119$ sec^{-1} (27) are in a similar range to that observed for other systems. The ratio between these rates ($k_{12}/k_{21} = K$) is in good agreement with the equilibrium constant determined by fluorescence and equilibrium dialysis methods (26). Early kinetic measurements of normally induced, heterogeneous antibody populations (4-6) resulted in mechanistic conclusions which were later verified by measurements on homogeneous myeloma proteins (7). The specific rates determined for the heterogeneous preparations are average values which obviously cannot be used for correlations of the nature described above. Still the availability of antibody preparations which could be fractionated by elution with a homologous series of structuraly related ligands raised the question to what extent kinetic parameters of these different fractions may be correlated with the structure of the ligands and with the nature of the eluate. Two systems have been studied until now: The dynamics interaction of 1-(m-nitrophenyl) Flavazoles of isomaltose oligosaccharides with purified antidextran antibodies (28) and more extensively those of 1-(dansyl) ethane diamine derivatives of oligoalanines with antipolyalanine fractions (15). The interaction of the haptens with the antibody binding sites were followed by measuring the fluorescent energy transfer from the excited protein tryptophanes to the dansyl side chain attached to the alanine hapten. In figure 5 the fluorometric titration of the ala_2 eluate of antipolyalanine HSA with the $\underline{D}$-ala-diaminoethane-dansyl ligand, is illustrated. The protein emission is quenched upon binding whereas the emission of the dansyl bound by virtue of the D-ala residue is increasing. Table 4 summarizes the data obtained in collaboration with Mr. Arie Licht on this system. The variation in both specific rates do not show the same trend for the two eluates. Moreover, their variation is limited to a range of less than an order of magnitude. It is, however, interesting that the rates of binding (k_{12}) are all within one to two orders of magnitude slower than those observed for the k_{12} values of the binding of DNP ligands to heterogeneous anti DNP antibodies (4,5). The specific rates of dissociation are within the range found in most other cases. The reason for the intriguingly slow rate of binding of these haptens is unclear and may have to do with the different chemical nature of the oligoalanine hapten as compared with DNP.

ACKNOWLEDGMENT

The studies reported in this paper have been supported by a research grant from the Volkswagenwerk foundation which is gratefully acknowledged.

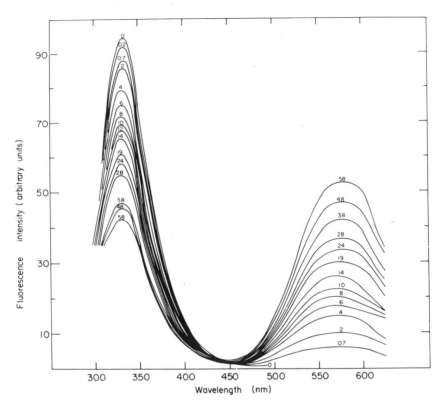

Figure 5. Fluorometric titration of ala$_2$ eluate of anti-
bodies against poly D-alanine HSA with $\underline{D}$-Ala-$\underline{N}$-(CH$_2$)$_2$ $\underline{N}$-
dansyl at 25°C pH 7.2 phosphate buffered saline.
Excitation wavelength 280nm. (Numbers refer to μl added of
1 x 10^{-3} M hapten solution.)

Table 4

Dynamics of interaction of alanine peptides with fractionated anti-polyalanine antibodies

Hapten	Antibody	$k_{12}M^{-1}sec^{-1}$	$k_{21}sec^{-1}$	$k_{12}/k_{21} = K_M^{-1}$
$\underline{\underline{D}}$(Ala)HN-(CH$_2$)$_2$-NH-dansyl	$\underline{\underline{D}}(Ala)_2$ eluate	4.6×10^5	3.1	1.5×10^5
"	$\underline{\underline{D}}(Ala)_3$ eluate	5.7×10^6	2.0	2.9×10^6
"	$\underline{\underline{D}}(Ala)_4$ eluate	3.0×10^6	1.5	2.0×10^6
$\underline{\underline{D}}(Ala)_2$-HN-(CH$_2$)$_2$-NH-dansyl	$\underline{\underline{D}}(Ala)_2$ eluate	4.1×10^6	1.2	3.4×10^6
"	$\underline{\underline{D}}(Ala)_3$ eluate	4.3×10^6	1.8	2.4×10^6
"	$\underline{\underline{D}}(Ala)_4$ eluate	1.7×10^6	3.8	4.5×10^4

All experiments carried out on a temperature-jump spectrofluorometer at 25°C pH 7.2 phosphate buffer saline. Excitation wavelengths 280nm, cut off at 400nm.

33

REFERENCES

1. R.J. Poljak, L.M. Amzel, H.P. Avey, L.N. Becka and A. Nisonoff, Nature New Biol. 235, 137 (1972).
2. E.A. Padlan, D.M. Segal, T.E. Spande, D.R. Davies, S.R. Rudikoff and M. Potter, Nature New Biol., 245, 165 (1973).
3. R.J. Poljak, L.M. Amzel, H.P. Avey, B.L. Chen, R.P. Phizackerley and F. Saul. Proc. Natl. Acad. Sci., U.S.A., 70, 3305 (1973).
4. A. Froese, A.H. Sehon and M. Eigen, Cand. J. Chem., 40, 1786 (1962).
5. L.A. Day, J.M. Sturtevant and S.J. Singer, Ann. N.Y. Acad. Sci., 103, 619 (1963).
6. A. Froese, Immunochemistry, 5, 253 (1968).
7. I. Pecht, D. Givol and M. Sela, J. Mol. Biol., 68, 241 (1972).
8. D. Haselkorn, S. Friedman, D. Givol and I. Pecht, Biochemistry, 13, 000 (1974).
9. G.G. Hammes, Adv. Protein Chem., 23, 1 (1968).
10. I. Pecht, D. Haselkorn and S. Friedman, FEBS Letters, 24, 331 (1972).
11. D. Haselkorn, A. Yaron, M. Sela and I. Pecht, to be published.
12. H.S. Eisen, E.S. Simms and M. Potter, Biochemistry, 7, 4126 (1968).
13. I. Schechter, B. Schechter and M. Sela, Biochim.Biophys. Acta, 127, 438 (1966).
14. S.F. Schlossman and A. Yaron, Ann. N.Y. Acad. Sci. 169, 108 (1970).
15. A. Licht and I. Pecht, to be published.
16. U. Hartmann, J. Schlessinger and I. Pecht, Proc. 6th Meeting Israel Immunol. Soc., Israel J. Med. Sci. (in press).
17. I. Schechter, Nature 228, 639 (1970).
18. R. Pollet and H. Edelhoch, J. Biol. Chem., 248, 5443 (1973).
19. I.Z. Steinberg and A. Gafni, Rev. Sci. Inst. 43, 409 (1972).
20. I.Z. Steinberg, in "Concepts in Biochemical Fluorescence" R. Chen and H. Edelhoch (eds.) Marcel Dekker N.Y. (1974).
21. L. Stryer and O.H. Griffith, Proc. Natl. Acad. Sci. U.S.A 54, 1785 (1965).
22. J.C. Hsia and L.H. Piette, Arch. Biochim. Biophys., 129, 296 (1969).

23. J.C. Hsia and J. Russell Little, FEBS Letters, 31, 80 (1973).
24. M. Potter and M.A. Leon, Science, 162, 369 (1968).
25. M.A. Leon and N.M. Young, Biochemistry, 10, 1424 (1971).
26. R. Pollet and H. Edelhoch, J. Biol. Chem., 248, 5443 (1973).
27. U. Hartmann and I. Pecht, unpublished.
28. E.A. Kabat and I. Pecht, unpublished.

MULTISPECIFICITY OF THE ANTIBODY COMBINING REGION AND ANTIBODY DIVERSITY

John K. Inman

Laboratory of Immunology
National Institute of Allergy and Infectious Diseases
National Institutes of Health
Bethesda, Maryland 20014

ABSTRACT. Evidence is accumulating that individual antibody species are capable of binding many structurally dissimilar haptens. If individual antibody species arising from an immunization usually do not share their alternate (disparate) specificities, and if cross reactions can be detected only above a reasonable threshold, then it can be shown with a probability model that heterogeneously populated antisera can indeed exhibit a high degree of specificity. Thus, the model substantiates the hypothesis that a limited repertoire of antibody species can, in various portions and combinations, populate specific antisera to an essentially unlimited number of antigens. The model further suggests that the required number of distinct combining regions (V_H x V_L pairs) may fall in the range of 10^4 to 10^6 if nature has followed a conservative course. Specific antibodies from unimmunized animals ("natural" antibodies) can best be explained on the basis of disparate multispecificities. The levels of such antibodies can then be related to the probability model and to estimates of an animal's total antibody combining region repertoire.

INTRODUCTION

Considerable evidence indicates that individual animals, when appropriately immunized, can produce a specific antiserum against almost any natural or synthetic substance. The classical studies of Landsteiner (1) showed that, with very few exceptions, an antiserum will react better with the immunizing hapten than with similar or dissimilar structures. The very high specificity of an antiserum has usually been attributed to a similar degree of specificity residing with the constituent antibodies. Such an assumption leads to the notion that most antibody species fit uniquely well to a determinant structure of the eliciting antigen. However, the number of possible chemical structures of combining site size, or even the number of groups sharing an immunodominant feature with similar substructures, will likely exceed any diligent estimate. The idea that a stable antigen-antibody complex requires a perfect fit between two complementary configurations thus demands an enormous antibody repertoire and places a huge burden on any theory of antibody diversity.

MULTISPECIFICITY

In a paper published in 1959 David Talmage (2) questioned the above concepts and proposed instead the following ideas: 1) A stable antigen-antibody complex will result in any case where it is possible for enough simultaneous, short-range interactions to occur. Or, by whatever mechanisms which might apply, a minimum binding energy is exceeded. 2) Many different antigenic determinants should be able to combine with the same antibody molecule. Lack of fit in one area can be compensated by increased binding elsewhere in the combining region. 3) The specificity of an antiserum containing many different antibody species will be greater than that of any single species. This results from the probability that the number of reactivities common to most of the species is greatly diminished compared with the number of reactivities possessed by a single antibody molecule. In other words, the heterogeneity of the antibody population has the effect of reducing the concentration of each individual species so that chance reaction with an unrelated antigen would be below the threshold of detection. Figure 1 illustrates the proposed situation. For the purpose of this discussion, an antibody species refers to a structurally distinct combining region without regard for differences in constant region structures which do not play a role in antigen binding. All h species of the hypothetical antiserum react with the immunogen determinant A by definition. A similar hapten, A', and a slightly less similar one, A", react with many and with fewer species, respectively. Such behavior agrees straightforwardly with the serological studies of Landsteiner (1) and many others. What is being proposed is that each individual species has its own characteristic reactivities against a range of dissimilar haptens, and that these diverse specificities are largely unshared. Thus, when the serum is tested against hapten G, only species #3 reacts. Less often, as with hapten D, two species will react. If h is large, then a negative serological reaction will be recorded for G and possibly also for D. Instead, had the animal donating the Figure 1 antibodies been immunized against hapten G, species #3 might have been a component of the resulting anti-G.

Recently, Varga et al. (3) reported that cross reactions

ANTIBODY SPECIES RAISED AGAINST
HAPTEN A

No.	1	2	3	4	5 · · · · · · · h	
	A	A	A	A	A	A
	A'	A'	A'		A'	A'
Specificities	A"		A"	A"		A"
	B	C	F	J	(D)	T
	E	(D)	G	W	H	L
	Q	M	R	X	P	Y
	V	S	N	K	Z	U
	:	:	:	:	:	:

Fig. 1. Specificity profiles of individual antibody
species in a hypothetical antiserum illustrating the concepts
of multispecificity (both familial and disparate). The
letters stand for determinant-sized haptens which, in each
vertical column, represent the potential reactivities or
specificities of an individual antibody molecular species.
A' and A'' are closely related in structure to the immunogen
hapten A (A' more so than A''). The other haptens are, for
the most part, structurally unrelated to A or to one another.
The disparate reactivities are largely unshared between different antibody species. Species numbers 2 and 5 share D-
reactivity and may provide for a weakly positive serological
reaction to hapten D in a suitable test system.

can occur with disparate structures and normally raised antibodies. Four such cross reactions were found after screening
rabbit anti-DNP antiserum with 144 diverse compounds using a
sensitive radioimmunoassay. More recently, Varga et al. (4)
found a binding frequency of about 1 in 200 upon screening
10 myeloma proteins with nearly 400 compounds. The lower
limit for the binding constant in keeping with this frequency
fell in the range of 10^4 to 10^5 1/mole. Merchant, Inman et
al. (5) have detected numerous disparate cross reactions by
the hemolytic plaque assay using red cells sensitized with
haptens of somewhat different structure than the immunizing
one.

PROBABILITY MODEL FOR SEROLOGICAL SPECIFICITY

Talmage (6) and later Schimke and Kirkpatrick (7)
attempted to explain in quantitative terms how high degrees
of serological specificity for all antigens can be attained
with a limited repertoire of multispecific antibodies. Their
use of combinatorial logic was valid and useful in as far as
they carried it. Possibly, because data was lacking on disparate multispecificity, and because the model used for ex-
plaining their approach was confusing, the ideas expressed
so clearly in Talmage's 1959 paper (2) went largely unheeded.
These ideas were revived in 1970 by A.N. Glazer (8) in an
interesting paper describing unexpected cross reactions at
enzyme binding sites, and also, in that same year, by Hood
and Talmage (9). The same principles were stated again in
1972 by Williamson (10) and, with special clarity, by
Rosenstein et al. (11).
    Recently, I have developed a quantitative model which
provides a means for calculating the probability of serological cross reactions within a system of multispecific antibodies. Again, combinatorial principles were applied, but
the model allows a more general handling of factors affecting
specificity than do the formulae of Talmage (6) or Schimke
et al. (7). The parameters of the model are the following:
n, the total number of structurally different combining
regions or V_L x V_H pairs an animal can make (the total
repertoire); h, the number of different combining regions
present in an antiserum (the heterogeneity factor); d, the
number of different combining regions in the total repertoire
that can potentially react with a randomly selected (disparate) hapten; P(i), the probability that i different combining regions in an antiserum will cross react with the
randomly selected hapten.
    An approach to the model is diagrammed in Figure 2, and

40

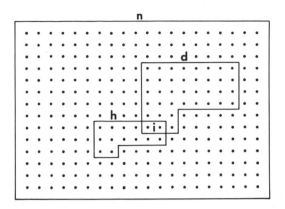

Fig. 2. A set diagram used in developing the probability model. Each dot represents a separate antibody combining
region species (or V_L x V_H pair). Out of all n of these, d
can potentially react with a randomly chosen structure. An
antiserum to a given hapten has h combining region species.
There are a priori probabilities that no overlap or various
degrees of overlap will occur involving i species (that is,
i species in the antiserum reacting with the randomly chosen
structure).

is based on a random drawing of $\underline{h}$ things from $\underline{n}$ distinguish-able objects. An unrelated subset of $\underline{d}$ objects exists in the total pool. There is a calculable $\underline{a\ priori}$ probability of drawing 0, 1, 2, or some number, $\underline{i}$, objects belonging to the subset of $\underline{d}$. The desired probability is given by an ex-pression of combinatorials sometimes referred to as the hypergeometric distribution. In terms of the above para-meters it is written

$$P(i) = \frac{\binom{d}{i} \cdot \binom{n-d}{h-i}}{\binom{n}{h}} = \frac{h! \, d! \, (n-h)! \, (n-d)!}{n! \, i! \, (h-i)! \, (d-i)! \, (n-h-d+i)!}$$

The factorial terms, which are too large to evaluate directly, are expanded into several series of products of non-factorial terms for calculating $P(0)$. Higher terms can be obtained by a simple reiterative computation as indicated below.

$$P(0) = \frac{\displaystyle\prod_{j=0}^{j=d-1} (n-h-j)}{\displaystyle\prod_{k=0}^{k=d-1} (n-k)} \qquad \text{and} \quad P(i+1) = R(i) \cdot P(i)$$

$$\text{where} \quad R(i) = \frac{(h-i)(d-i)}{(i+1)(n-h-d+i+1)}$$

No approximations are used. A computer program for the above expressions was written by Dr. David Alling, and various probability terms were calculated over reasonable ranges of $\underline{n}$, $\underline{h}$, and $\underline{d}$ values for a hypothetical immunological system. The first noteworthy feature of the results is the extent to which successive probability terms diminish. A typical re-sult is shown in Table 1 for a system with 400,000 total combining regions, including 400 which react with a dis-parate test hapten, and an antiserum with 40 antibody species. In this case, successive terms decrease about 70-fold. The importance of a threshold for detection is in-dicated. The threshold for a positive serological reaction is then defined as a minimum number of cross-reacting com-bining regions, i, required for detection. The probability of a positive reaction between an antiserum and a randomly chosen test hapten is, accordingly

$$\text{cumP}(i) = P(i) + P(i+1) + P(i+2) + \cdots\cdots P(h)$$

The specificity of an antiserum may be defined as the average

TABLE 1

INDIVIDUAL PROBABILITY TERMS FOR $n=400,000$, $h=40$, $d=400$

i	P(i)
0	0.961
1	0.0385
2	7.49×10^{-4}
3	9.45×10^{-6}
4	8.69×10^{-8}
5	6.07×10^{-1c}

number of randomly chosen test haptens required to yield one detectable serological reaction. Thus, Specificity = 1/cumP (i).

The number of combining region species in an antiserum, h, may reasonably lie between 10 and 100. Values for d, the disparate hapten repertoire, are more difficult to guess. A reasonable assumption is that nature is conservative. Accordingly, an average d value should not be more than several orders of magnitude larger than a typical h value. The quantity, h, will be less than d for the corresponding hapten due to maturation of the response and to random effects stemming from the animal's immunological history. I have customarily taken d to be 10 to 20 times h. The value of d would, of course, depend heavily upon the choice of binding constant defining the lower limit of a specific antigen-antibody interaction.

Figure 3. illustrates how the detection threshold affects the relationship between serological specificity and the total combining region repertoire. The values h=40, and d=400 are chosen as being typical. Extensive trials with a very sensitive screening assay which would detect any cross-reacting species would yield the dashed curve. However, if only one cross-reacting species is missed, and two or more are detectable, specificity is greatly increased. If 3 out of 40 species are just detectable, then much higher specificity can be realized. With n=200,000, over 10,000 randomly chosen substances would have to be screened to find one, probably weak, serological cross reaction. The same i=3, d=400 curve is shown again in Figure 4. along with i=3 curves for 4 times smaller and larger d values. The figures for d represent an average repertoire of antibodies reacting with the various test haptens in the hypothetical screening experiment. The less conservative value of d=1600 is compatible with a specificity of over 10,000 for a total repertoire of still less than one million. Cell surface determinants, which are probably complex, rigid and extended structures, may be represented by somewhat fewer antibodies in the repertoire. Behavior more like that shown by the d=100 curve may pertain. Small d values in such cases would help in preventing self-tolerance from rendering useless a major portion of the total repertoire.

The principal point made by Talmage (2) and Rosenstein et al. (11) was that a heterogeneous population of antibodies is much more specific than its components if a finite test threshold is allowed. Figure 5. clearly illustrates this thesis for a modest repertoire of 400,000 species. Specificity is plotted against serum heterogeneity, h. Threshold in terms of relative numbers of species just detectable is

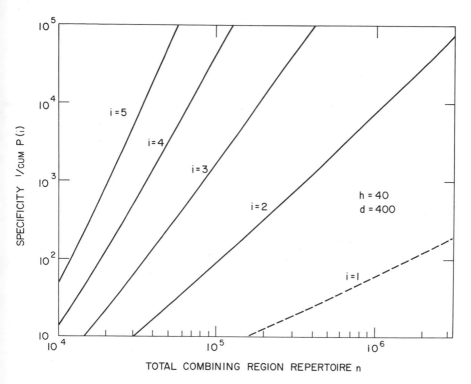

Fig. 3. The relationship between specificity of an antiserum containing 40 components and the total repertoire as affected by different test thresholds. Specificity, as defined on the ordinate, can be viewed as the average number of test haptens in a hypothetical screening experiment required to yield one detectable serological reaction. $\underline{d}$ is an average repertoire value for the test haptens used. In this figure $\underline{i}$ refers to the threshold number of cross-reacting antibody species, the number just detectable. Note that both scales are logarithmic.

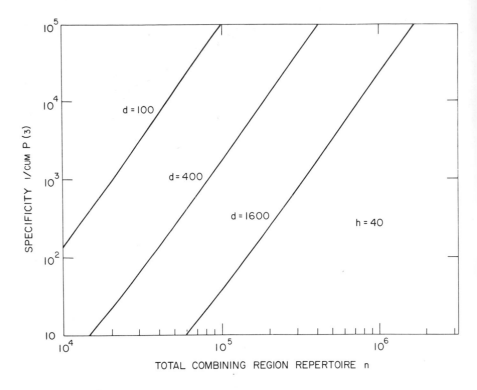

Fig. 4. Serological specificity for a serum containing 40 components vs. the total repertoire as affected by different assumed values for an average d. Threshold is exceeded with 3 or more cross-reacting species. For additional explanation see Fig. 3 legend.

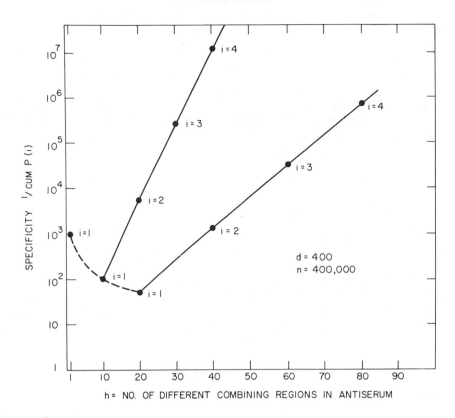

Fig. 5. Specificity as a function of antiserum hetero-geneity. The threshold for each point on a given curve is held constant in terms of the fraction (i/h) of species crossreacting that will give a positive serological reaction. The left-hand curve is set up for i/h = 0.1 (10% threshold); for the right-hand curve i/h = 0.05 (5% threshold). See Fig. 3 legend for additional explanation.

held constant. The left-hand curve is constructed for $i=h/10$ and the right-hand one for $i=h/20$, that is, for a 10% and 5% threshold, respectively. In this example, if an antiserum were composed of a single antibody species, a specificity of 10^3 would be realized. But, as h increases above 20 or so, the specificity achieved is much greater than that for $h=1$. The increase in specificity is then rapidly exponential. Restricted antisera would give a poor showing regarding specificity.

NATURAL ANTIBODIES AND ANTIBODY DIVERSITY

Disparate multispecificity may offer the best explanation for so-called natural antibodies. Sera from unimmunized animals have been shown to contain low levels of immunoglobulins reactive with a variety of natural and synthetic antigens (12). For most synthetic substances tested, there is no a priori basis for suspecting a structural relationship with any environmental antigen to which the donors may have been exposed. Therefore, it is tempting to believe that natural antibodies result from disparate cross reactions with certain individual antibodies raised in response to unintentional stimuli.

Jormalainen et al. (13,14) have shown that natural antibody titers vary widely from one individual to another within a strain or species, but that averages of these titers are meaningful in as much as they allow consistent interstrain or interspecies differences to be assessed. A relative natural antibody level against a given hapten in a large pool of normal sera should approximate the level of antibodies with that specificity from a representative sampling of the entire repertoire. Thus, the relative amount (i.e., fraction of total immunoglobulin) of a natural antibody should likewise approximate the value d/n for that hapten. Not many estimates of natural antibodies are available in terms of actual or relative amounts, instead of dilution titers, since such measurements are quite difficult to do reliably. Moroz, et al. (15) reported levels of 0.04 to 0.2% of the total immunoglobulin for anti-keyhole limpet hemocyanin in normal human sera. Farah (16) found, on the average, about 0.4% anti-DNP in human immunoglobulin. Winkler et al. (17) isolated anti-azobenzoate and anti-azobenzenesulfonate from normal rabbit sera in yields corresponding to initial levels of around 0.01% of the Ig. Natural antibody levels ranging from less than 0.01% up to 1% may be expected. The geometric mean of the above figures is around 0.07%, suggesting a typical d/n ratio of 7×10^{-4} for rabbit or man. If $d{=}400$, based on the assumption that nature is conservative, is divided by this value of d/n, a combining region repertoire of 570,000 is obtained which is in agreement with the range required for serological specificity.

The only attempt to estimate the value of d experimentally was made by Kreth and Williamson (18). Four inbred mice were immunized against the NIP (3-iodo-4-hydroxy-5-nitrophenylacetyl) hapten. Individual antibody species were identified and enumerated by comparative isoelectric focusing of sera in gel slabs with radioautographic visualization of NIP-binding components. The sera were taken from a large number of syngeneic recipients of limited cell transfers from the immunized donors. In this, way errors due to complex patterns and overlaps were avoided. From the frequency of identical antibody species occurring between individual donors, an estimate of the anti-NIP repertoire in the CBA/H strain of mice was made using statistical calculations (19). The most probable value was surprisingly large, around 8,000 antibody species or about 5,000 combining region species, but had a broad range of likely values. The actual number of combining regions could be lower if carbohydrate heterogeneity and unsuspected constant region subclasses had played a part in increasing electrophoretic heterogeneity. Recently, I have estimated the level of anti-NIP in a normal serum pool from 23 CBA/H mice by measuring specific binding and elution of radioiodinated 7S immunoglobulin using an immunoadsorbent column. The value found was approximately 0.09% which, taken with the estimate of 5,000 for d, points to a total combining region repertoire (V_L x V_H pairs) for the strain of nearly 6 million.

The number of variable sequences required to generate 600,000 or 6,000,000 combining regions will depend on what assumptions one makes concerning the relative abundance of V_H and V_L sequences and about constraints on random pairing. If one makes the assumption that there are r times as many V_H as V_L sequences possible, and there are g equal groups of V_H and V_L, within and only within which pairing occurs, then the total of potential variable regions for both chains is given by

$$\left(\sqrt{r} + \frac{1}{\sqrt{r}} \right) \cdot \sqrt{gn}$$

for a combining region repertoire of n. For example, if $r{=}3$ and $g{=}6$, then there are 4,382 variable regions required for $n{=}600,000$ and 13,856 for $n{=}6,000,000$.

CONCLUDING REMARKS

The above considerations highlight the importance of further studies of disparate structure multispecificity at the level of individual antibody species. Regarding this phenomenon, I would like to present one final model to replace the conventional complementary surface diagram for the antigen-antibody interaction. Large numbers of different haptens can react singly with an antibody combining region if different but mostly overlapping areas for contact are allowed. A simplified picture of a "combinatorial" site model is presented as Figure 6. Different selections of atoms from the same antibody combining region are shown forming multiple contacts with either of two distinctly different antigens. Many atoms in the variable region amino acid residues are potentially contactable by external structures. Only a portion of these atoms need to be contacted simultaneously for adequate binding to occur. For any successful binding, fortuitous geometry and modes of flexibility in both partners are required. The main point to be made is that the number of possible combinations (meaning selections) of contacted atoms within the combining region can be very large. Each selection represents the potential for binding a different structure. In the actual situation I estimate that something like 10 or more simultaneous short-range interactions are required for binding, and that at least 200 atoms in the combining region are potentially available. Now, the number of combinations of 200 things taken 12 at a time is 6×10^{18} and taken 14 at a time is 1×10^{21}. Such a large potential for multispecificity is essentially what is demanded of a sensibly limited antibody repertoire that can accomodate all possible chemical structures.

ACKNOWLEDGMENT

I wish to express my gratitude for the help given by Dr. David W. Alling of the National Institute of Allergy and Infectious Diseases in checking the mathematical operations and in setting up and performing computer evaluations of the probability model.

REFERENCES

1. Landsteiner, K., The Specificity of Serological Reactions, Harvard University Press, Cambridge, Mass., rev. ed., 1945.

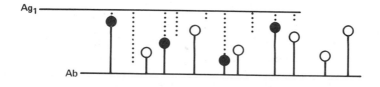

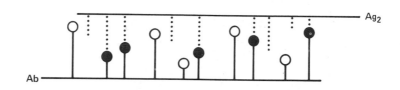

Fig. 6. A combinatorial concept of a highly multispecific antibody combining region. The same antibody is
represented in the upper and lower portions of the diagram.
The atoms of the antibody which are contactable by external
structures are shown as circles. Darkened circles are antibody atoms interacting with atoms of an antigen. The configuration of available atoms of an antigen is represented
by the terminal dots of dotted lines. The two different
antigens, Ag_1 and Ag_2, interact with the involvement of
different selections of atoms in both partners. A minimum
number of simultaneous interactions (contacts) would be
required for adequate binding to occur.

2. Talmage, D.W., Science 129, 1643 (1959).
3. Varga, J.M., Konigsberg, W.H. and Richards, F.F., Proc. Nat. Acad. Sci. U.S. 70, 3269 (1973).
4. Varga, J.M. and Richards, F.F., personal communication.
5. Merchant, B., Inman, J.K. and Srivastava, R.C., unpublished observations.
6. Talmage, D.W. and Cohen, E.P., Immunological Diseases Samter, M. and Alexander, H.L. (Eds.), Little, Brown & Co., Boston, 1965, p. 87.
7. Schimke, R.N. and Kirkpatrick, C.H., Immunologic Deficiency Diseases in Man (Vol. IV, No. 1 of Birth Defects Original Article Series), Bergsma, D. (Ed.) The National Foundation, New York, 1968, p. 328.
8. Glazer, A.N., Proc. Nat. Acad. Sci. U.S., 65, 1057 (1970).
9. Hood, L. and Talmage, D.W., Science 168, 325 (1970).
10. Williamson, A.R., Biochem. J. 130, 11 (1972).
11. Rosenstein, R.W., Musson, R.A., Armstrong, M.Y.K., Konigsberg, W.H. and Richards, F.F., Proc. Nat. Acad. Sci. U.S. 69, 877 (1972).
12. Boyden, S.V., Advances in Immunology, Vol. 5, Dixon, F.J. and Humphrey, J.H. (Eds.), Academic Press, New York, 1966, p. 1.
13. Jormalainen, S. and Mäkelä, O., Eur. J. Immunol. 1, 471 (1971).
14. Jormalainen, S., Eur. J. Immunol. 2, 483 (1972).
15. Moroz, L.A., Krygier, V. and Kotoulas, A.O., Immunol. 25, 441 (1973).
16. Farah, F.S., Immunol. 25, 217 (1973).
17. Winkler, M.H., Adetugbo, K. and Lehrer, G.M., Immunol. Commun. 1, 51 (1972).
18. Kreth, H.W. and Williamson, A.R., Eur. J. Immunol. 3, 141 (1973).
19. Wybrow, G.M. and Berryman, I.L., Eur. J. Immunol. 3, 146 (1973).

POLYFUNCTIONAL ANTIBODY COMBINING REGIONS

Frank F. Richards,* L.M. Amzel, W.H. Konigsberg,*
B.N. Manjula,* R.J. Poljak, R.W. Rosenstein,*
F. Saul, and Janos M. Varga*

Yale University School of Medicine *
New Haven, Connecticut 06510

Johns Hopkins University School of Medicine
Baltimore, Maryland 21205

Supported by Grants #AI-08614, AI-08202, AM-1003,
GM-12607 from the USPHS; GB-7870 and GB-1655 from
the NSF; by the American Heart Association, and by
a NIH Research Career Development Award, AI-70091,
to R.J. Poljak.

INTRODUCTION

The central theme of this study is an attempt
to resolve the apparent paradox presented by the
almost unlimited range of observed antibody combining specificities and the almost incredible
ability of an elicited antibody population to discriminate among very closely related antigens. It
is this specificity that is the most striking feature of an immune serum. For instance, an immune
serum will distinguish between two proteins having
as little as a single amino acid difference between them. It can also discriminate between two
steroids differing in a single functional group,
between D and L amino acids and between many other
closely related compounds. Landsteiner and his
collaborators (1), as well as other investigators,
have, over a period of thirty years, set out a
conceptual framework which has been generally accepted by immunologists and can be stated as
follows: 1. Antibodies are specific for the antigen used to elicit the immune response, 2. The
binding specificity of an individual immunoglobulin is determined by its amino acid sequence (3).
Antibodies may or may not bind antigens which are
structurally closely related to the eliciting antigen. When they do bind, it is with interaction
energies which are usually, but not always, lower

53

for the related antigen than for the eliciting antigen. The humoral immune response is usually heterogeneous. Many classes and groups of immunoglobulins are elicited in response even to a single antigenic determinant. The affinity of these antibody species for a simple antigenic determinant covers a wide range, indicating that many different types of antibody combining sites, complementary to the eliciting haptenic determinant, are present in the serum. From the evidence on which these propositions are based, a critical conclusion has been drawn, namely; that if the immunoglobulin population constituting the immune serum is highly specific for an antigen, so must be the individual immunoglobulins included in that population. This inference underlied a number of genetic and structural arguments concerning antibodies, especially those arguments related to the number of genes needed to code for the enormous number of immunoglobulins necessary to provide the observed range of antigenic specificities. This inference is still a keystone in much genetic and structural thinking about immunoglobulins (2), and it is the validity of this conclusion that we have challenged.

Quite early in the history of immunochemistry, the question was asked whether or not an antibody population raised against one hapten could in addition bind a second hapten (3). The conclusion from this and later studies (4) was that for a pair of determinants picked at random, there is little evidence that the same antibody population binds more than one determinant. Nevertheless, a number of studies suggested that the idea that a single immunoglobulin is directed against one determinant or against a group of structurally related determinants might have to be modified. Experiments were performed which suggested that there were in one animal of the order of 10^4 antibodies directed against a single small hapten (5). Since literally millions of small organic molecules which are presumptive haptens (6) have been described, the gene number required by a "monospecific" hypothesis would be very large indeed. Another approach has suggested that in small animals capable of hapten-specific humoral immune responses, there are not enough lymphocytes to account for the range of antibody specificities observed (7,8,9). Also, the many research groups who have measured the size of the antibody combining region have concluded that it measures perhaps 20-30 x 10-15 x 6 Å (10). Since there is good reason to believe that several areas within such a combining region enter into contact with the different determinants forming a relatively large antigen (10,11), the question arises whether such an antibody is in fact capable of binding many small determinants. Interpretation of such studies on antibody populations has not been easy, since it is difficult to distinguish between multiple binding to single immunoglobulins and single binding to multiple immunoglobulins. The advent of homogeneous myeloma immunoglobulins which bind haptens has simplified hapten binding studies (13). It is interesting that it has been noted from early studies with such proteins that they bound more than one type of hapten. Since, however, such binding is competitive and since the molecules used as haptens share some common structural features, it was possible that they bound to a common set of contact amino acids in the immunoglobulin (13).

The first direct evidence for spatially separated polyfunctional combining regions was obtained when we investigated protein 460, a mouse γA myeloma protein which binds the haptens, $\varepsilon 2$, 4 dinitrophenyl-L-lysine (εDnp lys) and 2 methyl 1,4 naphthoquinone (Menadione), with affinity constants of 1 x 10^5 Liters/Mole and 2 x 10^4 Liters/ Mole, respectively. In the course of these studies we found that there was a "hidden" sulfhydryl group whose properties affected the hapten binding of protein 460. In protein 460 this -SH group was alkylated very slowly by iodoacetic acid or by iodoacetamide. but reacted rapidly with Dnp-S-S-Dnp. The rapid rate of reaction depends on the fact that the Dnp group is first bound at the combining site prior to reacting with the free -SH group. After the formation of the covalent bond with protein 460, it no longer competes with the binding of ε Dnp lysine, but does interfere with Menadione binding, suggesting that the binding sites for

these two ligands may be spatially separated. The
ligating functions of protein 460 for εDnp lysine
and Menadione can be differentially inactivated by
the addition and removal of 4.3 $\underline{M}$ guanidine HCL.
After refolding, the capacity for Dnp binding was
greatly reduced while the affinity for Menadione
remained unchanged. Treatment of protein 460 with
2% dimethyl sulfoxide had the opposite effect. It
reduced Menadione binding but left Dnp binding intact (14).

   While these results suggest that some separation exists between the two binding sites, it does
not reveal the extent of the separation. To determine this it is necessary to measure the distance
between the ligand binding sites. One established
method for estimating distances of the order found
within protein molecules, is to measure the radia-
tionless transfer of energy from a donor molecular
probe molecule excited by a nanosecond pulse of
light. Such an excited probe gives off fluorescent light which is capable of being absorbed by a
second acceptor probe. The efficiency of energy
transfer (E) is related to the donor-acceptor distance,r , by the relationship:

$$E = \frac{r^{-6}}{r^{-6} + R_o^{-6}}$$

where R_o = the distance at which E=50%. It is
possible to measure energy transfer by nanosecond
fluorimetry and to calculate the distance r (15).
For us, this elegant technique had one major difficulty. Dnp and Menadione compete for binding to
the protein, hence; it is possible to bind only
one of these ligands to protein 460 at a time.
This makes direct energy transfer experiments impossible. We solved this problem by attaching a
donor probe to a third reference point and then
measuring successively the distance from donor to
Menadione. The unique -SH group associated with
the combining region of protein 460 after substitution with a suitable donor probe served as a
third reference point. We used two different dyes
as energy donors (N-iodoacetyl-N[1] -(1-sulfo-5-
naphthylethylenediamine) and N-(5-dimethylamino-
1-naphthalenesulfohydrazinyl-methyl-maleimide).

For acceptor probes we used both Dnp and Menadione
as well as fluorescein conjugated εDnp lysine.
Measurement of distances between donor and acceptor
probes is subject to the limitation that they have
no directional vectors and are thus expressed as
spheres centering on the donor probe. One sphere
is obtained for each -SH donor-hapten acceptor
distance. Therefore, it is possible to measure the
minimum distance which separates any two points
located on the surface of these two spheres. This
minimum distance between the Dnp and Menadione
binding sites proved to be 17 ± 3 Å, indicating
clearly that the closely overlapping site model is
incorrect in this instance; that there is substantial spatial separation between the sites, and that
the two ligands, Dnp and Menadione, presumably
have different sets of contact amino acids (16).
    While this work was in progress, collabora-
tion was begun with Dr. Roberto Poljak's group at
Johns Hopkins Medical School. This group had completed the 2.8 Å structure of the Fab fragment of
protein NEW (17). Protein NEW was not known to
bind any antigen, and since we wished to look at
the structure of the combining region at atomic
resolution, we needed to find a hapten. Therefore,
we tested protein NEW for ligand binding activity
using a rapid screening technique (18). In this
method, polyserine chains are attached to small,
activated, nylon discs and protein NEW is coupled
with glutaraldehyde to the polyserine chains fixed
to the nylon (Fig. 1). Protein NEW, attached to
these "polyserine whisker discs," was incubated
with individual members of a small battery of radioactive compounds, and then washed with buffer
for 1-2 seconds. The retained radioactivity was
then counted. Protein NEW bound uridine, and the
K_o as measured by equilibrium dialysis was approximately 1×10^3 L/Mole^{-1}. In the second step of
the assay over 300 non-radioactive compounds were
tested for their ability to displace uridine. This
assay has so far detected two structurally diverse
ligands which bind with K_o in excess of 1×10^5
L/Mole.
    A crystalline complex has now been obtained
of NEW Fab fragment and the first of these ligands,
a γ hydroxy derivative of Vit. K$_1$. Difference
Fourier diagrams at 3.5 Å resolution have been

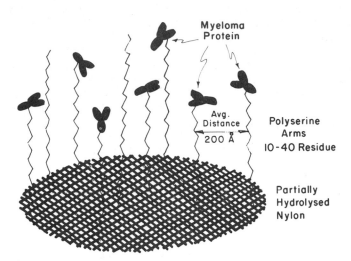

Figure 1

Polyserine Whisker Discs. Nylon net is partially hydrolyzed with HCl. The exposed amino
groups are used as initiators for formation of
polyserine whiskers from serine N-carboxy anhy-
dride. Immunoglobulins are coupled to the
polyserine strands with glutaraldehyde.

constructed and atomic models of the complex have
been built. These show for the first time the detailed structure of at least one part of the antibody combining region (19). The Vit. K_1 derivative
is located in a shallow depression between the
light (L) chain and the heavy (H) chain of the immunoglobulin (Fig. 2). One limb of the L-shaped
cleft is surrounded by the "hypervariable" loops
from the variable regions of the L and H chain. In
the upper portion of this limb of the cleft, deep
and at an oblique angle, lie the methylnaphthoqui-
none rings of Vit. K_1. The phytyl side chain loops
forwards and upwards, then turns and runs downward
making contact with both the H and L chain (Fig.3).
Approximately twelve amino acid residues appear to
be in contact with the ligand. From comparative
binding studies, using only the aromatic ring portion of the molecule, we know that the rings provide approximately 50% of the total binding energy
($K^0=1.7$ x 10^5 L/Mole^{-1}) while the phytyl side
chains provides the remainder. The longest dimension over which binding takes place is approximately 15 Å. Thus far, binding of even one hapten
has shown that a considerable portion of the binding cleft (one limb of which measures approximately 20 x 15 x 6 Å) is involved and that quite separate regions bind the ring portion and the
phytyl side chain. A second hapten, carminic acid
($K_0=1.4$ x 10^5 L/Mole^{-1}), has been found and difference Fourier maps of this hapten-Fab NEW complex are presently being obtained.

Although these studies on individual immunoglobulins do suggest that the combining region is
capable of binding structurally diverse haptens,
it could be argued that binding of only one of the
haptens has any functional significance in terms
of antibody production. We know that one of the
triggering responses for the "B" cell replication
and antibody production, is the binding of hapten
to the cell surface antibodies of the B cell. Such
cell surface antibodies are known to have the same
ligand binding specificity as the antibodies produced by the cell itself. The following question
can then be asked: When two diverse carrier bound
haptens, A and B, bind to a single cell surface
receptor immunoglobulin, are both these haptens

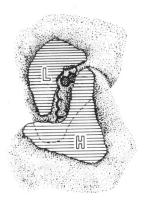

Figure 2

Block diagram of the shallow depression between the Heavy and Light chain of myeloma protein NEW which forms the combining region. The approximate location of one ligand Vit. K_1OH is indicated.

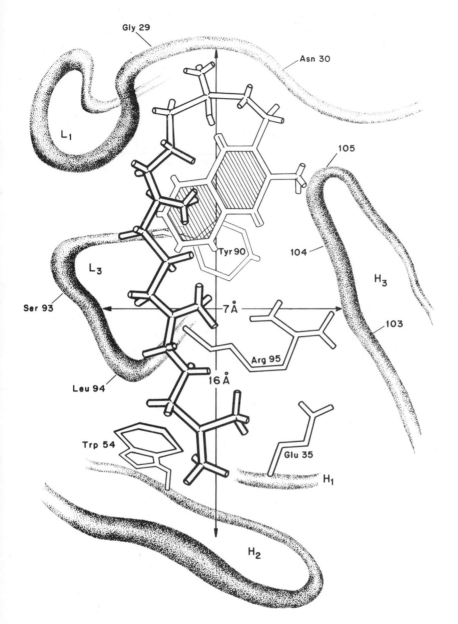

Figure 3 Schematic drawing of Vit. K_1OH bound to the combining region of IgG NEW (after a drawing by Irving Geis). L_1 and L_3 indicate the approximate location of the first and third hypervariable regions of the L chain. H_1, H_2, and H_3 designate hypervariable regions of the H chain. L chain residues Tyr 90 and Arg 95 are at the bottom of the shallow groove or crevice between the H and L chains. Trp 54 (an invariable residue in human H chain sequences) and Glu 35 (tentative assignment, not based on actual sequence data) are in close contact with the end of the phytyl chain of Vit. K_1OH.

capable of inducing production of the immunoglobulin which binds both haptens?

We tested this question in the following way:
A rabbit is injected with hapten A on a protein
carrier. From the immune serum we isolated the
anti-A antibodies and subjected them to isoelectric focusing (IEF) on polyacrylamide gels. We
identified the anti-A bands by treating the gel
with a radioiodinated derivative of hapten A, and
then washed and radioautographed the gel. A duplicate IEF gel is treated with a dissimilar radioiodinated hapten B. Bands were found which bound
both A and B. Mutual inhibition tests were then
carried out using non-radioactive A or B to see if
competition, characteristic of binding to a single
protein in the IEF band, could be demonstrated
(20). Hapten pairs, A and B, if chosen at random,
seldom bind to single IEF bands. The reasons for
this will be discussed later.

In order to maximize our chances of finding
"double-binding" antibodies, we chose hapten pairs
that we knew from the literature would bind either
to homogeneous immunoglobulins such as MOPC 460 or
that we knew gave anomolous cross reactions in
sera. Menadione, uridine, inosine, ribonuclease,
and Vit. K_1 were among those grouped in the hapten
A class. Hapten B was the Dnp group. A rabbit
immunized with uridine-BGG may show perhaps 100-
300 anti-uridine bands on IEF. Three or four of
these bands will also bind hapten B. These bands
represent the immunoglobulin products of between
1-2 clones of cells which are capable of being
stimulated by both antigens A and B. When the binding constant of the A + B binding bands is examined
as might be expected, the affinity of the immunoglobulins in the bands for hapten A is always higher than that for hapten B since these double-
binding immunoglobulins were selected by hapten A.
When the rabbit is subsequently challenged by hapten B, we noticed that the first immune response
is almost entirely that of cells producing A + B
binding antibodies. IEF bands corresponding to
such products may increase 80 fold in density and
no IEF bands binding A only showed similar increases. Later on, after hapten B challenge, more
anti-B bands appear and these do not cross-react
with hapten A. They also have a higher K_O for

hapten B than the A + B binding bands. Eventually
a complex anti-B response appeared, consisting
principally of anti-B bands with no anti-A activity (but presumably cross-reacting with other determinants). The A + B binding bands are still
present late in the immune response, but form a
progressively smaller proportion of the total
antibodies formed against hapten B.

The results of these experiments can be summarized as follows: Certain structurally unrelated
haptens bind to single immunoglobulins. When one
of these haptens is used for immunization and the
other used for boosting there is an early restricted response where antibodies against both haptens
are found. We interpret this as evidence that
immunocompetent cells have membrane receptors
which resemble the individual immunoglobulin in
their ability to bind more than one hapten and
that this binding stimulates the cell to proliferate with the result that more of the double-
binding antibodies are produced. Even with these
results there is still one more link missing in
the argument that the induced "double-binding"
antibodies are equivalent to the homogeneous myeloma proteins in their functional properties. An
objection can be raised that the apparent "double-
binding," leading to the production of these antibodies is due to stimulation of the same cells,
but that there is only one functional binding site.
If this were the case then one would expect that a
single functional site would not correspond in its
binding constants for both haptens to those which
are found in the myeloma protein. Moreover, if the
structure of the double-binding myeloma protein
binding region were different from its counterpart
in a "natural" antibody population, it would not
be expected that they would share idiotypic determinants which are known to be located in and
around the hapten binding region (21). Yet we have
been able to show that when a rabbit is sequentially immunized with Menadione-BGG and then with
Dnp-BGG, double-binding immunoglobulins are induced which share binding constants and idiotypic
determinants with protein 460, a myeloma protein
which binds both Menadione and Dnp (22). These
results and similar ones obtained with the myeloma
protein NEW suggest that: 1) The combining regions

of myeloma proteins and their "naturally induced" counterparts resemble each other, 2) In protein 460, Menadione and Dnp binding sites are widely separated, 3) Anti-hapten sera contain individual immunoglobulins which bind at least two structurally diverse haptens and that the production of such immunoglobulin species is induced by immunization with both haptens, 4) Reaction with anti-idiotypic sera, and measurement of hapten affinities suggest that the combining regions of "double-binding" myeloma proteins and their "naturally occurring" antibody counterparts resemble each other.

Taken together with the indirect data, which suggested the existence of multiple binding or polyfunctional antibody combining regions, there is considerable evidence that these are biologically important. We therefore have to see how well their existence fits with the known facts about the high specificity of immune sera.

If a single cell is capable of being stimulated by a variety of different antigenic determinants, it may be asked why the immune serum produced against an antigenic determinant shows such a high degree of specificity against the eliciting antigen. It is known that antigen binds to antibody producing cell precursors having suitable receptors on their surface. Hence, an antigen A will select those cell receptors which have anti-A specificity. We suggest that such cell receptors may be complementary to a large number of determinants. Thus, many specificities may be present in a single combining region of an antibody, but these will not necessarily be the same from cell to cell. Hence, the only quantitatively important specificity in the serum will be the one which is common to all the cell receptors and secreted immunoglobulins; i.e., the specificity towards the eliciting antigen. The other specificities will also be present, but will be diluted out by the fact that they differ from cell to cell (23). It is interesting that Talmage, in a perceptive theoretical paper in 1959, forecast that this type of mechanism might operate in antibody populations (24). Thus, in an immune serum we would expect a large quantity of highly specific antibodies and much smaller quantities of antibodies of many different specificities - including those to antigens with which the animal has had no previous contact. There is ample evidence for the existence of the latter group of "natural" anti-bodies. Perhaps, the most satisfying aspect of polyfunctional combining sites is that it would bring the binding properties of antibodies in line with those of other proteins. Most enzymes, for instance, bind a number of structurally unrelated compounds in their binding cavities or clefts. Thus, although they are often specific for a certain substrate, by virtue of the double require-ment of binding to a certain site, followed by correct alignment for catalysis, enzymes rarely if ever bind only a single substrate. It seems likely that antibodies follow the same general pattern, and that individual antibodies are not specific in binding only single antigens. Specificity of an immune serum may then be thought of as a population phenomenon, produced in many different antibodies by selection of different sub-sites capable of binding the eliciting antigen. Thus, for single immunoglobulins no new principles for binding single determinants need to be postulated. It seems likely that the antigen selects from among the available species, all those which have suit-able complementary binding sites. That such species also have other binding activities may become lost from view because the spectrum of such binding activities will vary from cell to cell, and will be diluted out by the great multiplicity of antibodies. The exquisite specificity of an immune serum can therefore be regarded as a phenomenon of the entire population of antibodies, and is not necessarily the property of each indi-vidual immunoglobulin.

Finally, the concept of polyfunctional anti-bodies, if true, would greatly reduce the number of antibodies needed to encompass the entire range of the immune response. It has been estima-ted that 10^4 - 10^6 heavy-light chain pairs might suffice (25) thus reducing the number of V region genes for light and heavy chains to around 100-500. If this is so, then no unusual genetic mechanism need be postulated to explain the gener-ation of diversity.

REFERENCES

1. Landsteiner, K., The Specificity of Serological Reactions, Revised Ed., Dover Publications, N.Y. (1962).
2. Gally, J.A., and Edelman, G.M., Nature (London) 227: 341 (1970).
3. Haurowitz, F., J. Immunol. 43: 331 (1942).
4. Knight, K.L., Lopez, M.A., and Haurowitz, F., J. Biol. Chem. 241: 2286 (1966).
5. Williamson, A.R., Biochem. J. 129: 1 (1973).
6. Wiswesser, W.J., Aldrichemica Acta 6: 41 (1973).
7. DuPasquier, L., Curr. Topics Microbiol. and Immunol. 61: 37 (1973).
8. Haimovich, J., and DuPasquier, L., Proc. Nat. Acad. Sci. (USA) 70: 1898 (1973).
9. Eisen, H.N., Little, J.R., Osterland, C.K., and Simms, E.S., Cold Spring Harbor Symposium on Quantitative Biology, Vol. XXXII, p. 75 (1967).
10. Kabat, E.A., J. Immunol. 97: 1 (1966).
11. Parker, C.W., Gott, S.M., and Johnson, M.C., Biochemistry 5: 214 (1966).
12. Richards, F.F., Pincus, J.H., Bloch, K.J., Barnes, W.T., and Haber, E., Biochemistry 8: 1377 (1969).
13. Eisen, H.N., Progress in Immunology 243 (1971) and Schubert, D., Jobe, A., and Cohn, M., Nature (London) 220: 882 (1968).
14. Rosenstein, R.W., Musson, R.A., Armstrong, M., Konigsberg, W.H., and Richards, F.F., Proc. Nat. Acad. Sci. (USA) 69: 877 (1972).
15. Wu, C-W, and Stryer, L., Proc. Nat. Acad. Sci. (USA) 69: 1104 (1972).
16. Manjula, B.N., Richards, F.F., and Rosenstein, R.W., J. Mol. Biol., submitted (1974).
17. Poljak, R.J., Amzel, L.M., Avey, H.P., Chen, B.L., Phizackerley, R.P., and Saul, F., Proc. Nat. Acad. Sci. (USA) 70: 3305 (1973).
18. Varga, J.M., Lande, S., and Richards, F.F., J. Immunol. in press, (1974).
19. Amzel, L.M., Poljak, R.J., Saul, F., Varga, J.M., and Richards, F.F., Proc. Nat. Acad. Sci. (USA) 71 April 1974.

20. Varga, J.M., Konigsberg, W.H., and Richards, F.F., Proc. Nat. Acad. Sci. (USA) 70: 3269 (1973).

21. Inbar, D., Hochman, J., and Givol, D., Proc. Nat. Acad. Sci. (USA) 69: 2659 (1972).

22. Varga, J.M., Rosenstein, R.W., and Richards, F.F., Federation Proceedings 33: 810 (1974).

23. Richards, F.F., and Konigsberg, W.H., Immunochem. 10: 545 (1973).

24. Talmage, D.W., Science 129: 1643 (1959).

25. Inman, J.K., Fed. Proc. 32: 957 (1973).

A STUDY OF V REGION GENES
USING ALLOTYPIC AND IDIOTYPIC MARKERS

T. J. Kindt, A. L. Thunberg,
M. Mudgett and D. G. Klapper

The Rockefeller University
New York, New York 10021

ABSTRACT. Allotypic and idiotypic markers of homogeneous rabbit antibodies to streptococcal carbohydrates have been employed to study genes controlling biosynthesis of antibody variable regions. Hapten prepared from Group C streptococcal carbohydrate inhibited binding of the antibodies to idiotypic antisera but not to group a allotypic antisera. The inheritance of idiotypic markers was supported by studies with partially inbred rabbits. Linkage between idiotype and group a allotype was observed in this study. Examination of the idiotypic determinants of homogeneous antibodies suggested that genes encoding antibody binding sites may be distinct from those encoding group a allotypes and other V region determinants. Antibodies with identical or crossreactive idiotypes but differing in other V region markers including group a allotype and V_L region structure have been observed.

INTRODUCTION. The mechanism underlying the biosynthesis of antibody binding sites is unprecedented in its adaptability. An individual is able to synthesize a large number of antibody molecules, each with a different specificity for one of many antigens including carbohydrates, proteins, nucleic acids, lipids, and a great variety of small molecules. The underlying question, therefore, becomes what is actually present in the genome of the organism that encodes such a large group of different molecules? Although theories describing the enigmatic genes are much discussed, there are few hard facts concerning genes that code for antibody binding sites.

One reason for this shortage of information is that at this time genetic material cannot be

directly examined. We are forced to rely for our
information on a study of antibodies rather than
on the genes themselves. Nevertheless by this indirect approach the molecular nature of antibody
diversity has been elucidated. Studies which combine the information obtained in structural studies
with that obtained by use of genetic markers will
further our knowledge on the nature of antibody bio-
synthetic mechanisms. Such a combined approach is
being used in studies on human proteins by Kunkel,
Capra, Kehoe (1,2,3) and their associates, and in
the mouse by Weigert and Cohn (4,5), Potter and
Nisonoff (6,7), and their associates. Our laboratory has been attempting similar analyses in the
rabbit (8). The results from these structural and
idiotypic studies may result in a reevaluation of
current theories or may force new theoretical for-
mulations. At the moment there appears to be little doubt that speculation will stay well ahead of
the substantiated facts.

Three major theories of antibody synthesis are
presented in Table 1. Listed for each theory are
the number of genes which are required for V_H and
V_L regions, and the number of these genes which are
involved in synthesis of a single binding site.
These numerical analyses assume that an individual
requires 10^6 binding sites and that any combination
of V_H and V_L regions may be used to produce useful
antigen binding sites. For the multiple germ line
gene theories (9,10), an individual must have 10^5
genes per V region of each chain. One gene would
encode a single V region. One complete V region
of approximately 110 residues would be encoded by
each gene. It should be pointed out, however, that
if all H-L combinations are allowed, each germ line
V gene may serve in as many as 10^3 combinations to
form binding sites.

Somatic mutation theories (11,12), on the
other hand, require as few as 10 V genes per individual. As with the germ line theory, 1 V region
(approximately 110 residues) is encoded by each
gene. However, the mutant progeny of each gene
may serve for as many as 100 V regions and for as
many as 10^5 binding sites.

If more than one gene encodes a single V region (13), a great deal of diversity can be encoded with fewer V genes in the germ line than are required by the germ line model. In Table 1 we have shown the number of genes that would be required for 10^6 binding sites if two or three genes, each encoding a segment of a V region, interact to synthesize the complete V region. If any combination of two genes can interact to form a single V region then 33 genes for each segment are required. If three genes interact, 10 are required. Although the number of amino acids encoded by each gene may vary, we have assumed in this formulation that each is equal. In gene interaction theories each of the various V region genes would be used in different combinations to synthesize many binding sites.

Our experimental approach has been aimed at the determination of the number of genes involved in the synthesis of a single V region. An answer to this question would certainly influence considerations on the total number of genes required for antibody diversity. Our studies have employed markers for the constant portions of V_H and V_L regions in combination with the idiotype as the marker for binding sites (hypervariable regions).

We will first describe the V region markers used: for the V_H region, the group a allotype; for the V_L region, the V_κ subgroups; for the binding site, the idiotypes. Next, data on inheritance of idiotype and linkage to allotypes will be presented, and third, we will discuss studies which suggest that idiotypes and other V region markers may be the products of separate genes. Finally we will discuss a model that attempts to explain these data.

Allotypic markers of rabbit I_gG H chains: Figure 1 depicts the rabbit I_gG molecule and molecular localization of the allotypes. First, consider the V_H region of an a positive I_gG. In this area there are three allotypes, a1, a2, a3. (14). Ninety percent of the H chains possess the group a markers. In addition to the group a markers, there exist what are known as a negative or a blank molecules which may be broken down into at

Table 1

Numerical Aspects of Antibody Genetics [1]

Theory	No. of genes		No. amino acid residues per gene	No. V regions per gene
	per Individual per chain	per single V region		
Multiple germline genes	10^3	1	110	1
Somatic mutation	10	1	110	10^2
V gene interaction [2]	33 (×2) 10 (×3)	2 3	55 37	33 10^2

1. This analysis assumes that 10^6 binding sites are required and that any V_H - V_L combination will give rise to a functional binding site.

2. These numbers further assume that any combination of interacting V region genes is allowable.

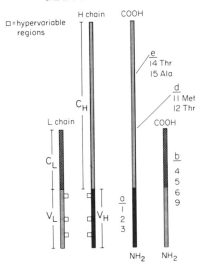

Fig. 1. Allotypes of rabbit lgG.

least two separate groups on the basis of genetic studies by Kim and Dray (15) and structural studies by Prahl, Todd and their associates (16-18). The group a V_H allotypes are encountered in all classes of rabbit immunoglobulins and while they are close-ly linked to the constant region of the rabbit H chain, crossovers between V_H and C_H genes have been documented (19,20). The groups d and e genetic markers are present in the C_H region and have been correlated with single amino acid substitutions (21,22).

Genetic markers of rabbit κ chains. Allotypes of the group b, that is b4, b5, b6 and b9 are loca-ted in the constant region of the L chain (23, 24, 25). The allotypes of the group b are not linked to allotypes of the group a nor to groups d or e. This suggests that the L chains and the H chains are encoded on separate chromosomes.

While there is no allotypic marker analogous to the group a allotype for the V_L region, the N-terminal sequences of the L chains of homogeneous antibodies are useful as markers for the V_L region. In Table 2 it can be seen from the compiled se-quences of L chains from streptococcal antibodies that they break down into five major groups, $V_{\kappa I}$, $V_{\kappa II-a}$, $V_{\kappa II-b}$, $V_{\kappa III-a}$, $V_{\kappa III-b}$. The L chains that are blocked at the N-terminus may com-prise one or more additional subgroups. While there are considerable sequence differences at some positions within some of these groups; for example, position 2 of the $V_{\kappa IIb}$ group, one group can be differentiated from another on the basis of the sequence at the beginning of the N-terminus and the length of the chain. These differences in chain length are based on alignment for maximum homology (26). The V_κ subgroups will be used as a marker for the V region of the L chain. These V_L markers are not allotypes, but more properly iso-types.

Idiotypic markers for binding sites. The other V region marker to be employed here is call-ed an idiotypic marker (32,33). An idiotypic marker consists of antigenic determinants in the hypervariable regions of both H and L chains of a

Table 2

Comparison of N-terminal Amino Acid Sequences of L Chains from Rabbit Antibodies Raised by Immunization with Streptococci

Rabbit	Antigen*	Allotype L chain	Vκ subgroup	0	1	2	3	4	5	6	7	8	9	10	11	12	13	14	15	16	17	18	19	20	21	22	23	24	25	Ref.
4135	C	4	I	A	D	I	V	M	T	Q	T	P	A	S	V	S	E	P	V	G	G	T	V	T	I	K	C			27
3521	C	4	I	—	N	—	—	—	—	—	—	—	—	—	—	—	G	A	—	—	—	—	—	X	—	N	—			28
2711	C	4	I	—	—	V	—	—	—	—	—	—	—	—	—	—	—	—	—	—	—	—	—	—	—	—	—			29
4136	C	4	II-a	( )	—	V	—	—	—	—	—	—	X	—	—	E	—	—	—	—	—	—	—	—	—	—	—			30
2990	C	4	II-a	( )	—	V	—	—	—	—	—	P	T	A	—	—	—	—	—	—	—	—	—	—	—	—	—			29
3013	A	4	II-b	( )	A	Y	D	—	—	Z	—	—	—	—	—	—	T	—	—	—	—	—	—	—	—	—	—			29
3547	A	4	II-b	( )	A	Y	D	—	—	—	—	S	—	—	—	—	T	A	—	—	—	—	—	—	—	N	—			25
2436-1	C	4	II-b	( )	A	F	Z	L	—	Z	—	—	—	—	Z	—	A	A	—	—	—	—	—	—	—	—	—			26
2461-1	C	4	II-b	( )	A	F	Z	L	—	Z	—	—	—	—	T	—	A	A	—	—	—	—	—	—	—	—	—			26
2461-Ia	C	4	II-b	( )	A	A	Z	L	—	Z	—	—	—	—	—	Z	—	A	V	—	—	—	—	—	—	—	—			29
2461-Ib	C	4	II-b	( )	A	L	Z	L	—	Z	—	—	—	—	—	—	A	A	—	—	—	—	—	—	—	—	—			29
4182-1	C	9	II-b	( )	A	L	Z	L	—	—	—	—	S	—	T	X	A	A	—	—	—	P	—	—	—	—	—			31
2869-II	C	9	II-b	( )	A	V	—	L	—	—	—	—	S	—	X	—	A	A	—	—	—	—	—	—	—	N	—			31
3412	C	4	III-a	( )	A	—	—	L	—	Z	—	—	X	P	—	X	A	A	—	—	—	—	X	—	L	—				26
2690	C	4	III-b	( )	—	—	—	L	—	Z	—	—	S	—	X	—	V	A	—	—	—	—	X	—	I(L)	—				
3113	A	4	III-b	( )	—	—	—	—	—	Z	—	—	S	—	X	—	V	A	—	D	—	X	—	N	—	X	A	31
3413	C	4	III-b	( )	—	—	L	—	—	—	—	—	X	S	K	S	V	—	—	D	—	—	—	N	—	Q	A	
4153-1	C	9	III-b	( )	—	V	—	—	—	—	—	—	S	—	T	A	A	—	—	E	—	—	—	N	—				31
4153-II	C	9	III-b	( )	—	V	—	—	—	—	—	—	S	—	T	K	A	A	—	E	—	—	—	B	—				31
2869-I	C	9	III-b	( )	—	—	L	—	—	—	—	—	S	—	T	X	A	A	—	E	—	—	—	N	—				
4035	C	4		Blocked																										
3664	C	4		Blocked																										
3660	A	4		Blocked																										

Position

* A indicates Group A streptococci was used for immunization; C indicates Group C streptococci was used for immunization.

74

homogeneous antibody or paraprotein. The idiotypic determinant includes the binding site of the
molecule. Figure 2 shows the method by which rabbit idiotypic antisera are prepared. Highly purified homogeneous antibody is injected into a rabbit which has the same allotypic combination as the
rabbit from which the antibody was isolated. The
antisera prepared in this manner are highly specific for determinants on the antibody associated
with the binding site.

RESULTS

Antigenic distinction between allotypic and
idiotypic determinants: Structural studies carried out using pooled IgG (32,33), specific antibodies, and myeloma proteins have indicated that
there are at least three, perhaps four, hypervariable regions in the antibody H chain. These
hypervariable regions are involved in the antigen
binding site and presumably also in the idiotypic
determinants. Structural studies on rabbit antibodies carried out by Porter, Mole (32,33) and
Koshland (34) have indicated that amino acid substitutions correlating with group a allotypic markers are present in the V region and some substitutions may be contiguous with those associated
with the hypervariable regions or the idiotypic
determinants.

Because the idiotype and group a allotypes
overlap in the structural sense, it is possible
that their antigenic determinants might also overlap. Data to the contrary was obtained by haptenic inhibition studies that underscore the distinction between idiotypes and allotypes. To examine
this question,a small hapten prepared by limited
acid hydrolysis of the Group C carbohydrate (35)
was used in inhibition of idiotypic and allotypic
binding reactions. This hapten contains N-acetyl-
galactosamine linked to rhamnose units. Its exact
size and structure has yet to be determined. A 0.4%
solution of hapten completely inhibited the reaction between Group C antibody and Group C carbohydrate antigen. Hapten inhibition of the binding
reaction between various Group C antibodies and
idiotypic and allotypic antisera is depicted in

Figure 3. The top frame shows that reactions between idiotypic antisera and the antibodies against
which they are directed are 25-50% inhibited by the
hapten. Reactions with the proband antibody, that
is, the one against which the anti-idiotypes were
prepared, as well as reactions with cross reactive
antibodies were inhibited by the hapten. When
two antisera had been prepared against the same
antibodies (as is the case with antibody 3412) reactions with both antisera were inhibited by the
hapten. In contrast to the results obtained with
idiotypic antisera, the middle part of the figure
shows that binding reactions of these antibodies
to the group a allotypic antisera were not inhibited to any extent by the hapten. This result suggests that although the group a allotype and the
idiotype are both in the V region, they have distinct antigenic determinants. As would be predicted, the hapten did not influence the binding to
group b antisera.

Earlier experiments (38) had indicated that
differences in the binding sites of the homogeneous antibodies may influence the allotypic determinant. These studies showed that the group a
allotypic specificities present on some homogeneous
antibodies could be differentiated from each other
and from the specificities present in an allotypically matched pool of I$_g$G. In spite of this atten-
uation of allotypic specificities by substitutions
associated with specific binding sites and the
structural proximity of the allotypic and idiotypic
correlates, it appears from the hapten inhibition
studies that the antigenic determinants associated
with the two markers are distinct.

Genetic association between idiotypes and
group a allotypes: The inheritance of the idiotype of a homogeneous Group C antibody was revealed by a survey of Group C antisera from related
and non-related rabbits (39, 40, 41). Streptococcal antisera were tested for the presence of this
idiotypic marker. The test system involved inhibition of the binding reaction between an idiotypic antisera and a cross reactive streptococcal
antibody. The specificity of this reaction has
been well documented. The results indicated that

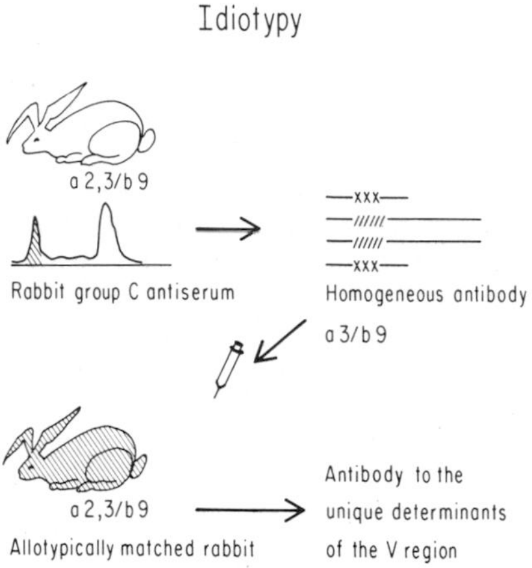

Idiotypy

a 2,3/b 9

Rabbit group C antiserum

Homogeneous antibody

a 3/b 9

a 2,3/b 9

Allotypically matched rabbit

Antibody to the
unique determinants
of the V region

Fig. 2. Preparation of idiotypic antisera.
A purified homogeneous antibody is absorbed onto
streptococcal cells, emulsified in incomplete
Freund's adjuvant and injected into a second
rabbit, matched allotypically to the donor.

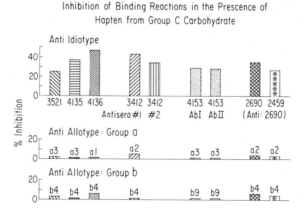

Inhibition of Binding Reactions in the Prescence of
Hapten from Group C Carbohydrate

Fig. 3. Inhibition of idiotypic and allotypic reactions by 0.4% (w/v) concentration of
hapten prepared from Group C streptococcal carbohydrate. Inhibitions were carried out at 50% of
maximum binding. This value was predetermined
for each antibody and antiserum.

77

58% of the related rabbits expressed the proband idiotype while it was detected in only 1% of the streptococcal antisera from non-related rabbits. The relationship between the group $\underline{a}$ allotypes of the related rabbits and this idiotype is shown in Table 3. The allotype of the proband antibody was a2/b4 and it was produced in an $\underline{a}2$, $\underline{a}3$ rabbit. Of $\overline{47}$ $\overline{r}$abbits with allotype $\underline{a}2$, $\underline{a}2$, $\overline{}$thirty-three or 70% were positive for thi$\overline{s}$ id$\overline{i}$otype. Of 49 hetero-zygous rabbits with allotype $\underline{a}2$, $\underline{a}3$, twenty-six or 53% were positive. In contra$\overline{s}$t, $\overline{o}$f the 23 rabbits with the allotype $\underline{a}3$, $\underline{a}3$, only 1 (4%) was idiotyp-ically positive f$\overline{o}$r t$\overline{h}$is marker. Correlation of this idiotype with the allotype $\underline{a}2$ is statistically significant at the 0.001 level. $\overline{}$All the related rabbits involved in this study had the L chain al-lotype $\underline{b}4$.

Structural and binding site correlates of idiotypically cross-reactive antibody: It became apparent that idiotypically cross reactive anti-body was only one of several components in the streptococcal antisera. Several cross reactive antibody components were isolated on the basis of their binding affinity for a Group C immunoadsor-bent column. The same relative binding affinity was observed for each antibody component from each antiserum which gave idiotypic cross reaction. These antibody components with similar affinities were further checked for the V_L region marker, that is, their V_κ subgroup (44). Results of these findings are summarized in Table 4. First it was noted that all cross reactive antibodies required the same strongly acidic conditions to be eluted from the Group C affinity column. The cross reac-tive fractions from this column comprised small percentages (5 - 20%) of the total antibody pre-sent in the cross reactive antisera. Quantitative amino acid sequence analyses of the N-terminals the L chain of these antibodies including the pro-band, indicated that Ile-Val-Met (subgroup $V_{\kappa III b}$) was the major sequence in all the fractions. Pre-immune serum from several of the rabbits from which the idiotypically cross reactive antibodies were isolated, were checked for the presence of the Ile-Val-Met sequence. In these animals, as in the b4 $I_g G$ pool (25), the expression of this sequence was

Table 3

Group a Allotypes of Related Rabbits Tested For
Idiotypic Cross-Reaction to an a2 Antibody

| Allotype | No. Tested | Idiotypically positive | |
		No.	%
a2a2	47	33	70
a2a3	49	26	53
a3a3	23	1	4

Table 4

Idiotypically Cross-Reactive Fractions
Isolated From Sera of Related Rabbits

Rabbit	elution pH of Fx	% of total Ab	N-terminal L chain sequence[2]
2690 [1]	- - -	90	IVM
2459	2.8	20	IVM
2662	2.8	14	IVM (60%)
3413 [3]	2.8	11	IVM
3419	2.8	5	-

1. Proband antibody was isolated from this serum.
2. Determined as described previously (25).
3. L chain sequence data of a different, non
    cross reactive antibody from this serum is
    listed in Table 2.

at the 2-5% level. These considerations suggest that this idiotype is associated with the subgroup V_κ IIIb.

Antibody molecules with the same idiotype but different V region markers: Examination of idiotypic determinants on rabbit antibodies have uncovered several examples of identical or cross reactive idiotypes on molecules with differences in other V region markers. Three such observations have been made. These idiotypic cross reactions between molecules with structural or allotypic differences have several features in common. All of the antibody pairs have similar specificity for an antigen, and the idiotypic reactions as well as the cross reactions were inhibitable by the antigenic hapten described above. Each idiotype was dependent on a specific heavy-light combination for expression. That is to say, the idiotype was not detectable on recombinant molecules prepared from the H or L chains of the antibody with L or H chain from I_gG pools or other non cross-reactive antibodies.

The first observation of idiotypically similar antibodies with different V region markers came from a pair of antibodies isolated from the same rabbit,3521. The antibodies were very similar in specificity and electrophoretic mobility. The light chains were identical for the first 25 amino terminal residues and indistinguishable by electrofocusing (28, 42). One antibody, however, had the allotype a3 while the other lacked any group a allotype. The V_H allotype difference was confirmed by structural analysis of peptides from the amino terminals of the antibody H chains(28). In spite of this difference in the V_H allotype, the molecules had identical idiotypes. This was shown by radiobinding and radiobinding inhibition experiments. Two different idiotypic antisera were used and gave identical results in this comparison (42).

The second cross-reaction involved two antibodies, one from each of two siblings(4135 and 4136). These antibodies had different group a allotypes, one was a3 (4135) and the other was a1

(4136) and different L chain subgroups, $V_{\kappa 1}$ and
$V_{\kappa}II$-b. In Table 2 is depicted the amino terminal
light chain sequences of these two antibodies.
There are six differences in the first twenty residues of these chains.

The idiotypic cross-reaction of the two antibodies first observed by hemagglutination was verified by radiobinding experiments depicted in Figure
4. Both 4135 and 4136 antibodies bound to idiotypic
antisera prepared against 4136. Antisera prepared
against antibody 4135 on the other hand, did not
react with antibody 4136 in either the hemagglutination or in radiobinding assays. Figure 4 also
shows that both the reaction and the cross-reaction
were inhibitable by the hapten antigen.

The third example of idiotypic cross reaction
between two antibodies was observed recently by
Thunberg (8, 30). These two antibodies 4153I and
4153II were isolated from one rabbit. Group a allotype of these antibodies is a3 and the L chains are
of V_{κ} III-b subgroup with a $\overline{V}$al N-terminus (Table
2). They were quite different by electrophoresis.
An idiotypic antiserum was prepared against a highly
purified preparation of one of them. While the two
antibodies gave a strong idiotypic cross reaction
with this antiserum, they did not give identical reactions. Diagrammed in Figure 5 are recombinant
molecules prepared utilizing the H and L chains of
each of the two molecules in combination with the H
or L chain of the other. Inhibition of radiobinding experiments using the recombinants localized
the idiotypic difference between the two molecules
to the H chains. The L chains were idiotypically
indistinguishable. Further comparison of these
light chains by gel electrophoresis shows considerable difference, and not only are they different
electrophoretically, but N-terminal sequence analysis showed that although they are the same $V_{\kappa}III$-b
subgroup (Table 2), a difference was found in the
first 23 residues. There is a Ser-Lys interchange
at position 12. This finding further documents
that two antibodies can have idiotypic similarity
or even idiotypic identity despite differences in
other V region parameters.

Table 5

V Region Characterization of Three Different
Pairs of Idiotypically Cross Reactive Antibodies

Pair	Rabbit/ab	Group a Allotype	V_κ Subgroup	Idiotypic Characterization
1	3521 Ab 3	a3	$V_\kappa 1$	Identical
	3521 AbN	a	$V_\kappa 1$	H and L
2	4135 Ab	a3	$V_\kappa 1$	Cross Reactive
	4136 Ab	a1	$V_\kappa IIa$	
3	4153 AbI	a3	$V_\kappa IIIb$	L Chain Identical
	4153 AbII	a3	$V_\kappa IIIb$	H Chain Cross Reactive

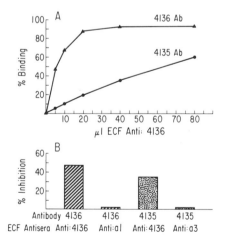

Fig. 4. A. Binding of radiolabeled 4136
and 4135 antibodies to an idiotypic antiserum
prepared against 4136 antibody.
B. Inhibition of the binding re-
actions between 4136 anti-4136 and 4135 anti-4136
by hapten from Group C streptococcal carbohydrate.
The binding of neither antibody to group a anti-
allotype sera was inhibited.

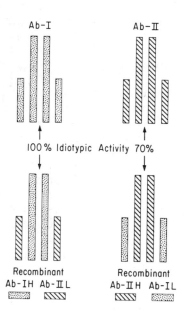

Fig. 5. Recombinant molecules prepared using H and L chains of 4135-I and 4135-II in all combinations. These recombinants were tested for their ability to inhibit the binding reaction between radiolabeled 4153 I and anti-4153 I.

DISCUSSION Idiotypic cross reactions were detected among 58% of the Group C streptococcal antisera from related rabbits, while this same idiotypic specificity was present in antisera of only 1% of similarly immunized, unrelated rabbits. Linkage was observed between this idiotype and the allotype a2. Further studies indicated that cross reactive antibodies were similar in specificity for antigen and that these antibodies selected light chains from the same V_K subgroup. There is accumulating evidence from our laboratory and others (45) to suggest that idiotypes and other V region markers are not necessarily products of the same gene. Different antibodies may have identical or similar idiotypy despite differences in other V region markers. An analogous finding has been reported by Hopper (45) who found idiotypic cross reactivity between two myeloma proteins that differed in class, L chain type and V_H subgroup! How can these results be explained?

The most straightforward explanation is that two or more genes code for the V region of a single antibody. Our results and those of Hopper could be interpreted as follows: the amino acid residues specifying the idiotype and the amino acid residues specifying the group a allotype (or V_H or V_L subgroup) are encoded on separate genes. These separate genes in some way interact to code for synthesis of a single V region. Linkage of these gene segments is indicated by studies with idiotypes and group a allotypes. There is evidence that V region subgroups, allotypes and idiotypes are all products of germ line genes; therefore, the gene segments are in the germ line. Whether the genes interact in a cis or trans fashion (46) is not yet known, but the question is open to test by a study of idio typy in rabbits heterozygous for the V_H allotypes of groups a, x and y. (15)

In Table 1 it is suggested that a gene segment codes for 37 or 55 amino acid residues; or approximately 1/3 or 1/2 of a V region. This is an obvious oversimplification. But it should be possible to determine the specific number of amino acids encoded by each gene through a structural examination of H and L chains from antibodies with appropriate

combinations of idiotypes and other V region markers for which the amino acid correlates have been
determined.

The model is also oversimplified by the assumption that all combinations of genes may be used.
Data on the variable expression of different V_H
allotypes would suggest that all combinations of V_H
allotype and binding sites are not equally utilized.
This point may be further complicated by question-
ing the assumption that all H-L chain combinations
give rise to useful binding sites. The net result
of such incompatibilities would be an increase in
the number of genes needed to encode the necessary
binding sites.

The precedent for gene interaction models may
be taken from studies on the genes that code for
V and C regions. (19, 20, 46) This precedent was
invoked in the somatic recombination model put
forth by Gally & Edelman (47). The postulated
translocation which serves to connect a small number of C regions with a large number of V regions
might be used in the present instance to translo-
cate a few allotypes into many idiotypes. Another
possibility for gene interaction would involve episomes that insert the information for binding sites
into the three or four hyper variable regions of
the antibody H or L chain. This type of model has
been used by Wu & Kabat (13) to explain hypervariability in L chains. The present situation would
require that the episomes are inherited and that
certain episomes preferentially insert into certain
variable regions. The latter point could be partially explained if allotypic genes and the episomes specifying idiotypes in a cis configuration
most frequently interact with one another.

In summary, data have been presented that suggest that antibody binding sites are encoded by
genes separate from those encoding other V region
markers. An explanation for these data has been
given in the form of gene interaction models. Further experiments to test such a model have been
outlined.

ACKNOWLEDGEMENTS. This work was supported by
National Institutes of Health Grants AI-08429 and
AI-11995, and a grant-in-aid from the American
Heart Association. T. J. K. is an Established
Investigator of the American Heart Association.
The authors thank Dr. R. M. Krause for his support
and encouragement and for his careful review of
this manuscript. We gratefully acknowledge the
astute criticisms of Dr. L. E. Mole. The techni-
cal assistance of Ms. Rochelle Seide, Messrs.
Rostyk Kutny, Henry Lackland and Juan Irizarry
lightened our work load considerably.

REFERENCES.
1. Kunkel, H. G., Agnello, V., Joslin, F. G.,
       Winchester, R. J., and Capra, J. D., J.
       Exp. Med., 137, 331 (1973).
2. Capra, J. D., Kehoe, J. M. Winchester, R. J.,
       Kunkel, A. G., Fed. Proc. No. 4337
       (Abstr)., 1973.
3. Kunkel, A. G., Winchester, R. J., Joslin, F.
       G., and Capra, J. D., J. Exp. Med., 139,
       128 (1973).
4. Carson, D. and Weigert, M., Proc. Nat. Acad.
       Sci., 70, 235 (1973).
5. Sher, A. and Cohn, M., Europ, J. Immunol.,
       2, 319 (1972)
6. Pawlak, L. L., Mushinski, E. B., Nisonoff, A.
       and Potter, M., J. Exp. Med., 137, 22
       (1973).
7. Rudikoff, S., Mushinski, E. B., Potter, M.,
       Glaudemans, D. P. J. and Jolley, M. E.,
       J. Exp. Med., 138, 1095 (1973).
8. Thunberg, A. L. and Kindt, T. J., Submitted
       for Publication, 1974.
9. Wigzell, H., Scand. J. Immunol., 2, 199
       (1973).
10. Hood, L., Stadler, Symp. Vol.5 (1973). Univ.
       Mo., Columbia, p. 73.
11. Cohn, M., in the Biochemistry of Gene Ex-
       pression in Higher Organisms, Pollak, J.
       K. and Lee, J. W., eds., E. Reidel
       Publishing Co., Dordrecht, Holland, pp.
       574-592.
12. Jerne, N. K., Eur. J. Immunol., 1, 1 (1971).

13. Wu, T. T. and Kabat, E. A., J. Exp. Med, 132, 211 (1970).
14. Oudin, J., J. Cell. Physiol., 67, Sup. 1, 77-108 (1966).
15. Kim, B. S. and Dray, S., J. Immunol., 111. 750 (1973).
16. Tack, B. F., Feintuch, K., Todd, C. W. and Prahl, J. W., Biochem., 12, 5172 (1973).
17. Tack, B. R., Prahl, J. W. and Todd, C. W., Biochem., 12, 5178 (1973).
18. Prahl, J. W., Tack, B. F. and Todd, C. W., Biochem., 12, 5181 (1973).
19. Mage, R. G., Young-Cooper, G. O. and Alexander, C., Nature, New Biology, 230, 63 (1971).
20. Kindt, T. J., and Mandy, W. J., J. Immunol., 108, 1110 (1972).
21. Prahl, J. W., Mandy, W. J. and Todd, C. W., Biochem., 8, 4935 (1969).
22. Appella, E., Chersi, A., Mage, R. G. and Dubiski, S., Proc. Nat. Acad. Sci., 68, 1341 (1971).
23. Frangione, B., FEBS Letters, 3, 341 (1969).
24. Appella, E., Rejnek, J. and Reisfeld, R. A., J. Mol. Biol., 41, 473 (1969).
25. Kindt, T. J., Seide, R. K., Lackland, H. and Thunberg, A. L., J. Immunol., 109, 735 (1972).
26. Hood, L. Eichmann, K., Lackland, H., Krause, R. M. and Ohms, J. J., Nature, 228, 1040 (1970).
27. Chen, K. C. S., Kindt, T. J. and Krause, R. M. Proc. Nat. Acad. Sci.,(U.S.) 1972, in press.
28. Waterfield, M. D., Prahl, J. W., Hood, L. E., Kindt, T. J. and Krause, R. M., Nature, New Biology, 240, 215 (1972).
29. Hood, L., Waterfield, N. D., Morris, J. and Todd, C. W., Ann. N. Y. Acad. Sci., 190, 26 (1971).
30. Thunberg, A. L., Doctoral Dissertation, The Rockefeller University, 1974.
31. Thunberg, A. L., Lackland, H. and Kindt, T. J. J. Immunol., 111, 1755 (1973).
32. Kunkel, H. G., Mannik, M. and Williams, R. C., Science, 140, 1218 (1963).

33. Oudin, J. and Michel, M., J. Exp. Med., 130, 595 (1969).
34. Mole, L. E., Jackson, S. A., Porter, R. R. and Wilkinson, J. M., Biochem. J., 124, 301 (1971).
35. Porter, R. R., Annal. Immunol., 125, 85 (1974).
36. Koshland, M. E. , Davis, J. J. and Fujita, N. J., Proc. Natl. Acad. Sci. (U.S.), 63, 1274 (1969).
37. Shulman, S. and Ayoub, A., J. Immunol., (1973).
38. Kindt, T. J., and Seide, R. K., Tack, B. F. and Todd, C. W., J. Exp. Med., 138, 33 (1973).
39. Eichmann, K. and Kindt, T. J., J. Exp. Med., 134, 532 (1971).
40. Kindt, T. J., Seide, R. K., Bokisch, V. A. and Krause, R. M., J. Exp. Med., 138, 522 (1973).
41. Kindt, T. J. and Krause, R. M., Annal. Immunol. 125, 369 (1974).
42. Kindt, T. J., Klapper, D. G. and Waterfield, M. D., J. Exp. Med., 137, 636 (1973).
43. Weigert, M., Raschlke, W. C., Carson, D., Cohn, M., J. Exp. Med., 139, 137 (1974).
44. Klapper, D.G., Fed. Proc., 33, 2991, (Abstr.), 1974.
45. Hopper, J. E., Fed Proc., 32, 989, (Abstr.) 1973.
46. Kindt, T. J., Mandy, W. J. and Todd, C. W., Biochem., 9, 2028 (1970).
47. Gally, J. A. and Edelman, G. M., Nature, 227, 341 (1970).

FIRST ORDER CONSIDERATIONS IN ANALYZING
THE GENERATOR OF DIVERSITY

Melvin Cohn, Bonnie Blomberg, William Geckeler, William
Raschke, Roy Riblet and Martin Weigert

The Salk Institute
Post Office Box 1809
San Diego, California 92112

and

The Institute for Cancer Research
7701 Burholme Avenue
Philadelphia, Pennsylvania 19111

I. THE HYPOTHESIS

We will present arguments testing the following
theory of diversification: Each animal expresses on the
order of $10^2 V_L$- and $10^2 V_H$-germ-line genes or 10^4 germ-line
antibodies upon which somatic selection operates. The
germ-line V-genes are selected upon as coding non-self
specificities of survival value to the animal when it first
encounters pathogens (viral, bacterial, etc.). The
selection on germ-line V-genes for combining specificity
operates on only about 10^2 out of the 10^4 germ-line antibodies ($V_L V_H$ combinations). Thus selection on $\sim 10^2$
pairs of $V_L V_H$ genes assures that the total number of
$V_L V_H$ combinations, 10^4, will be functional as immunoglobulin. The somatically expressed V-genes vary by
mutation and are selected upon stepwise and sequentially
by antigen so as to increase the number of somatic variants of a given germ-line V-gene about ten-fold i.e.
$10^3 V_L \times 10^3 V_H = 10^6$ antibodies. This might be considered
to be the minimum level of diversification expected of a
mature immune system.

Virgin antigen-sensitive cells generated from stem
cells during development and throughout life express germ-
line encoded receptors as a majority population and mutants as a minority population. As antigenic selection
is imposed, the mutant population is increased relative to
the germ-line population so that the mature animal

expresses the mutant as a majority population and the germ-line as a minority population.

II. FRAMEWORK AND COMPLEMENTARITY-DETERMINING RESIDUES

We will assume that the V-region of any L or H sub-unit can be divided according to function as being framework or complementarity-determining. Amino-acid raplacements in the framework are due principally to mutation and selection of germ-line V-genes whereas replacements of complementarity-determinants are due principally to mutation and selection of somatically derived V-genes.

III. PATTERN OF VARIATION OF A SINGLE GERM-LINE V-GENE

We have searched for a way to study the somatic descendents of a single germ-line V-gene. It seemed reasonable to sequence the λ chain of the inbred mouse because it is expressed as a minor population. If the κ/λ ratio in serum immunoglobulin reflects the V_κ/V_λ germ-line gene ratios, then the number of germ-line V_λ-genes should be few (even one) and as a consequence the pattern of somatic variation should be discernible easily. This turns out to be correct.

Eighteen BALB/c mouse λ-chains have been sequenced (Figure 1). Twelve are identical (λ_0), four have one amino acid replacement (one base change, λ_1), one has two replacements (two base changes, λ_2), one has three replacements (four base changes, λ_4). The nine amino acid replacements (ten base changes) are all in the hypervariable regions and are believed therefore to be complementarity-determining.

We interpret this pattern as follows:

1. The twelve λ_0 chains of identical sequence are coded by one germ-line V_λ-gene.
2. The variation is due to mutation and selection only for those with replacements in complementarity-determining residues[a].
3. Each germ-line V-gene yields on an average ten somatic variants in each individual[b].

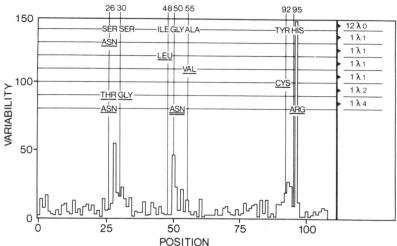

Figure 1.   The summary of the replacements in V_λ.

All positions outside of those indicated are identical in the eighteen sequenced chains. The under-lining of the amino acid residue indicates the number of bases required to account for the replacement compared to λ_o. The numbering of the position is that used by Wu and Kabat (25) in constructing the plot of VARIABILITY versus POSITION. The sequence of λ was compared with that of κ to optimize the homology and thereby best determine the position number.

$$\text{VARIABILITY} = \frac{\text{Number of different amino acids}}{\text{Frequency of the most common amino acid}}$$

At any one position, VARIABILITY has a minimum value of one when the position is invariant and a maximum of four hundred when all twenty amino acids are expressed in equal proportions.

The myeloma proteins sequenced were:

λ_o - HOPC-1(γ2a),MOPC104(μ),J558(α),J698(α),
       H2061(α),MOPC511(α),W3159(α)Y5431(BJ),
       Y5485(BJ),Y5830(BJ),Y5669(BJ).

λ_1(ASN)   - S176(α)

λ_1(LEU)   - RPC20(BJ)

λ_1(VAL)   - Y5606(γ3)

λ_1(CYS)   - Y5444(γ2a)

λ_2 - H2020(BJ)

λ_4 - S178(BJ)

The data are taken from (26) and unpublished.

IV. ESTIMATE OF TOTAL NUMBER OF GERM-LINE V_L-GENES

The next step in the argument is to use this minimal hypothesis accounting for the variability of the λ-gene, to count the total number of germ-line V_K-genes which are expressed. We recall the rule that for any given V-sequence, replacements in framework residues define germ-line V-genes. If two V-sequences differ in framework residues then two germ-line V-genes code for them. If two V-sequences are identical in framework but differ in complementarity-determining residues then one germ-line V-gene has given rise to two somatic variants. For an inbred population like the BALB/c mouse, the number of germ-line V-genes in the population equals that in the individual. Ideally the number of sequences available for analysis should be so large that any additional sequence would be identical in the framework region to a previously studied chain. The total number of germ-line V_K-genes could then be counted directly as the total number of V_K-sequences differing in framework residues. Unfortunately the number of sequences is not large enough to be ideal and a way of estimating the total number of germ-line V_K-genes from the limited data is needed.

We propose the following as a rough order of magnitude calculation.

N = total number of randomly chosen known sequences.

G = total number of somatically expressed germ-line V-genes.

m = N/G

It can be calculated from the Poisson distribution that the proportion of the total number of sequences which will be found once (singles) or twice (doubles) is

$$\text{Singles} = me^{-m}$$

$$\text{Doubles} = \frac{m^2 e^{-m}}{2}$$

The $\dfrac{\text{Singles}}{\text{Doubles}} = \dfrac{2}{m} = \dfrac{2G}{N}$

$$G = \frac{N}{2} \ X \ \frac{singles}{doubles}$$

The available data are collected in Figure 2. Only the first twenty-three positions have been sequenced for a large enough number of kappa chains.

1. For the estimation of the total number of germ-line V_K-genes, immunoglobulins of known antibody activity cannot be used because they are not randomly chosen, thereby tending to minimize the calculation of the total number of germ-line genes. However, they can be used to count germ-line V_K-genes directly. At least thirty-five germ-line V_K-genes are known and can be counted directly from the total number of known sequences which is fifty-five. These V_K-genes are indicated by Roman numerals in Figure 2.

2. There are a total of thirty-five randomly chosen sequences (see Figure 2). The number of times that a particular sequence has been found distributes as follows:

	MAXIMUM	MINIMUM
SINGLES	21 (21)	16 (16)
DOUBLES	5 (10)	6 (12)
TRIPLES	0 (0)	1 (3)
QUADRUPLES	1 (4)	1 (4)
N = TOTAL SEQUENCES =	(35)	(35)
G =GERM-LINE GENES	73	46 AVERAGE = 60

The distribution actually found gives the maximum value of G. The minimum value of G is calculated assuming that two sequences differing by only one amino acid are in error and they are actually identical. In any case the rough calculation places the number of V_K-genes in the germ-line (G) around sixty. Since only the N-terminal twenty-three amino acids have been used in the calculation, the value of G must be corrected for the remainder of the sequence. The total number of framework residues in the V-region is around ninety, four times the number analyzed. We estimate for the total sequence

V$_\kappa$-GENE	#	1	2	3	4	5	6	7	8	9	10	11	12	13	14	15	16	17	18	19	20	21	22	23	PROTEIN
(consensus)		ASP	ILE	VAL	MET	THR	GLN	SER	PRO	ALA	SER	LEU	SER	VAL	SER	LEU	GLY	GLU	ARG	VAL	THR	ILE	SER	CYS	
I	1								SER				MET	GLN	ALA		ILE			LYS					LPC1
II	1							THR	(ASX)	PHE		LEU				ALA		?						THR		MOPC35
III	1								GLN	SER	PHE	MET			THR		VAL	ASP			SER	VAL	THR			TEPC157
IV	1								SER	PHE	MET	VAL(THR)			VAL		(GLX)	?		?	?	?			MOPC379
V	1							THR	LYS	PHE	MET				THR		VAL	(LYS)			SER		THR			HOPC5
VI	1		ASN						LYS				MET		MET	VAL						LEU	THR			MOPC21
VII	1		ASN		LEU									ALA				GLN	ALA							MOPC63
VIII	1			GLN					THR	THR	SER				ALA			ASP	?					THR		MOPC173
IX	1			GLN							SER				ALA						SER	LEU	THR			MOPC41
X	1			GLN						ASP	TYR				ALA	VAL		THR					THR			MOPC149
XI	1			GLN		ILE				SER				MET	PHE	ALA		ILE	ASP	GLX	SER					McPc600
XII	1				LEU				?				THR	?			THR(THR)	ASX	?					?		MOPC316
XIII	1				LEU									ALA				GLX	LYS	ALA						BFPC61
XIV	1			VAL					THR	LEU	THR				THR	ILE		PRO	ALA	SER	[LEU]					McPc674
XV	1			VAL					THR	LEU	THR				THR	ILE		PRO	ALA	SER						McPc843
XVI	1	GLU	VAL	LEU								ILE	MET		ALA			GLN			SER	MET				TEPC29
XVII	1	GLU	VAL						THR			LEU			ALA			?	GLX	ALA	SER	?	?			MPC47
XVIII	1	GLU	ASN		LEU							ILE	MET		ALA	PRO						MET	THR			MOPC29
XIX	1	GLU	ASN		LEU							ILE	MET		ALA	PRO		ASX				MET	THR			TEPC153
XX	1			VAL	LEU				THR			LEU			PRO	(SER)		ASP	GLU	ALA	?			?		MPC37 (1)
XXI	1			GLN											VAL						?					M
XXII	2			GLN										ALA	VAL									THR		MOPC31c, MOPC178
XXIII	2									HIS(?)	LYS(?)	PHE	MET		THR			VAL	ASP			SER		THR		MPC11 (2), 641
XXIV	2			GLN											VAL			THR(?)						THR		TEPC173, RPC23
XXV	2	GLU	THR	THR	VAL								MET	ALA	ILE			LYS								MOPC265, MOPC773
XXVI	2				LEU								THR			THR	PRO	ASP	SER	ASX	SER	LEU				MOPC46 (3), MOPC172
XXVII / XXVIII	4				LEU									ALA				GLN	ALA							TEPC124, MOPC321 (4), BFPC32, MOPC70
XXIX	1			VAL					THR	LEU				THR				ASP	ALA	SER						MOPC460 [DNP]
XXX	2			VAL	VAL				THR	GLY	LEU			PRO			MET	ASP			SER					W3129 [α(1→6) DEXTRAN], W3434
XXXI	2				ILE				GLU	LEU			LYS	PRO			THR	SER		SER		SER				MOPC167 [CHOLINE], MOPC511
XXXII	2			GLN							SER				ALA			ASP	THR				MET	THR		W3082 [LEVAN], J606
XXXIII	3										SER				ALA				LYS				MET			McPc603 [CHOLINE], McPc870 [MANNOSE], MOPC384 [GALACTOSE]
XXXIV	4								THR	PHE		ALA			THR	ALA	SER	LYS	LYS							S63, TEPC15 [PHOSPHORYL-CHOLINE], S107, HOPC8
XXXV	6	GLU			LEU							ILE	THR	ALA	ALA								THR			S10, X24, X44 [β(1→6) GALACTAN], T191, J539, J1

Figure 2. See legend on page 95.

Figure 2. The sequences of the N-terminal twenty-three positions of all known mouse V_K-chains.

The numbering of the V_K-genes is discussed in the text, V_K-genes, IXXVIII are not associated with any known antibody specificity whereas V_K-genes, XXIX-XXXV are associated with the indicated specificities.

The residues enclosed in a box indicate that the corresponding bracketed myeloma proteins differ by only one amino acid in the N-terminal twenty-three residues and this difference may be an error.

The data for this figure has been taken from (8, 9, 20, 27, 28, 29).

(1) MOPC467 [anti-wheat] has same sequence as MPC37(XX).

(2) MPC11 has extra N-terminal 12 amino acids (count as separate gene?)

(3) S23 [anti-DNP] has same sequence as MOPC46 and MOPC172(XXVI).

(4) V_K-genes XXVII and XXVIII code for the same N-terminal residues but differ elsewhere and are discussed as part of figures 3, 4, and 5. The four myeloma proteins TEPC124,MOPC321,BFPC32 and MOPC70 are split into two groups as indicated.

that G will be two to four times larger than the calculated value of sixty. The total number of germ-line V_K-genes is then $120 < G < 240$.

This estimate that the value of G calculated from the N-terminal twenty three residues must be multiplied by about two in order to obtain the total number of germ-line V_K-genes, has been verified experimentally (Figure 3). The two germ-line V_K-genes XXVII and XXVIII code for the identical N-terminal sequence (see Figure 2), certainly up to position 26, the beginning of the first complementarity-determining region and probably through it to position 34. The question posed is whether the remainder of the V-sequence of each of the four proteins, TEPC124, MOPC321, BFPC32 and MOPC20 will be identical in framework residues. The answer is that they fall into two groups; V_K-gene XXVII coding TEPC124 and MOPC321; V_K-gene XXVIII coding BFPC32 and MOPC20. This can be seen first by looking at framework residues at positions 34,36,58,72-85 and 100 where the replacements define the two groups. In the complementarity-determining regions, positions 26-32, coded by germ-line V_K-genes XXVII and XXVIII appear to be identical, whereas regions 50-54 and 92-96 again fall into two groups, confirming the conclusion derived from framework residues that two germ-line V_K-genes are involved. In fact the simplest assumption to explain these sequences is that a cross-over occurred at codons 33-34 between either V_K-gene XXVII or V_K-gene XXVIII and another V_K-gene. This would generate the two V_K-genes XXVII and XXVIII identical to position 33 but differing from position 34 to the end (position~110) of the V_K-gene. These data are illustrated again in Figures 4 and where the most likely germ-line encoded sequence is shown and the pattern of replacement limited to the complementarity determining regions of each V_K-gene XXVII and XXVIII is illustrated (Figure 4). The average number of replacements in complementarity-determining regions is ≤ 3 (Figure 5).

These results confirm for V_K the conclusions arrived at from the study of the variation in V_λ (Figure 1).

This analysis justifies the use of a correction factor of about two by which the value of G calculated from the N-terminal twenty-three residues must be multiplied in order to obtain the total number of germ-line V_K-genes. If the two V_K-genes XXVII and XXVIII were

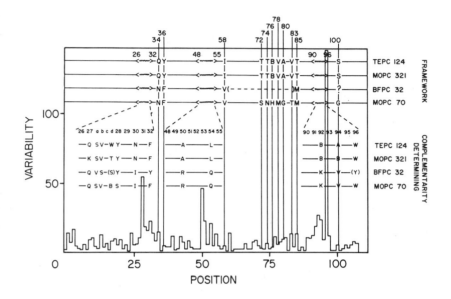

Figure 3. The complete sequence of the proteins coded by V_K-genes XXVII and XXVIII which are identical up to position 23 (see Figure 2) are illustrated by separating framework from complementarity-determining residues. The sequences are superimposed on the Wu-Kabat plot (see Figure 1). Data taken from (20,27).

CODE   A(ALA), B(ASX), C(CYS), D(ASP),

E(GLU), F(PHE), G(GLY), H(HIS), I(ILE),

K(LYS), L(LEU), M(MET), N(ASN), P(PRO),

Q(GLN), R(ARG), S(SER), T(THR), V(VAL),

W(TRP), Y(TYR), Z(GLX).

POSTULATED SEQUENCES CODED BY GERM-LINE V_κ-GENES XXVII AND XXVIII

POSITION / GENE	27	27a	27b	27d	28	30	32	34	36	50	54	58	72	74	76	78	80	83	85	92	94	96	100
GERM-LINE XXVII	GLN	SER	VAL	SER	TYR	ASN	PHE	GLN	TYR	ARG	LEU	ILE	THR	THR	ASX	VAL	ALA	VAL	THR	ASN	ASP	TRP	SER
SOMATIC TEPC124				TRP																	ALA		
SOMATIC MOPC321	LYS			THR																			
GERM-LINE XXVIII	GLN	SER	VAL	SER	TYR	ILE	PHE	ASN	PHE	ALA	GLN	VAL	SER	ASN	HIS	MET	GLX	THR	MET	LYS	VAL	TRP	GLY
SOMATIC BFPC32		VAL	GLX				TYR						(		?				)			(TYR)	
SOMATIC MOPC70				ASX	SER																		

POSITIONS NOT NUMBERED ARE IDENTICAL IN XXVII AND XXVIII FOR THE FOUR KAPPA CHAINS, TEPC124, MOPC321, BFPC32, MOPC70 WITH THE EXCEPTION THAT POSITIONS 59-84 HAVE NOT BEEN ANALYZED FOR PROTEIN BFPC32.

<COMPLEMENTARITY-DETERMINING RESIDUES>

Figure 4. The most likely sequence coded by germ-line V_κ-genes XXVII and XXVIII and the replacements in the complementarity-determining residues.

Underlining indicates number of base changes to account for replacements in the myeloma proteins TEPC124, MOPC321 and BFPC32 and MOPC170. In comparing framework residues, germ-line V_κ-gene XXVII is used as a reference and in comparing complementarity-determining residues the V_κ-genes XXVII or XXVIII are used as references respectively.

Data taken from (20, 27).

SUMMARY OF BASE DIFFERENCES BETWEEN GERM-LINE V_K-GENES XXVII AND XXVIII

TOTAL BASES TRANSLATED FROM V_K-mRNA $\sim$ 330 (110 AMINO ACIDS)

NUMBER OF BASES CODING FOR COMPLEMENTARITY-DETERMINING RESIDUES...$\sim$ 45

NUMBER OF BASES CODING FOR FRAMEWORK RESIDUES.....................$\sim$285

TOTAL BASES $\sim$ 330

NUMBER OF BASE DIFFERENCES BETWEEN GERM-LINE V_K-GENES XXVII AND XXVIII

    FRAMEWORK   = 13

    COMPLEMENTARITY DETERMINING = 6

                 TOTAL = 19

NUMBER OF SOMATIC MUTATIONAL STEPS FROM GERM-LINE V_K-GENE XXVII FOR

        TEPC124   = 2

        MOPC321   = 2

NUMBER OF SOMATIC MUTATIONAL STEPS FROM GERM-LINE V_K-GENE XXVIII FOR

        BFPC32 $\leqq$ 6

        MOPC70   = 3

Figure 5. Summary of replacements in framework and complementarity-determining residues of V_K-genes XXVII and XXVIII (see figures 3 and 4).

99

derived by recombination then the value of two is high depending on how frequent such an event is compared to variation by mutation. Further, if calculations based on the variation in the N-terminal twenty-three residues come within a factor of two of predicting total variation, then the evolution of the system must involve stepwise duplication and variation of framework residues by frequent mutational substitutions[c].

It might be well to ask at this point what factors might increase or decrease the number of germ-line V-genes estimated. The major factor leading to an underestimate would be non-randomness of the myeloma population studied. The assumption here is that only a subpopulation of germ-line V_L or V_H genes are expressed in myelomas. We have no way to evaluate this except to point out that no one has proposed a satisfactory relationship which associates given V_L-genes with transformation to neoplastic. The major factor leading to an overestimate would be the assumption that all framework residue differences are germ-line V-gene encoded. This extreme assumption is supported by the finding that of the twenty λ light chains sequenced, ten mutations have been expressed in complementarity-determining residues and none in the framework. There is no simple model of random mutation coupled to the assumption that most framework replacements are neutral which would reduce our estimate significantly, i.e. more than a factor of two. Consequently we will use for our discussion the estimate of 10^2 germ-line V_L-genes. Although it is premature to make a similar estimate for germ-line V_H-genes it does not seem to be different.

IV. ANTIBODY SPECIFICITIES CODED BY GERM-LINE V-GENES

We have postulated that the selection pressure on germ-line V-genes is for specificities of maximum survival value at birth. Each V-gene be it V_L or V_H is maintained because when expressed complemented with one or two appropriate partners, it codes for the required specificity. Given $10^2 V_L$ and $10^2 V_H$ genes it is not possible to select simultaneously on all $10^4 V_L V_H$ combinations because a mutation leading to a replacement in a complementarity-determining residue of a given germ-line V_L-subunit for example, will change the specificity of all other germ-line antibodies resulting from the 100 germ-line V_H-sub-units with which it is complemented. Consequently it is expected that the antibody activities selected upon to be coded by germ-line V-genes would be limited to roughly 100-200 $V_L V_H$ combinations i.e. for each determinant $1V_L +$ $1V_H$ or $1V_L + 2V_H$ or $2V_L + 1V_H$. This selection on $\sim 10^2$ out of 10^4 possible germ-line $V_L V_H$ combinations assures that all are functional as immunoglobulin.

We will illustrate this with the specificity for the determinant, $\alpha(1\rightarrow 3)$ glucoside, and extend the argument to $\beta(1\rightarrow 6)$-D-galactan, phosphorylcholine and $\alpha(1\rightarrow 6)$ glucoside, all of which seem to be coded in the germ-line.

The response to $\alpha(1\rightarrow 3)$ dextran has the following characteristics (1-3).

1. Certain mouse strains e.g. BALB/c and 129, respond rapidly with an antibody uniquely of the $\lambda\mu$ class and of a restricted idiotype. This idiotype is borne by all BALB/c myeloma immunoglobulins with anti-$\alpha(1\rightarrow 3)$ dextran activity e.g. J558. These strains are referred to as high responders.

2. Certain mouse strains e.g. C57BL/6, respond slowly with antibody of the κ class and of an unrelated idiotype. These are referred to as low responders.

3. The F_1 hybrid between high and low responder strains has the high responder phenotype.

4. The response difference between low and high responders both with respect to rate and idiotype is determined by a gene linked to within 0.4% recombination units of the known heavy chain allotype markers of the C_H-genes.

The interpretation of these findings is that the high responder has germ-line V_H-genes, absent in low responders, which in complementation with the germ-line V_λ-gene codes for $\alpha(1\rightarrow 3)$ dextran specificity[d]. Low responders may not have any germ-line $V_L V_H$-gene combination coding this specificity. They may however, respond slowly in the kappa class to the same determinant on $\alpha(1\to3)$ dextran presumably as a consequence of somatic mutation and selection. Anti-$\alpha(1\to3)$ dextran is one example of a germ-line encoded specificity.

The point being illustrated here is that an animal which possesses structural germ-line V-genes coding for recognition of a given determinant may be distinguishable from one lacking these genes by both the rate of the response and the sequence of the induced antibody. This can be seen by mapping the response difference to a known locus coding for immunoglobulin subunits.

The experimental argument that other specificities are germ-line gene encoded is more tenuous because it must be made in the absence of response difference genetics and largely from studies with idiotype markers; sequence data covering complementarity-determining regions are limited. Responsiveness to antigen is an important marker because it is the only primary definition we have of the combining site.

The idiotypic determinant which most uniquely defines a given antibody molecule is one which is ligand-modifiable (4). When the addition of the ligand inhibits the reaction between the antibody and its anti-idiotype, the idiotypic determinant is referred to as ligand-modifiable. Even an antiserum which recognizes a ligand-modifiable idiotypic determinant may not be able to distinguish antibody molecules which differ by only one or two replacements in the complementarity-determining residues (5). In any case, reasonable likelihood arguments that other specificities are germ-line gene encoded, can be made from the combination of partial sequence and idiotype. Let us review the argument.

If induced myeloma immunoglobulins arise repeatedly with specificity towards a given determinant and if these proteins had identical V_L and V_H sequences, the likelihood would be that this specificity is germ-line gene encoded. The suggestion is strengthened if a unique antibody identical to the repeat myeloma proteins, is induced normally by immunogens bearing the given determinant. The next step is to search for animals which although they respond equally well to the given determinant, do so with homogeneous antibodies. If the sequence of these antibodies differed in framework residues, we would conclude that the animals differed in their germ-line V-genes. If every member of an inbred population responds identically with one type of antibody whereas every member of another inbred population responds identically with the other type of antibody, the specificity of these antibodies is likely germ-line V-gene encoded. A genetics of the sequence difference would map the V_L- or V_H-genes involved. If the sequences of both V_L and V_H differed between the strains it would not be possible to tell without extensive genetic analysis which difference was due to an allele and which had resulted from somatic selection for the complementary partner.

If "ligand-modifiable idiotype" is substituted for "sequence" in the above analysis the conclusion is still reasonable but weaker. However, experimentally, the study of the ligand-modifiable idiotype is so much easier that it is most often used. The best established case in this second category (only because it lacks responsiveness genetics) is the anti-phosphorylcholine specificity which is found repeatedly in BALB/c myeloma proteins (6, 7). These proteins have indistinguishable idiotypes. Further, antibody of BALB/c mice to the phosphorylcholine determinant carries the same idiotype. The sequences of the myeloma proteins with indistinguishable idiotype are identical through the first complementarity-determining regions of both the L (κ) and H-chains (8). From this we extrapolate to the induced antibody and assume that it too has the same sequence because the idiotype is indistinguishable from the myeloma protein counterpart. We presume that anti-phosphorylcholine specificity is germ-line gene encoded because 1) various inbred strains which respond equally well, do so with antibody of unrelated idiotype whereas each member of a given inbred strain responds with an indistinguishable idiotype and 2) the idiotype difference maps linked to the allotype marker of the heavy chain locus.

Since as yet genetic studies has not been carried out, the argument is weaker for the germ-line gene encoding of the $\beta(1\rightarrow6)$ D-galactan specificity (9) and with still decreasing experimental solidity, for the $\alpha(1\rightarrow6)$ dextran and levan specificities (10)[e].

V. SOME CONSEQUENCES OF THIS MODEL OF THE GERM-LINE V-GENE PROPERTIES

It is quite reasonable that the specificities selected for in the germ-line be directed largely against carbohydrate determinants. These are the essential constituents of the surface of pathogens and are most difficult to modify by mutation. On the one hand it is almost impossible to change the specificity of an enzyme by mutation without loss of function and on the other hand changing of the carbohydrate surface by inactivating an enzyme alters the virulence e.g. the smooth to rough mutation of pneumococci. If germ-line V-genes are selected upon for the specificities they code, then the postulate of a special somatic mechanism to generate before immunogen encounter all of the possible specificities a mature immune system can express is gratuitous. Any germ-line encoded specificity would have no selective advantage in evolution if the equivalent group of specificities could be generated somatically from germ-line genes before immunogen were encountered[f]. Two questions must be discussed:

1) What determines the size of the family of germ-line genes from which an individual's immune system develops?
2) What determines the effectiveness of the somatic mechanism which increases the range of the initial diversity?

The lower limit of the size of the germ-line V-gene pool is set by two factors:1) the requirement for immediate protection against the most likely pathogens encountered at birth and 2) the requirement for a minimum number of different clones upon which somatic selection can operate initially to increase the immune system's range of diversity sufficiently rapidly. The upper limit of the germ-line V-gene pool size is determined by the accumulation of essentially redundant specificities upon which evolutionary selection cannot operate efficiently. This leads to the accumulation of inactivated V-genes which are expressed in antigen-sensitive cells that are wasted$^{(f)}$. Further, special mechanisms to maintain as well as regulate the expression of many similar genes must simultaneously evolve$^{(g)}$.

An increasing rate of diversification in the soma is selected upon by the need for maximum diversification in a minimum time. However there is a counter selective pressure, for above a certain threshold any further increase in rate no longer provides a selective advantage and in addition requires the evolution of special complex mechanisms. This threshold rate seems to be an average of ten somatic variants from each germ-line V-gene in the first month following immunogenic encounter. This rate is equivalent to a turnover of 10^7 cells per day and a mutation rate of 10^{-7}/base pair/generation(11).

Any mechanism which increases differentially the mutation frequency particularly of complementarity determining codons or the number of generations/day, shortens the time for somatic selection to yield a mature immune system. If the mutation rate of complementarity-determining codons is that found as maximal in bacteria (10^{-5}/base pair/generation), antigenic selection would have to be stepwise on single step mutants as they appear because it would still not be high enough to generate the total diversity in the absence of selection. The more likely estimate of mutation rates close to 10^{-7}/base pair/generation are compatible with present data on the mature immune system which puts the average number of somatic replacements per V-sequence around two with a maximum value close to five.

The more direct evidence favoring sequential selection has been analyzed carefully elsewhere (12,13). However a general comment must be made concerning the nature of the selection by immunogenic encounter. Induction requires recognition of the antigen not only by the antigen-sensitive cell but by the cooperating thymus-derived system using a recognition unit which is in part coded by a locus (IR-1) linked to the major histocompatibility complex. Since a known structural V_H-gene can control responsiveness, it is a reasonable assumption that IR-1 codes for a new structural V-gene locus which when complemented with known V-loci results in an immunoglobulin functioning as this recognition unit (14)[h].

VI. THE RELATIVE IMPORTANCE OF SEQUENCE

The question we need to answer is how many germ-line V-genes are expressed somatically in a way which can be selected upon by antigen? The number of germ-line V-genes carried as functionless or inactive is an important second order consideration.

If framework replacements permit the counting of germ-line V-genes and complementarity-determining residues the counting of somatically derived variants of germ-line V-genes then the general properties of the immune response which we have analyzed is valid. The numbers of complete sequences and of cases of V-gene controlled responsiveness are too limited at present to do better than get order of magnitude values as to the relative contributions of somatic and germ-line V-genes to diversity.

However, there does not seem to be a totally independent competing methodology. For example, mRNA-DNA hybridization cannot be substituted for sequence in counting functional germ-line V-genes. On the one hand answers which put the number of hybridizable V-genes per locus in tens of thousands (15) do not tell us how many are functional. If counting by amino acid sequence puts the number expressed in the hundreds, then all that such hybridization data would tell us, is that there are many functionless V-genes. On the other hand hybridization studies which put the number at close to one per mRNA hybridized (16, 17) requires some kind of estimate, based on sequence, of the factor by which to multiply to get the total number of germ-line V-genes. One critical study (16), interprets a reiteration frequency of 200 found for about 20% of the κ-chain mRNA as being due to non-translated nucleotides which might have various regulating functions common to all V_K-genes. Even if this interpretation were correct it does not permit an independent count of functional V-genes. It is the agreement of hybridizable count and sequence count which supports the above interpretation and implies that virtually all germ-line V-genes are somatically expressed in a way which can be selected upon by immunogenic encounter. There is little or no waste, an expectation of the model in which individual germ-line V-genes are selected for by the specificities they code.

Clearly we need a more accurate estimate of the number of germ-line V-genes expressed in a way which can be selected upon somatically. This is one answer to "why more sequences?"

FOOTNOTES

(a) Somatic mutations which introduce replacements in framework residues are either neutral or affect adversely the functioning of the subunit in the immunoglobulin molecule and for this reason are not found. The situation is the same as that one must postulate to explain why replacements in the C-region are not seen.

It is reasonable, in fact likely, that there is a differentially higher mutation rate in complementarity-determining regions but this is a second-order consideration only if the differential rate is not so high that all possible variants appear before immunogenic selection is imposed. If the mutation rate were constant throughout the V-gene and if mutations in about 10% of the bases lead to amino acid replacements in complementarity-determining residues, in the absence of selection, the probability that all ten replacements would be in complementarity-determining residues is 10^{-10}.

(b) Seven different V_λ-sequences have been found thus far and two more are implied as intermediates in a sequential selection process making a total of nine. This is a rough approximation for we are considering the BALB/c mouse population as an individual. If the mature immune system expresses somatically 10^6 antibodies ($10^3 V_L \times 10^3 V_H$) and the germ-line, 10^4 antibodies ($10^2 V_L \times 10^2 V_H$), then the estimate is reasonable that each germ-line V-gene yields on an average ten somatic variants.

There is another way to look at these data. If the average number of amino acid replacements in the germ-line V_λ-sequence were two, then there could be as many as 100

V_λ-sequences somatically derived in the BALB/c population. If this is extrapolated to all germ-line V-genes then the population could express 10^8 antibodies ($10^4 V_L \times 10^4 V_H$) but an individual likely expresses much less, $\sim 10^6$. The average number of replacements in the V_λ-sequence is at minimum, 1.5 replacements per sequence (nine replacements in six sequences).

It might be added parenthetically that the postulate of a special somatic mechanism to generate all variation before the animal is exposed to foreign antigens is not needed if somatic genes differ on an average from germ-line genes by only one or two mutations.

(c) Another experimental estimate of the factor for extrapolation from twenty-three to ninety framework residues can be made as follows (Figure 2):

Number of N-Terminal Residues Considered	V_K-genes Counted	V_K-genes Calculated (G)
1	3	-
6	12	-
12	24	46
23	27	73

If less than twenty-three residues are considered, it can be seen that the number of genes actually counted is nearly the same if only the first twelve residues had been available. The calculated number as one doubles the number of residues under consideration, increases not quite doubling as one goes from a consideration of twelve versus twenty-three residues. For the total chain this gives a maximum extrapolated value of four or a more likely value of two since the plateauing values as more residues are considered shows that replacements are often linked.

(d) The alternative possibility is that the anti-dextran V_H-gene is identical in BALB/c and C57BL/6 but the V_λ-genes differ. This requires close linkage of the λ and heavy chain genes. If the responsive difference were due to λ-genes, not V_H-genes, then in a (BALB/c x C57BL/6)F_1 mouse the effective BALB/c λ chain ought to be expressed with heavy chains of both parental types. In fact this is not found; only BALB/c heavy chains are detectable in the

purified anti-dextran antibody. This analysis would prove
that the difference is in the heavy chain V-genes except
for one possibility. If λ were in fact closely linked to
the heavy chain it might be allelically excluded with it
thus giving only parental λ-heavy combinations. To resolve
this issue λ must be mapped to some other unlinked
location in the genome or shown by sequence to be identical
in the two strains.

(e) Generalizing from models made by Jerne (18) and
Bodmer (19), it might be proposed that germ-line V-genes
are selected upon uniquely for anti-self specificities.
This is to be contrasted with our proposal that the specificities selected for are essentially non-self.Occasional
cases might arise where germ-line V-genes encoding a given
antibody are put into an animal which has the corresponding determinant as a self-component. If the genetics
of the population were such that they always remained
together, we could expect the germ-line encoded antibody
to be lost because it is not expressed in a way which can
be selected upon. In this respect a unique paradox
should be illustrated. If anti-idiotype (anti-I or anti-
(anti-S)) directed against an antibody with self-speci-
ficity (anti-S) is under analysis then anti-I will be
expressed with a behavior imitating that seen in the case
of all dominant immune response genes (IR-genes). The
response difference will map linked to the genes determining the expression of S. If S-genes happen to be
linked to any of the known immune related loci, a
difficulty of interpretation arises. Consequently, the
genetics of anti-idiotypic responsiveness cannot be used
to analyze immune responsiveness unless it is known that
the specificity of the antibody carrying the idiotype is
not directed against a self-component which is tolerogenic.

(f) Starting with the assumption that the total diversity
is generated prior to antigenic selection e.g. all V-genes
are in the germ-line (no somatic diversification exists),
the reverse argument has been made by Hood (20) as follows:

It is known that the specificity coded by a given
antibody V-gene overlaps with those of many other antibody
V-genes. Given this heterogenity, selection cannot

operate on individual V-genes if many other V-genes code
similar specificities. Accordingly natural selection cannot operate on individual V-genes but must "operate on
families of V-genes taken as a whole" (20).

The meaning of the concept "selection on the whole
family" is too imprecise to be of value at this point in
our analysis. However the above problem posed by multigenic system of V-genes is precisely the reason that we
have analyzed a model in which the number of V-genes carried in the germ-line is limited at a maximum determined
by the selection on individual V-genes. When redundancy
sets in the excess is lost keeping the number of functionless V-genes low. Overlapping specificities are a result
of somatic not germ-line selection. In this way the
population does not have to conserve in the germ-line a
large number of V-genes which an individual never uses
[see (21) for discussion]. Our model requiring germ-line
selection on individual V-genes is supported by the findings with responsiveness to $\alpha(1\rightarrow3)$ dextran (see text).

(g) If there are $\sim10^2 V_L$- and V_H-genes in the germ-line, two
problems are now raised which have embarrassed but never
been accounted for by those who believe that all V-genes
are in the germ-line. These are: 1) the rabbit V_H-allo-
type markers and 2) the phylogenetically-associated
residues marking V_H-genes.

    1.   Rabbit V_H-allotype markers.

The precise paradox arises not in a consideration of
the allotype defined as a serological marker but in the
allotype defined as an amino acid marker [see (21) for dis-
cussion]. The paradox arises only if it is claimed that the
identical amino acid marker is coded by all (or most) V_H-
genes of one locus and another amino acid marker is coded
by all (or most) V_H-genes of the allelic locus. If a given
amino acid marker is coded by a small number of the V_H-genes
in one locus, no problem arises as we know that V-genes can
be duplicated and it is reasonable that mutation in a framework codon would create an allelic V-gene which was later
duplicated. In other words the allelic amino acid difference
precedes the duplication. There are no data today which show
that an identical amino acid marker is coded by the majority
(a large number) of V_H-genes of one allelic locus and

another amino acid marker is coded by the majority (a large number) of V_H-genes at another allelic locus (22). In fact it is predictable that this will not be found.

2. "Phylogenetically-associated" residues marking V_H-genes.

The question here is identical to that posed for the rabbit V_H-allotype markers. How does one count the absolute not relative number of V_H-genes carrying a given phylogenetically-associated marker? If the absolute number is small no special problem arises; if it is large the many paradoxes of the evolution of a multigene system are posed.

The experimental analysis is limited in the same way as that discussed for rabbit V_H-allotype associated residues. The sequences coded by at least sixteen germ-line V_H-genes are known (29). The prototype sequence is that determined on unblocked serum V_H-chains (23, 24) in which each residue was found in $\geq$ 95% of the total. It is clear in comparing the prototype sequence with the sequences coded by different germ-line V_H-genes, that many of them do not code for the "phytogenetically associated" residues. For the inbred BALB/c mouse six known V_H-genes code the linked residues Lys-Lys at positions 3 and 19 suspected of being phylogenetically-associated (23). The number not carrying this pair of residues is ten. The total number of known V_H-genes coding unblocked N-terminal residues is sixteen. The actual number could be twice this (assuming 10^2 V_H-genes; 0.2 unblocked N-terminal; then there are a total of 20 V_H-genes coding unblocked H-chains; $\sim$10 of these are known). The evolution of about $10V_H$ genes carrying phylogenetically associated residues is not very paradoxical if duplication and deletion are a major pathway of their evolution.

A similar situation is encountered if the "restricted" antibodies induced in rabbit are analyzed for the allotypically associated residues (22).

(h) The responsiveness to $\alpha(1\rightarrow 3)$ dextran is controlled by structural V_H-genes. In most cases which have been studied responsiveness is determined by alleles at the IR-1 locus unlinked to the H-locus. The IR-1 locus contributes in part to the structure of the receptor of the cooperating thymus-derived system required for induction. To most polydeterminant antigens a response difference would not be detected, if a mutation were to alter the affinity of a unique receptor. First of all the recognition of the antigen could occur in many ways so that the loss of one recognition would go unnoticed and secondly if polymeric antigens are used, a decrease in affinity may not be revealed because of the polyvalent interaction with the receptor. Antigens which fall into this latter category are termed colloquially "thymus-independent". Since $\alpha(1\to3)$ dextran is such an antigen and since the λ-locus does not determine the responsiveness difference, it is surprising that regulation of responsiveness by another gene, in addition to V_H-dextran, is indicated.

There are certain mouse strains e.g. A/HeJ which are non-responders i.e. $\log_2$ titer 3. The (A/HeJ x 129/J)F_1 is a high responder. A backcross between (A/HeJ x 129/J)F_1 and A/HeJ is illustrated in Figure 6. The F1 mice which are classified as low responders in Figure 6 actually fall into two equal groups, non-responders and low responders. The kinetics of these responses are illustrated in Figure 7. The non-responders never show a detectable $\log_2$ titer. The low responders reach peak $\log_2$ titer of 9-10 in 25 days which is the value high responders reach in 5 days. The high responder by 14 days plateaus at a $\log_2$ titer of 12. A second locus revealed by this cross could be either the kappa or IR-1 locus. Assuming for illustration that the second locus is IR-1 the interpretation would be as follows (see Figure 8):

A non-responder must have the low response alleles at both loci (Group I). In this situation an antibody response to $\alpha(1\to3)$ dextran cannot get started because it is not possible to exert a sufficient somatic selection pressure on either the V_H-locus or the IR-1(?) locus. However, if a high response allele is present at the IR-1(?) locus (Group III) then the somatic selection is sufficiently strong to permit the appearance of anti-$\alpha(1\to3)$ dextran activity but it is in the kappa class since the V_H-dextran gene which complements with λ is missing. The slow rise in this kappa activity to a high level (Figure 7)

112

LINKAGE OF ANTI-DEXTRAN RESPONSE TO HEAVY CHAIN ALLOTYPE LOCUS

BACKCROSS (129/J X A/HeJ) X A/HeJ

A/HeJ Non-Responder
129/J High Responder

		PRESENCE OF STRAIN 129 ALLOTYPE +	PRESENCE OF STRAIN 129 ALLOTYPE -
Anti Dextran Response Characteristics	High titer and Reference idiotype (J558)	79	0
	Low titer and Lacking reference Idiotype	0	100

Figure 6. Linkage of anti-dextran response and the heavy chain allotype loci in (129/J x A/HeJ)F_1 x A/HeJ backcross mice.

129/J high responder carrying reference idiotype of myeloma protein J558

A/HeJ non-responder.

The low and non-responder phenotypes in the offspring both lack the 129/J allotype and are pooled in the data(i).

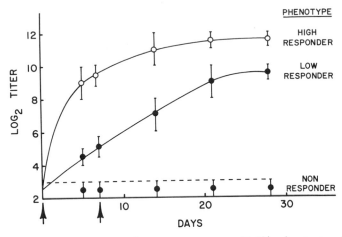

Figure 7. Kinetics of response to $\alpha(1\rightarrow3)$ dextran in progeny of a backcross (A/HeJ x 129/J)F$_1$ x A/HeJ. [Footnote (i)].

	IR-1(?)	V$_H$-dextran gene
A/HeJ	1/1	1/1
129/J	h/h	h/h

		(A/HeJ x 129/J)F$_1$					
		IR-1(?) V$_H$		IR-1(?) V$_H$		IR-1(?) V$_H$	IR-1(?) V$_H$
A/HeJ		1 1		1 h		h 1	h h
IR-1(?) V$_H$- dextran 1 1		1/1 1/1		1/1 h/1		h/1 1/1	h/1 h/1
		I		II		III	IV
Phenotype of response		Non-responder		High responder in reference idiotype(J558)		Low responder lacking reference idiotype(J558)	High responder in reference idiotype(J558)
Mouse Strain showing phenotype		A/HeJ		BALB/c		C57BL/6	129/J

Figure 8. An interpretation of the phenotypes revealed in the (A/HeJ x 129/J)F$_1$ x A/HeJ backcross.

1 = low response allele

h = high response allele

114

is interpreted to reflect the somatic selection of antigen-sensitive B-cells expressing those germ-line encoded $V_K V_H$ receptors which by a single amino acid replacement acquire a detectable anti-$\alpha(1\rightarrow3)$ dextran specificity.

If a high responder allele is present at the heavy chain locus (V_H-dextran) (Groups II and IV) then a high response in the reference idiotype is found. The reason that groups II and IV cannot be distinguished easily by the tests thus far used is because the antigen is a repeating polymer. However, attempts are being made to distinguish groups II and IV by studying the class of the response, IgM or IgG, using TNP-dextran in which dextran is used as a carrier and anti-TNP is measured. Group IV may switch to IgG while Group II remains in the IgM class. There are indications that this occurs. Group III shows that once a minimum threshold level of cooperating activity is present in the strains being analyzed, differences in responsiveness determined at V_L or V_H loci are revealed provided that their effect makes the B-cell response limiting. The strains under analysis could vary widely in their germ-line determined levels of cooperating activity (IR-1) as long as this variation operates above a threshold level necessary to permit a response defined as "high" in one of the strains.

ACKNOWLEDGMENTS

This work was supported by grant (A-105875) and training grant (CA-05213), both from the National Institutes of Health to Dr. Melvin Cohn, and grant (GM-18263) from the National Institutes of Health to Dr. Martin Weigert.

REFERENCES

1. B. Blomberg, W. Geckeler and M. Weigert, Science 177, 178 (1972).
2. B. Blomberg, D. Carson and M. Weigert, In Specific Receptors of Antibodies, Antigens and Cells. Third Int. Convoc. Immunol., eds. D. Pressman, T. B. Tomasi, Jr., A. L. Grossberg, N. R. Rose. S. Karger, Basel, pg. 285 (1973).

3. R. Riblet and M. Weigert, unpublished.

4. B. Brient and A. Nisonoff, J. Exp. Med. 135, 951 (1970).

5. D. Carson and M. Weigert, Proc. Nat. Acad. Sci. U.S. 70, 235 (1973).

6. R. Lieberman, M. Potter, E. Mushinski, W. Humphrey and S. Rudikoff, in press (1974).

7. A. Sher and M. Cohn, Eur. J. Immunol. 2, 319 (1972).

8. P. Barstad, S. Rudikoff, M. Potter, M. Cohn and L. Hood, Science 183, 962 (1974).

9. S. Rudikoff, E. Mushinski, M. Potter, C. Glandemans and M. Jolley, J. Exp. Med. 138, 1095 (1973).

10. M. Weigert, W. Raschke, D. Carson and M. Cohn, J. Exp. Med. 139, 137 (1974).

11. M. Cohn, In The Biochemistry of Gene Expression in Higher Organisms, eds. J. K. Pollak and J. W. Lee. D. Reidel Publishing Co., Dordrecht, Holland, pg. 574 (1973).

12. A. Cunningham, In Contemporary Topics in Molecular Immunol. 3 (in press) (1974).

13. A. Cunningham, Scandinavian J. Immunol. (in press) (1974).

14. M. Cohn, In Genetic Control of Immune Responsiveness, eds. H. McDevitt and M. Landy. Academic Press, New York, pg. 367 (1972).

15. E. Prekuman, M. Shoyab and A. R. Williamson, Proc. Nat. Acad. Sci. U.S. 71, 99 (1974).

16. S. Tonegawa, A. Bernardini, B. J. Weimarm and C. Steinberg, FEBS Letters (in press) (1974).

17. A. Bernardini and S. Tonegawa, FEBS Letters (in press) (1974).

18. N. K. Jerne, Eur. J. Immunol. 1, 1 (1971).

19. W. Bodmer, Nature 237, 139 (1972).

20. L. Hood, In Proc. Stadler Genetics Symp. 5 (in press) (1974).

21. M. Cohn, Ann. N. Y. Acad. Sci. 190, 529 (1971).

22. D. Braun and J. C. Jaton, In Current Topics in Microbiology & Immunol., (in press) (1974).

23. D. Capra, R. Wasserman and M. Kehoe, J. Exp. Med. 138, 410 (1973).

24. M. Kehoe and D. Capra, Proc. Nat. Acad. Sci. U.S., 69, 2052 (1972).

25. T. T. Wu and E. Kabat, J. Exp. Med. 132, 211 (1970).

26. M. Weigert, I. Cesari, S. Yonkovich and M. Cohn, Nature 228, 1045 (1970).
27. E. Appella and J. Inman, In Contemporary Topics in Molecular Immunol. V. 2, 51 (1974).
28. G. Smith, Science 181, 941 (1973).
29. L. Hood, this Symposium.

ANTIBODY DIVERSITY: AN ASSESSMENT

L. Hood, P. Barstad, E. Loh, and C. Nottenburg

Division of Biology
California Institute of Technology
Pasadena, California 91109

ABSTRACT.   Four propositions are discussed. 1. Selection[*] limits the variable regions expressed in the myeloma and normal pools of immunoglobulins. 2. Most antibody families have multiple variable genes in the germ line. 3. Hypervariable regions are predicted by a germ line theory. 4. New and unexpected amino acid sequence patterns suggest that many mysteries of antibody genetics, evolution and control remain yet to be unraveled.

INTRODUCTION

Genetic studies as well as detailed amino acid sequence analyses on immunoglobulins have revealed patterns which have provided important insights into the nature of genetic mechanisms responsible for antibody diversity, evolution and expression (1). Certain structural and genetic features appear common to all vertebrate immunoglobulins. First, all immunoglobulins are composed of two distinct polypeptides, light chains and heavy chains. Second, all antibody polypeptides are divided into two segments, the variable (V) and constant (C) regions. The variable regions of the antibody molecule encode the antigen binding site whereas the constant regions carry out various other functions. Third, antibody polypeptides are coded by three families of genes, two for light chains (λ and κ) and one for heavy chains (H), which are unlinked in the mammalian genome. The variable and the constant regions appear to be coded by separate but linked genes within each family. Fourth, a comparison of many variable regions from a given antibody family reveals three to four regions of increased variability which are termed "hypervariable" regions. The following will be a discussion of four propositions which are supported by sequence and genetic patterns derived from recent studies on vertebrate immunoglobulins.

I.   SELECTION LIMITS THE VARIABLE REGIONS EXPRESSED IN THE MYELOMA AND NORMAL POOLS OF IMMUNOGLOBULINS.

The clonal selection hypothesis suggests that at some

time in ontogeny and independently of antigen, individual lymphocytes become committed to responding to a single type of antigenic determinant, presumably through a single molecular species of antibody receptor on the lymphocyte cell surface (2). Presumably the interaction of surface receptor molecules and complementary antigen activates the specific lymphocytes and leads to clonal proliferation and the secretion of specific antibody (Figure 1). Daughter cells derived from clonal expansion are restricted to the synthesis of that same antibody. Thus, the only immunoglobulins which can be studied by current chemical and genetic techniques are those derived from cells which have been clonally expanded. Immunoglobulins derived from two distinct sources, normal heterogeneous immunoglobulins and homogeneous myeloma proteins, have been most thoroughly analyzed (3,4,5). The pool of normal (heterogeneous) immunoglobulin (i.e., variable regions) present in the serum of a given animal results from a particular history of antigenic exposure. A myeloma immunoglobulin is produced by the clonal expansion of a single antibody producing cell through neoplastic transformation. The neoplastic clone frequently expands to predominate over all other antibody producing cells and, accordingly, the homogeneous immunoglobulin produced by this cell line can constitute 95% or more of the serum immunoglobulin. Obviously, distinct myeloma tumors arise in differing individuals. The sequences from many different myeloma proteins can then be compared to assess the diversity of immunoglobulins from the myeloma pool. Because myeloma proteins have revealed most of the important patterns of antibody diversity and evolution, it is important to consider whether the myeloma pool reflects all of the diversity coded by the antibody genes of a given organism or whether the myeloma pool represents a selected subset from the actual pool of antibody diversity.

In Figure 2 are given the ratios of residue alternatives at each of the first ten positions for the myeloma (44 proteins) and normal pools of immunoglobulins from the inbred BALB/c mouse (6). Significant qualitative as well as quantitative differences are present. The myeloma pool has certain residue alternatives which are totally lacking in the normal pool (e.g., threonine at position 3, isoleucine at position 4, isoleucine at position 5, aspartic acid at position 6, etc.) and the normal pool has residue alternatives which are totally lacking in the myeloma pool (e.g., alanine or serine at position 6 and isoleucine at position 7). In each case the percentage of these residues is well within the limits of detection for our analytic system.

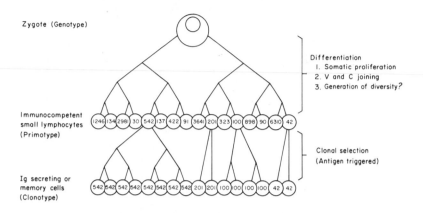

Zygote (Genotype)

Differentiation
1. Somatic proliferation
2. V and C joining
3. Generation of diversity?

Immunocompetent
small lymphocytes
(Primotype)

Clonal selection
(Antigen triggered)

Ig secreting or
memory cells
(Clonotype)

FIGURE 1. A model of somatic differentiation of antibody producing cells according to the clonal selection theory. This model suggests that there are two stages of development--differentiation which is independent of antigen and clonal expansion which is triggered by antigen. The different numbers signify the commitment of distinct lymphocytes to a different molecular species of antibody (adapted from 38). Accordingly, three different levels of information storage and expression are possible. First, the information for the antibody V genes is stored directly in the vertebrate genome (genotype). Second, V_L and V_H genes are expressed as antibody molecules on the cell surface of differentiated lymphocytes (primotype). Finally, certain lymphocytes undergo clonal expansion (by antigen or neoplastic conversion) to produce clones which synthesize the immunoglobulin molecules which are available for study by the immunologist (clonotype). The critical question has to do with whether or not only a small subset of the primotype is selected for clonal expansion by antigen or the myeloma process (see text).

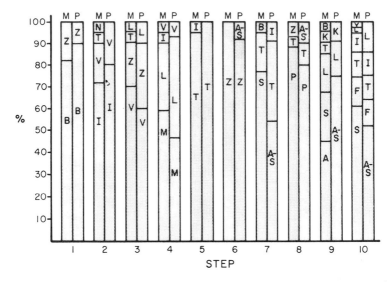

FIGURE 2. Comparison of the pooled data from BALB/c normal and myeloma κ chains. Step refers to the residue position beginning at the N-terminus. At each step the column labeled M refers to the percentage of each amino acid at that position in the myeloma pool whereas the column labeled P refers to the percentage of each amino acid at that position in the pool of normal κ chains. The κ myeloma pool is generated from the 44 sequences published in reference 15. The normal pool was isolated from serum taken from 50 normal BALB/c mice. The one letter amino acid code is given in the legend to Figure 4.

Second, the ratios of certain residue alternatives are strikingly different in the myeloma as compared to the normal pool (e.g., leucine at position 10). Similar data on mouse H chains (5, 7), human H chains (4, 5), and human κ chains (4,8,9) also suggest that qualitative and quantitative differences exist between the myeloma and normal pools. These differences suggest that certain variable region sequences are present in the myeloma proteins which are not seen in the normal pool and vice versa. Thus, it appears that both the myeloma and the normal pools are selected. The extent of this selection is, of course, unknown. However, generalizations about antibody diversity or evolution which are derived from either type of data must be interpreted with the reservation that both the myeloma and normal pools are windows of unknown size from which immunoglobulin genes are viewed.

II. MOST ANTIBODY FAMILIES HAVE MULTIPLE VARIABLE GENES IN THE GERM LINE.

A quest for the genetic mechanism for antibody diversity has been one of the driving forces of molecular immunology. Two alternative hypotheses for antibody diversity have been proposed--the germ line theory suggests that diversity arises in antibody genes during the evolution of the species, whereas the somatic theories propose that antibody diversity is created anew during the development of each individual (1,3,4,10). The principal insights into this controversy have come through the patterns observed from the detailed amino acid sequence analysis of homogeneous myeloma immunoglobulins. The first relevant pattern observed was that of V region subgroups, that is, the V_K regions of human immunoglobulins could be divided into three sets (subgroups) which were defined by linked amino acid residues and sequence gaps (11,12). Since individual V regions from differing subgroups differed from one another by 40-50% of their sequence, the important genetic inference was drawn that each subgroup must be encoded by a distinct V gene. The concept of V region subgroups has, however, outlived its usefulness and indeed has become impossible to apply to contemporary sequence data for two reasons. First, it has been possible to define sub-subgroups by sets of smaller numbers of linked residues which are apparent within the original subgroups (12). Thus arises the unanswerable question of how many linked residues are sufficient to define an additional sub-subgroup (i.e., additional germ line V gene). Second, with the accumulation of many V region sequences in a variety of

123

different antibody families, it appears that the spectrum of
diversity is more continuous than previously thought (e.g.,
note the mouse κ diversity described below). Once again it
becomes impossible to agree on a definition for subgroups.
The definition of a subgroup (i.e., germ line V-gene) for one
who believes in somatic mutation is quite different from that
of his counterpart who believes in a germ line basis for
antibody diversity--indeed, even the subgroup definitions for
those who believe in distinct somatic theories are quite different (compare 10,13,14).

Genealogic analysis appears to be the most fruitful procedure for analyzing the diversity of V regions (Figure 3).
Operationally the V region sequences in a hypothetical
example (level F - Figure 3) are related to one another by
a genealogic tree which determines a primordial gene (level
A - Figure 3) from which all V sequences can be derived with
a minimum of genetic events (single base substitutions, gene
duplication and codon insertions or deletions). The primordial L gene (level A - Figure 3) undergoes gene duplication and each daughter gene fixes five single base substitutions (indicated by the 5 on the branch joining levels A
and B) in evolving from level A to B. In addition, the
primordial V_K gene deletes codons 94-95 and 9 (indicated by
brackets with a subscript). Subsequent gene duplications,
nucleotide substitutions and codon deletions finally generate
the many distinct genes at level F. These genetic events can
occur in the germ line or during somatic mutation.

The fundamental question with regard to these theories
is what level on the genealogic tree is represented by germ
line genes. For example, all immunologists agree that the V_K
and V_λ regions are coded by separate germ line genes (Figure
3). The critical question is how many V genes of each family
are present in the germ line. In this regard, those who
believe in ordinary somatic mutation (i.e., no special mutational mechanism) have generally agreed that 1) the average
lymphocyte line undergoes a very limited number of somatic
mutations in its V genes (i.e., 1-4 single base substitutions) and 2) two or more identical V regions derived from
independent myeloma tumors are coded directly by germ line V
genes (10). Both of these concessions to the multigenic
nature of the antibody families tend to move the level of
germ line genes on the genealogic tree out to the more terminal twigs (e.g., level E or higher in Figure 3). Let us now
consider the actual V region sequence data from the antibody
families of the BALB/c mouse.

The BALB/c mouse strain is highly inbred and, accordingly, genetic polymorphisms which might obscure sequence

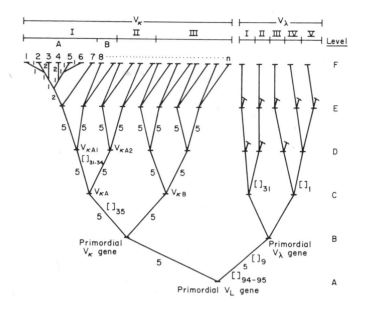

FIGURE 3. A hypothetical genealogic tree for human V_L regions. The tree is constructed from a set of proteins, such as human V_L regions, by generating a series of ancestral or nodal sequences (levels E, D, C, and so on) using the minimum possible number of "genetic events" (base substitutions, sequence insertions or deletions, and gene duplications). The genetic events responsible for generating this genealogic pattern could occur, in part, during somatic differentiation (somatic theory) or entirely during the evolution of the species (germ line theory). The V_K branch is divided into three subbranches (subgroups) designated I, II and III. The fact that each of these subbranches can be further subdivided is indicated by IA and IB. The fine details of one region of the genealogic tree are represented by V_K regions 1-8. (From reference 1).

patterns pertinent to the genetic mechanisms of antibody
diversity should be minimized, if not eliminated.

The kappa family. The N-terminal sequence of 62 BALB/c
kappa chains has been examined over their N-terminal 23 residues (15,16,17). Forty-three of the 62 proteins have distinct sequences in this region and indeed a majority of the
proteins clearly differ from one another by multiple nucleotide substitutions (Figure 4). A genealogic analysis of many
of these sequences demonstrates almost a complete spectrum of
diversity among these V regions (0-16/23 residues different)
making it somewhat difficult to define distinct V region
genealogic branches (18). At least 25 genealogic branches
are present which differ from most other branches by six or
more residues. Since the N-terminal 23 residues constitute
approximately 1/5 of the entire V region, the V_K regions in
distinct branches will probably differ by 30 or more residues
from one another. It is important to stress that the unselected BALB/c V_K sequences examined to date have demonstrated no saturation of diversity; that is, the first 20 V_K
sequences examined yielded approximately as many new genealogic branches as did the second 20 examined. Presumably,
the same would be true of a third set of unselected V_K sequences (the selected V_K sequences are those derived from
immunoglobulin molecules with binding activity for certain
haptens--see Figure 4). Because the V region diversity has
not saturated, we have reservations about certain statistical
approaches to the estimation of V_K gene diversity (10,20,21,
22,19).

It is important to consider the nature of sequence differences which exist among V_K regions which are very similar.
We analyzed the complete V region sequence of four κ chains
nearly identical at their N-terminus (M70, M321, M63, and
T124--Figure 4) (23,24). M70 differed from the other three
V_K regions by 20 to 21 residues; M63 differed from M321 and
T124 by about 8 residues and M321 and T124 differed from one
another by just three residues. The genealogic tree for
these V_K regions suggests that at least three germ line V_K
genes must encode these proteins (Figure 5). M70 must be
encoded by a separate V_K gene as it is distinct from the
others. It is unlikely M63 and the T124-M321 pair could be
generated from a single V_K gene (level B--Figure 5) as 3
identical (parallel) mutations would be required in the
mutation of two independent lymphocytic lines leading from
B to the synthesis of T124 and M321. No selective forces
are known which might employ random somatic mutation and
select from the many variants generated two V genes with

multiple identical substitutions--accordingly, separate V_K genes must be postulated for the M63 and the M321-T124 pair (note that this is the same reasoning used to argue that two or more identical V regions must be coded by germ line V genes). The unanswerable but provocative question is whether the M321-T124 pair are coded by the same or distinct germ line genes (see the λ data discussed below). Thus, four V_K regions, nearly identical at their N-terminus, apparently are coded by at least three germ line V_K genes.

One additional line of evidence also suggests that the V_K regions of the BALB/c mouse are coded by many germ line genes. In an examination of about 50 consecutive Bence Jones proteins (homogeneous urinary light chains derived from individuals with myeloma), one pair was observed which appeared to be identical by immunologic, peptide map, and electrophoretic criteria (25). The sequence analysis of both of these proteins is nearly complete and it appears that they will indeed be identical. A statistical calculation can be carried out to determine how large the pool size of different V_K regions must be such that a sample of 50 yields one identical pair. At the 90% confidence level the pool size ranges between 700 and 10,000 germ line V_K genes.

Thus, the extensive screen of amino terminal sequences, the examination of four similar V_K regions and even the examination of two apparently identical κ chains suggest that the κ family in the BALB/c mouse is coded by a large number of distinct germ line V_K genes. The mouse H family also appears to be coded by multiple V_H genes.

The heavy chain family. The N-terminal sequence of 28 BALB/c heavy chains has been examined over their N-terminal 20 residues (7). Seventeen of the 28 sequences differ by one residue or more. Genealogic analysis shows that these sequences fall into four major branches (Figure 6). The V regions within a branch differ from those on other branches by 40-50% of their sequence. The major branch, containing 18 V_H regions, is broken down into at least three smaller subbranches.

The variable region of the heavy chain is about 120 residues in length and hence the N-terminal 20 residues represent about 1/6 of the V_H region. Accordingly, a rough estimate of the number of amino acid differences between two V_H regions can be determined by multiplying the difference in diversity shown over the N-terminal 20 residues by six (this is an underestimate because no hypervariable regions are present at the N-terminus). Thus, the V_H regions in different branches will probably differ by 48 residues

	1 2 3 4 5 6 7 8 9 0 1 2 3 4 5 6 7 8 9 0 1 2 3	Specificity
Most common residue	D I V M T Q S P A S L S V S L G E R V T I S C	
613, BFPC32, M70, M321, T124	—— L ———————— A ————— A ———	
McPC603	————————— S ——— A ————— M —	P.C.
RPC23, M	— Q ——————————— V ———— T —	
MOPC31C	— Q ————————— A — V ———— T —	
TEPC173	— Q ——————————— V — T —— T —	
MOPC63	N — L ——————— A ———— A ———	
BFPC61	—— L ——————— A ——— Z K A ———	
MOPC384	————————— S ——— A — K — M ——	Galactose
McPC870	————————— S ——— A — K — M ——	Mannose
178, 313	— Q ——————— A — V — T ——— T —	
611	— Q ——— S — X ——— V — G ——— T —	
MOPC41	— Q ——— S ——— A ———— S L T —	
LPC1	——— A — M Q A — I — K ———	
MOPC21	N ——— K — L — M — V ——— L — T —	
149	— Q ——— D Y — A — V — T ——— T —	
47A, 47B	— Q ——— S — E E ——— V — G ——— T —	
MOPC35	——— T — B F — L — A — ? ——— T —	
MOPC149	— Q ——— B Y — A — V ——— T —	
MOPC460	— V ——— T — L — T ——— D — A S ———	DNP
MOPC46, 172	—— L ——— T ——— T P — D S — S L ——	
S23	—— L ——— T ——— T P — D S — S L ——	DNP
T15, H8, S107	——— T F — A — T A S K K ———	P.C.
MOPC173	— Q ——— T T S —— A ——— D ? ——— T —	
S10, X24, X44, T191, J539, JI	E — L ——— I T A A ————— T —	1,6 G
M265, M773	E T T V ————— M A I — K ——— [ ] —	
HOPC5	——— T K F M — T — V — K —— S — T —	
MOPC467, MPC37	— V L ——— T — L —— P ——— D E A S ———	
3129, 3434	— V — V — T G L —— P — M — D —— S ———	1,6 D
McPC843	— V——— T — L T ——— T I — P A S ———	
MOPC29	E N — L ——— I M — A — D ——— M T —	
TEPC29	E V — L ——— I M — A ——— L — S M ——	
3082, J606	— V Q — I ——— S ——— A ——— D I — M T —	Levan
MOPC316	—— L — ? — T ? — T T — B ?— ? ? —	
641	—— N ——— X X F M — T — V — D —— S — T —	
TEPC157	——————— Q S F M — T — V — D —— S V T —	
McPC674	— V ——— T — L T——— T I — P A S L ——	
TEPC153	E N — L ——— I M — A — P —— B — M T —	
MPC47	E V ——— T — L — A ——— ? Z A S M ——	
S194	? B — L ——— I M A A ——— K — M T —	DNP
McPC600	— Q — I ——— S — M F A — I — D Z — S ——	
MOPC167, MOPC511	—— I — B E L — B P — T S — E S — S — T —	Choline
MOPC379	——————— S F M V T — V — Z ? — ? ? ? —	

Figure 4. See legend on page 129

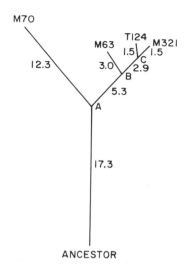

FIGURE 5. A genealogic tree of four mouse V_K regions with limited sequence differences (see text). Taken from reference 1.

FIGURE 4. Amino terminal sequences of myeloma κ chains from inbred BALB/c mice. The one letter amino acid code is used: A = Ala, R = Arg, D = Asp, N = Asn, C = Cys, Z = Glx, E = Glu, Q = Gln, G = Gly, H = His, I = Ile, L = Leu, K = Lys, M = Met, F = Phe, P = Pro, S = Ser, T = Thr, W = Trp, Y = Tyr, V = Val, ? = undetermined, [] = deletion. Abbreviations: DNP, dinitrophenyl; P.C., phosphorylcholine; 1,6 G, β- (1→6)-D-galactan; 1,6 D, α-(1→6)-dextran. Data is from references 15, 16, 17, and 10. Where there are conflicts in the published sequences we have generally listed data from reference 15.

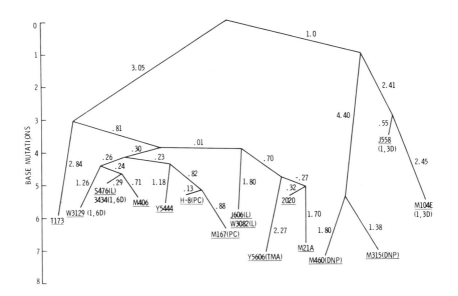

FIGURE 6. A genealogic tree of heavy chains from BALB/c myeloma proteins. This tree was constructed using only the N-terminal 20 residues. Many of the immunoglobulins from which these V_H regions were derived bind to one or more haptens. These specificites are shown below the tumor number. Abbreviations: DNP, dinitrophenyl; PC, phosphorylcholine; 1,6D, $\alpha 1{\to}6$ dextran; 1,3D, $1{\to}3$ dextran; L, Levan; TMA, trimethylamine (7). Not shown on this figure but constituting a separate major branch is the V_H sequence from tumor protein S176.

or more, whereas proteins within a major branch can, from
this estimate, differ by as many as 24 or more residues. A
comparison of the only two nearly complete mouse V_H sequences
from different branches (M315 and M173) is consistent with
the above extrapolations in that they differ by 10 residues
in the first 20 and by 62/104 residues and two sequence gaps.

Accordingly, the V_H regions in the BALB/c mouse also
display considerable variable region diversity, although
apparently somewhat less than their V_K counterparts. Whether
or not the V_H diversity is significantly less than the V_K
diversity is uncertain, however, because most of these V_H
sequences were derived from immunoglobulins selected because
they exhibited binding activity for various haptens. Thus,
these heavy chains constitute a highly selected subset of
the BALB/c heavy chain myeloma pool. It will be of considerable importance to determine whether unselected V_H regions exhibit considerably more diversity. In any case, the
overall conclusion is that the BALB/c heavy chain family
also exhibits substantial sequence diversity and presumably
is coded by multiple germ line V_H genes. The variability of
the H and κ families stands in striking contrast to the
highly restricted sequence diversity of the mouse λ family.

The lambda family. Eighteen mouse V_λ regions have been
examined. Twelve of the 18 appear to be identical and the
remainder differ from the major sequence by 1-4 base substitutions (10). Whether the minor variations in the V_λ sequences are due to somatic mutation or, in fact, are coded
by germ line genes, it appears that the sequence diversity
and presumably the number of germ line V_λ genes is highly restricted in the BALB/c λ as compared to the κ family. It
will, of course, be extremely important to assess the degree
of V_λ diversity present in the normal λ pool in order to
determine whether the myeloma process selects a small subset
of the actual V_λ gene library. This experiment is techni-
cally difficult because λ chains are expressed at the level
of a few percent in normal mouse serum.

From the assessment of the amino acid sequence diversity present in the BALB/c immunoglobulin families a number
of interesting conclusions can be tentatively drawn regarding theories of antibody formation.

1. The BALB/c kappa family is coded by multiple germ
line V genes. Most somatic theories now concede that there
are probably 100 or more V_K genes in the germ line of the
BALB/c mouse, although the definitions as to what constitutes evidence for a germ line gene differs widely (10,13).
It appears likely that this number will increase

significantly in the future as it has in the past with the
accumulation of additional sequence data (see successively
19,20,21,22,10). Indeed, the germ line and somatic estimates
of the lower limits on the V_K gene number are remarkably
similar to one another in some cases (see 1 and 10). In the
genealogic analysis (Figure 3) the level of germ line genes
has clearly been moved out to the most terminal twigs of the
branches. Thus, the somatic theory contends that there are
many V_K genes each of which can mutate a small amount to
generate new specificities whereas the germ line theory suggests that most of the distinct V sequences are coded by
corresponding germ line V genes. As more and more germ line
V genes are conceded by those who favor a somatic view point,
it will be increasingly difficult to distinguish these
possibilities experimentally. However, as the number of
germ line V genes increases, the requirement for functional
somatic mutation becomes increasingly unnecessary and ad hoc.
For example, 10^6 different antibody molecules can be coded
for by 1000 V_L and 1000 V_H genes if all L-H combinations are
functional (1000 x 1000 = 10^6). In addition, a single antibody molecule may interact specifically with a variety of
related and even unrelated antigens (see 26) to further reduce the total number of different antibody genes required.
Accordingly, it appears reasonable to suggest that the
somatic mutation which may occur in any multigene system can
occasionally improve the specificity of a particular antibody molecule, but that generally most specific antibody
molecules are coded directly by germ line genes.

   2. The mouse V_λ myeloma regions appear to be coded
by one or a few genes. This example is interesting because
it clearly delineates the mutational process occurring at
the terminal twigs of the genealogic tree. As noted above,
it will be difficult to distinguish between a germ line and
a somatic mutational mechanism at this level of diversity.
These data also raise several additional interesting questions. Do the V_λ myeloma proteins reflect the actual V_λ
gene diversity present in the BALB/c genome? Is the correlation between low serum levels of λ chain (>5%) and limited
sequence diversity significant; that is, will species with
a low level of a particular light chain type also demonstrate highly restricted V region diversity? Parenthetically,
it might be noted that the human λ family (expressed in
the serum at the 20-30% level) appears to be extremly diverse (even more so than the kappa family which constitutes
70-80% of the serum light chain).

3. <u>The mouse V_H family is also multigenic</u>. Most of the BALB/c myeloma heavy chains appear to have an unblocked α amino group whereas 78% of the serum heavy chains are blocked (5). This clear example of selection by the myeloma process raises serious questions about the extent of selection that occurs among all antibody families with regard to V genes (see proposition I) and how large the myeloma window of diversity actually is. If, for example, if only 5% of the V gene products were selected by the myeloma process, then our estimates of V gene diversity from myeloma data would have to be multiplied by an appropriate factor. The difficulty is that this factor will almost be impossible to determine.

4. <u>When somatic theories concede that antibody families are multigenic, they must explain species associated residues, rabbit V_H allotypes and other types of V region genetic markers</u> (1). These are the very arguments which have for years "rendered the germ line theory unlikely." All theories, somatic and germ line alike, are multigenic in nature and accordingly now appear to be in the same boat with regard to these issues. We suspect the solutions to these problems will be very similar for both types of theories (see 1).

5. <u>The amino acid sequence analysis of antibody V regions currently appears to be the most reliable method for counting antibody V genes</u>. In our opinion the other major approaches to antibody V gene counting - serology (27), isoelectric focusing (see 28), and RNA-DNA hybridization (see 29,30,31) - still provide indirect and often ambiguous results (e.g., compare 29 and 31). Let us now consider one special sequence pattern, the hypervariable region, which has, in our view, been over-zealously interpreted to favor somatic mutation.

III. HYPERVARIABLE REGION PATTERNS ARE PREDICTED BY
A GERM LINE THEORY

One intriguing sequence pattern has been the observation that light and heavy chains have three or four regions of extreme variability (constituting 25-35% of the V region) (32,33). These areas are designated hypervariable regions. Two theories have focused on the hypervariable regions as areas with a special role in generating antibody diversity. One theory proposes that strong selective forces expand out certain mutations in hypervariable regions because these areas are directly involved in antigen complementarity and mutations within these regions can improve the binding to

133

antigen (10). A second model suggests that hypervariable "episomes" are inserted into framework genes to generate antibody diversity (27). Both of these models appear somewhat ad hoc to us in that the following arguments will demonstrate that hypervariable regions are a reasonable expectation of a germ line model.

1. Why in a set of homologous proteins should there be regions with extensive sequence diversity and regions of limited sequence diversity? Let us consider all of the cytochrome c molecules which have been completely sequenced (34). Hypervariable clusters (i.e., residue positions at which 6 or more substitutions are seen in comparing 38 proteins) tend to appear on the outside of this molecule and at corners of helical bends (34, R. Dickerson, personal communication). Presumably these hypervariable clusters represent neutral mutations which do not fundamentally alter the structure of the cytochrome c molecule. In contrast, the area of the molecule which interfaces with the heme group and those regions believed to interact with the reductase and oxidase in the electron transport chain are highly conserved because of their precise complementarity requirements. Thus, to a first approximation the hypervariable regions appear to be regions where many substitutions are neutral and the conserved regions seem to be required for the precise shaping of certain regions of the cytochrome c molecule.

2. Might the same reasoning apply to the variability of antibody V regions? The three dimensional structure of a Bence-Jones dimer (urinary light chains) as well as Fab crystals suggests that there is a characteristic and highly conserved "antibody fold" which is found in V as well as C domains (35,36). Poljak estimates that more than 50% of the residues in a given V region must be highly conserved with regard to side chain properties in order to preserve the antibody fold. Thus, it is reasonable to expect that a large portion of the V region should be highly conserved. In contrast to the cytochrome c picture, however, antibody molecules have to code for many different antigenic sites and, accordingly, those regions of the chain forming the active site crevice should be extremely diverse. Indeed, the x-ray pictures of two Fab fragments with specific haptens in place suggest that three of the four heavy chain hypervariable regions fold to form a portion of the active site crevice as do two of the three light chain hypervariable regions (35, 37). What then is the role of the two hypervariable regions

outside the active site? One possibility is that they are
regions in which neutral mutations can occur (both are on
the outside of the molecule). Thus, some of the hypervariable regions may reflect the variability of the active site
whereas others may constitute a region where neutral mutations can be accepted. This latter viewpoint is supported
by the observation that the New protein has deleted the
nonactive site hypervariable region of its light chain and
still binds perfectly well to a particular hapten (35).
Accordingly, one cannot a priori argue that all hypervariable
regions are "complementarity determining residues" (see 10).
Obviously, if selective forces do not act on certain hypervariable regions, their extreme sequence variability suggest
that this diversity is coded in the germ line by many
different V genes. Thus, the hypervariable segments of antibody V regions may reflect regions contributing to active
site diversity, regions which can accept many neutral
mutations, or regions with other as of yet unnamed functional
requirements. It seems unnecessary at this point to postulate that hypervariable regions are coded by episomal genes
or other equally vague genetic mechanisms.

IV.   NEW AND UNEXPECTED AMINO ACID SEQUENCE PATTERNS
      SUGGEST THAT MANY MYSTERIES OF ANTIBODY GENETICS,
      EVOLUTION AND CONTROL REMAIN YET TO BE UNRAVELED.

Only cautious generalizations should be drawn about the
nature of antibody diversity from the few antibody families
which have been studied in detail to date. A number of
relatively recent and intriguing observations suggest there
is much to be learned.

1. The diversity of normal (heterogeneous) immunoglobulin κ chains from man and mouse is well documented (6,
8,9 - see Figure 2). At each of the N-terminal 10 residue
positions, two and often three or four residue alternatives
appear. Indeed, the N-terminal region of human and mouse
V_K regions is one of the more variable areas of the κ polypeptide chain. This diversity presumably reflects, at
least in part, the expression of many different V_K germ line
genes. In striking contrast, a careful quantitative analysis of the N-terminal 17 residues of pigeon light chain
demonstrates that twelve of the first 17 residues positions
express just a single residue. Indeed, the remaining five
positions have only a single minor residue alternative. Isoelectric focusing reveals a highly restricted electrophoretic pattern. Birds have a single major light chain class

135

(>95%) which is homologous to mammalian λ chains (39,40). The N-terminus of human λ chains, as noted earlier, is extremely heterogeneous (3) - thus the vertebrate λ gene family has the capacity to diversify. These observations raise a number of intriguing questions. Are avian V_λ regions highly restricted in sequence heterogeneity (or is the normal pool a highly selected subset of the true pigeon V_L diversity)? How is the diversity distributed in avian V_λ regions (is the diversity primarily in hypervariable regions or is the N-terminus of these chains highly conserved for functional reasons)? Is there additional diversity in the pigeon heavy chains to compensate for the apparent lack of diversity in the light chains? These questions are now under active investigation in our laboratory.

2. In the mouse the extreme V_κ diversity and V_λ sequence restriction correlates with the normal serum expression of these light chains in that the more diverse κ chain is expressed 20 times more frequently than the λ chain. As noted earlier, this association suggested to some that the serum ratios of these chains may crudely reflect the number of germ line V genes encoding each antibody family (see 1, 19). Gibson has recently isolated κ chains which are expressed at approximately the 5% level from normal pooled horse serum (41). Quantitative amino acid sequence analyses demonstrate that horse κ chains are quite heterogeneous. Again interesting questions are raised. Will _normal_ mouse λ chains be as heterogeneous as normal horse κ chains (i.e., is the myeloma λ pool highly selected in the mouse)? Do, indeed, quite distinct degrees of heterogeneity exist in various light chain families? Perhaps V_λ and V_κ genes in the mouse genome are equally diverse. Can the λ and κ families code for similar antibody specificities? Why does the serum expression of these light chain families vary so markedly in different mammals (see 11)? It will be important to document in considerable detail the extent and nature of heterogeneity which exists in antibody families from differing creatures at various stages of vertebrate evolution.

3. Attempts to correlate the rabbit V_H allotypes (the group a markers--al,a2,a3) with precise amino acid residues have been singularly unsuccessful. Early studies on pooled rabbit heavy chains suggested that multiple amino acid residues throughout the entire V_H region were characteristic of the al or the a3 molecules (42,43). Subsequent studies on homogeneous heavy chains from rabbit antibodies have suggested that most of these residues do not correlate

absolutely with allotype (44). If the V_H family is multi-genic, as appears to be true of mouse heavy chains, then the simple genetic explanation of one V_H gene for each group a allotype is untenable. Indeed, the apparent differences among V_H regions of differing allotypes appear remarkably similar to those seen among the three human V_K subgroups, each of which now appears to be coded by multiple V_K genes (see 1,12). Perhaps all rabbits have three groups of V_H genes which we designate as a1, a2, and a3, and a closely linked control mechanism determines which group is expressed in a particular rabbit. The actual chemical basis for the group a rabbit allotypes still remains as elusive as ever.

Yet another intriguing set of sequence patterns have come from the analysis of biclonal myeloma proteins (see 45, 46,1). These proteins promise to offer some very exciting insights into the control mechanisms which regulate antibody synthesis.

Hence it is our feeling that very important aspects of antibody diversity, evolution and control have yet to be elucidated by detailed amino acid sequence studies on the immunoglobulins from animals at various stages of vertebrate evolution.

V. ONE OF THE FRONTIERS IN MODERN GENETICS IS THE
STUDY OF MULTIGENE SYSTEMS.

The antibody V genes in most immunoglobulin families constitute a multigene family with at least two unusual evolutionary properties presumably requiring unusual evolutionary mechanisms (see 1). Other multigene families are known which share one or both of these evolutionary features (e.g., histones, 18S, 28S, 5S ribosomal genes). Most other multigene families, however, differ from the antibody families in that the individual gene members are identical or nearly identical. Accordingly, two issues can be raised. First, do all multigene families, irrespective of whether their members are (nearly) identical (histones) or just similar (antibodies) share common evolutionary mechanisms? Second, will other nonidentical (informational) multigene systems be described with properties similar to the antibody multigene families? The antibody system is an ideal model system for studying the genetics and evolution of multigene systems. First, it is the only known multigene system in which individual gene products can be obtained and characterized. Second, antibody molecules can be obtained in relatively large quantities. Third, antibodies can be obtained from animals throughout the vertebrate spectrum.

Fourth, an enormous variety of information already exists on the cell biology, genetics and biochemistry of the immune system. It is our feeling that in future years many new informational multigene systems will be described and of all the potential multigene candidates, the antibody system appears to afford the greatest opportunities for unraveling the mysteries of the evolution, genetics and control in multigene systems.

ACKNOWLEDGMENTS

Our work has been supported by grants from the National Institutes of Health and the National Science Foundation. L.H. has a Research Career Development Award from NIH. We thank our colleagues, C. Sledge, J. Silver, and V. Farnsworth, for stimulating discussions.

REFERENCES

1. L. Hood, Stadler Symposium of Genetics 5, 73 (1973).
2. F. M. Burnet, The Clonal Selection Theory of Acquired Immunity, Cambridge Univ. Press, London and New York, 1959.
3. G. Smith, L. Hood, and W. Fitch, Ann. Rev. Biochem. 40, 969 (1971).
4. J. Gally, The Antigens I, Academic Press, New York and London, 1973.
5. J. D. Capra, R. Wasserman, and J. M. Kehoe, J. Exp. Med. 138, 410 (1973).
6. E. Loh, R. Gendolfi, and L. Hood, in preparation.
7. P. Barstad, M. Weigert, M. Cohn, and L. Hood, in preparation.
8. J. A. Grant, and L. Hood, Immunochemistry 8, 63 (1971).
9. D. Gibson, V. Farnsworth, and L. Hood, in preparation.
10. M. Cohn, this volume.
11. L. Hood, W. Gray, B. Sanders, and W. Dreyer, Cold Spring Harbor Symposium 33, 353 (1967).
12. L. Hood, and D. Talmage, Science 168, 325 (1970).
13. J. Gally, and G. Edelman, Nature 227, 341 (1970).
14. C. Milstein, and J. Pink, Prog. Biophys. Mol. Biol. 21, 209 (1970).
15. L. Hood, D. McKean, V. Farnsworth, and M. Potter, Biochemistry 12, 741 (1973).
16. E. Appella, and J. Inman, Contemporary Topics in Molecular Immunology 2, 51 (1974).
17. P. Barstad, M. Weigert, and L. Hood, unpublished observations.

18. V. Farnsworth, and L. Hood, unpublished observations.
19. M. Weigert, I. Cesari, S. Yonkovich, and M. Cohn, Nature 228, 1045 (1970).
20. M. Cohn, Ann. N. Y. Acad. Sci. 190, 529 (1971).
21. M. Cohn, Cellular Immunol. 1, 461 (1971).
22. M. Cohn, The Biochemistry of Gene Expression in Higher Organisms, J. Pollak and J. Lee (Eds.), D. Reidel Pub. Co., Dordrecht, Holland, 1973, p. 572.
23. D. McKean, M. Potter, and L. Hood, Biochemistry 12, 749 (1973).
24. D. McKean, M. Potter, and L. Hood, Biochemistry 12, 760 (1973).
25. P. Barstad, M. Hood, P. Periman, and L. Hood, in preparation.
26. J. Inman, this volume.
27. T. Kindt, this volume.
28. H. Kretch, and A. Williamson, Eur. J. Immunology 3, 141 (1973).
29. E. Premkumar, M. Shoyab, and A. Williamson, Proc. Nat. Acad. Sci. U.S.A. 71, 99 (1974).
30. P. Leder, this volume.
31. S. Tonegawa, this volume.
32. T. Wu, and E. Kabat, J. Exp. Med. 132, 211 (1970).
33. J. M. Kehoe, and J. D. Capra, Proc. Nat. Acad. Sci. U.S.A. 68, 2019 (1971); Capra, personal communication.
34. R. E. Dickerson, Scientific American 226, 58 (1972).
35. R. Poljak, L. Anzel, H. Avey, B. Chen, R. Phizackerley, and F. Saul, Proc. Nat. Acad. Sci. U.S.A. 70, 3305 (1973).
36. M. Schiffer, R. Girleng, K. Ely, and A. Edmundson, Biochemistry 12, 4620 (1973).
37. E. Padan, this volume.
38. J. Gally, and G. Edelman, Ann. Rev. Genet. 6, 1 (1972).
39. J. A. Grant, B. G. Sanders, and L. Hood, Biochemistry 10, 3123 (1971).
40. C. Nottenburg, and L. Hood, unpublished observations.
41. D. Gibson, Biochemistry, in press.
42. J. Wilkinson, Biochem. J. 117, 3P (1970).
43. L. Mole, S. Jackson, R. Porter, and J. Wilkinson, Biochem. J. 124, 301 (1971).
44. J. Jaton, D. Braun, A. Strosberg, E. Haber, and J. Morris, J. Immunol. 111, 1838 (1973).
45. A. Wang, S. Wilson, J. Hopper, H. Fudenberg, and A. Nisonoff, Proc. Nat. Acad. Sci. U.S.A. 66, 337 (1970).
46. C. Sledge, and L. Hood, unpublished observations.

MOLECULAR AND FUNCTIONAL PROPERTIES
OF LYMPHOCYTE SURFACE IMMUNOGLOBULIN

John J. Marchalonis

Molecular Immunology Laboratory
The Walter and Eliza Hall Institute of Medical Research
Parkville, Victoria, 3052, Australia.

ABSTRACT. To provide direct information on the molecular and functional properties of membrane immunoglobulins of murine and human thymus-derived lymphocytes (T-cells) and bone marrow-derived lymphocytes (B-cells), surface proteins of lymphocyte populations were labelled with ^{125}I-iodide using the enzyme lactoperoxidase to catalyze the reaction. Immunoglobulin solubilized by metabolic release, organic solvents or nonionic detergents was specifically precipitated with antiglobulin antisera and analyzed by poly-acrylamide gel electrophoresis in buffers containing sodium dodecylsulfate. The predominant surface immunoglobulin of B lymphocytes was comprized of light chains and μ heavy chains joined by disulfide bonds. The intact unit had a mass of approx. 200,000 daltons. Surface immunoglobulin of thymus lymphocytes, peripheral T cells and $\Theta+$ thymoma lines also consisted of a molecule of M.W. approx. 200,000 and was comprized of light chains and heavy chains resembling μ chains in physical and antigenic properties.

Studies with murine T cells specifically activated to syngeneic tumor associated transplantation antigens and to foreign erythrocytes (helper cells) showed that an appreciable portion of the 7S IgM-like surface immunoglobulin possessed binding specificity for the activating antigen. These results were consistent with an antigen receptor role for T cell surface immunoglobulin. Moreover, certain $\Theta+$ cell lines synthesize immunoglobulin which appears to possess certain properties expected of collaborative T cell immunoglobulin. These results support a considerable body of indirect evidence which indicates that immuno-globulin consisting of light chains and μ heavy chains funct-ions as the receptor for antigen on B cells and on T cells which bind proteins, erythrocytes or haptens, function as specific helper cells in cell-cell collaboration or mediate delayed type hypersensitivity.

INTRODUCTION

Combination of antigen with specific lymphocyte surface receptors is crucial to the initiation of immune differentiation. The molecule nature of these receptors and their role in the activation of lymphocytes have been challenging problems to immunologists for over seventy years. Ehrlich, in 1900 (1), argued that since circulating antibodies showed exquisite specificity for antigen it was not necessary to invoke a separate recognition system for the antibody-forming cells. The problem of the receptor in antigen-recognition by lymphocytes became more complicated recently with the discovery of two distinct categories of lymphocytes, thymus-derived cells (T cells) and bone-marrow-derived lymphocytes (B cells), both of which exhibit specific surface receptors for antigen (2, 3). The same "Occam's razor" type of analysis first applied by Ehrlich would also apply to the question whether T and B lymphocytes express distinct specific receptors for antigen. A wealth of recent data obtained by inhibition of antigen-binding (4-12) and specific helper cell activity (13, 14) establish that T cells, as well as B cells, possess surface immunoglobulin which contains light chain and μ chain antigenic determinants (see 15, 16 for reviews). These studies do not, however, provide information on the state of association of these chains on the cell surface, or, indeed whether the detected antigenic determinants comprize intact polypeptide chains. Moreover, they do not unequivocally resolve the receptor issue because inhibition might result from steric obstruction if immunoglobulin occurs in close proximity to another molecule which is the true receptor for antigen.

In this paper I shall describe studies involving isolation of surface immunoglobulin of B cells, T cells and Θ+ thymoma lines which were designed to provide direct information on the molecular properties of this immunoglobulin and on its putative receptor function. Furthermore, I will provide data consistent with the hypothesis

(17, 18) that T cell receptor immunoglobulin serves as a specific collaborative factor in cooperative interactions between T cells, B cells and macrophages.

A BIOCHEMICAL APPROACH TO THE
LYMPHOCYTE RECEPTOR PROBLEM

To obtain direct information on the structure of lymphocyte surface immunoglobulin and on the receptor function of this molecule, it was necessary to have a means of isolating the molecule from the cell surface. Because membrane protein constitutes approximately 1.1×10^{-12} gm/cell (19) and a given receptor, e. g. immunoglobulin, might comprize only 1% of this figure, an extremely sensitive technique was required to facilitate physico-chemical analyses of membrane proteins. Use of radioisotopes of iodine, chiefly ^{125}I-iodide, had previously enabled study of antibodies produced by single cells (20), a problem which entailed sensitivity of comparable magnitude. In the present case, we adopted the lactoperoxidase-catalyzed radioiodination technique, first developed in this laboratory for the labelling of immunoglobulins (21), for use as a probe to label accessible surface proteins of normal and neoplastic lymphocytes (22). It was possible to attach ^{125}I-iodide covalently to tyrosines on surface proteins of living lymphocytes. The restriction of label to surface proteins was shown by two techniques; (a) electron microscopic autoradiography (22), and (b) direct isolation of membranes and comparison of specific activities of intact cells with those of isolated plasma membrane preparations (Crumpton, M. J. and Marchalonis, J. J., unpublished observations). The specific activity (counts ^{125}I per mg protein) was 30 to 55-fold higher for purified lymphoma plasma membranes than it was for the intact cells. This result agrees well with the fraction of lymphocyte mass which the plasma membrane comprizes (19). More than twenty-five membrane proteins are labelled in the lactoperoxidase-catalyzed radioiodination of intact, living lymphocytes. Studies from a number of laboratories have established the utility of lactoperoxidase-catalyzed radioiodination as a method for the surface labelling of erythrocytes (23), lymphocytes (22, 24, 25),

fat cells (26) and HeLa cells (27). I would emphasize, however, that different cell types require modified conditions
to obtain optimum uptake of ^{125}I-iodide, and rigorous
attention to detail is necessary to facilitate comparisons
among various cell types.

The labelling of surface proteins with radioiodine
is the first step in the proposed chain of biochemical
analyses of lymphocyte surface immunoglobulin. It is subsequently necessary to solubilize the radioiodinated protein
in such a manner that it retains its antigenic and functional
properties. We use a number of procedures to solubilize
labelled cells, including (a) metabolic release (28), (b) use
of organic solvents, e. g. acid-urea (29), (c) use of non-
ionic detergents, e. g. NP40 (24), and (d) various combinations of (b) and (c). The method of metabolic release is
especially useful because surface molecules released by
living cells maintained under short term tissue culture conditions generally show the least denaturation and degradation. As I shall illustrate in Table 3 below, all extraction
methods are not universally applicable to all lymphocyte
types. Immunoglobulin, and other components such as the
Θ (Thy, 1) alloantigen (30, 31) were identified and isolated
by specific immunological precipitation. Precise details
will be given in legends to figures and tables. The basic
experimental scheme for the analysis of ^{125}I-labelled cell
surface proteins followed throughout this paper is illustrated
by the flow sheet shown in Figure 1.

Surface immunoglobulin of B lymphocytes.

We have performed studies of B lymphocytes of mice
(29, 32), man (33) and chickens (Szenberg, A. , Cone, R. E.
and Marchalonis, J. J. , unpublished observations). I shall
use data obtained for human chronic lymphocytic leukemia
(CLL) cells, which are thought to represent neoplastic
monoclonal B lymphocytes (34, 35), to illustrate the isolation and partial characterization of B cell surface immunoglobulin. Figure 2 presents data illustrating the immunological precipitation of ^{125}I-labelled cell surface proteins,
solubilized using NP40, of two CLL preparations. The
counts at "0 washes" represent high molecular ^{125}I-labell-
ed proteins in the initial precipitation mixture. Subsequent

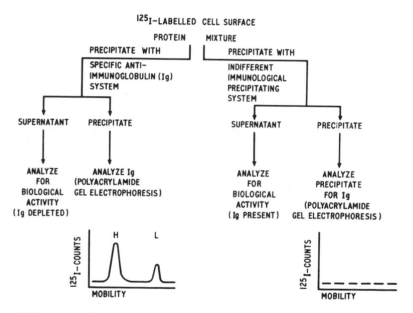

Fig. 1. Flow diagram illustrating sequence of events in the immunological and biochemical analysis of immunoglobulin present in extracts of ^{125}I-labelled lymphocyte surface protein mixtures.

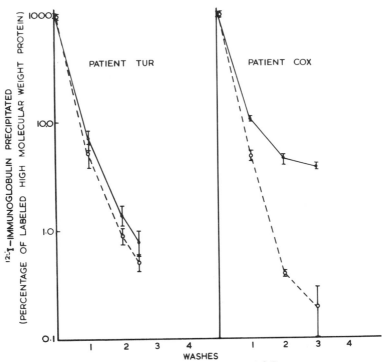

Fig. 2.   Wash loss analysis of ^{125}I-labelled cell
surface protein mixtures from chronic lymphocytic leukemia (CLL) cells of two patients TUR and COX.   Lymphocyte suspensions were labelled using the lactoperoxidase-
catalyzed method (22).   After washing, they were extracted with 0.5% nonidet P40 in phosphate buffered saline
pH7.2 for 15 minutes at room temperature.   The suspension was centrifuged and the supernatant dialyzed against
0.15M Tris-HC1.   The solutions containing non-dialyzable
^{125}I-labelled protein were coprecipitated to obtain immunoglobulin using rabbit antiserum directed again t K,λand
μ chains and sufficient carrier ("cold") IgM myeloma protein was added to ensure that >90% of the human immunoglobulin present was precipitated.   A control precipitation to assess the amount of counts nonspecifically trapped
by a precipitate of comparable mass consisted of "cold"
fowl IgG (Y) immunoglobulin and rabbit antiserum to this
protein.   Counts at "O washes" represent the initial
counts (here normalized to 100%).   Counts at "1 wash"
represent those in the first precipitate.   Subsequent counts
represent precipitates following resuspension and washing
with phosphate buffered saline. Taken from reference 33.

counts, at various "washes", are those in the precipitates. The specific system possessed antibody activity directed against human K, λ and μ chains and sufficient carrier IgM immunoglobulin to ensure >90% precipitation. The control system consisted of an indifferent immune precipitating system which brought down a comparable amount of protein; in this case, it consisted of fowl $\gamma G(Y)$ immunoglobulin (FγG) plus rabbit antiserum to this antigen. The curve obtained for patient TUR shows a clear-cut negative result, i. e. both curves drop rapidly and no significant difference between the specific and control systems was observed. In contrast, the curve for patient COX gives a typical positive result. After three washes the number of counts specifically precipitated is >10 times higher than that trapped in the control precipitate. In the study made (33), CLL cells of six of eight patients possessed surface immunoglobulin extractable by the Nonidet P40 (NP40) method. This result is in accord with the conclusion that most CLL cells are B cells (35). We have shown elsewhere that NP40 extraction serves quite well to obtain murine B cell immunoglobulin, but is unsatisfactory for T lymphocytes (31).

Table 1 presents results of a series of studies designed to quantitate ^{125}I-labelled surface immunoglobulins of B lymphocytes of murine, human and avian (chicken) sources. In all cases, 1-5% of counts in ^{125}I-labelled high molecular weight surface protein was specifically precipitated as immunoglobulin of murine and human B lymphocytes was predominantly IgM.

It is possible to ascertain many molecular properties of isolated surface immunoglobulin by dissolving the immunological precipitates in dissociating solvents and analyzing the soluble ^{125}I-labelled protein by techniques such as polyacrylamide gel electrophoresis (PAGE). Figure 3 illustrates ^{125}I-surface Ig of CLL cells of patient MAT resolved by PAGE in SDS-containing buffers. The unreduced immunoglobulin (Figure 3a) migrates predominantly as a single component which is retarded relative to IgG immunoglobulin. This mobility is consistent with that of the 7S subunit of IgM. In gel filtration experiments, we have determined a molecular weight of 180,000 - 200,000

TABLE 1

Isolation of ^{125}I-Surface Immunoglobulins of B Cells

Cell source	Extraction	Anti Ig System (cpm x 10^{-3})	Control System (cpm x 10^{-3})	% High M.W. Counts specifically precipitated
Spleen (nu/nu)	Turnover	MIG + ANTI-MIG	Hcyn + Anti-Hcyn	
		41.7 ± 2.3	2.8 ± 0.9	2.2
Spleen (nu/nu)	NP40	14.4 ± 0.7	0.3 ± 0.2	1.1
CBA Spleen (cell electrophoresis >99% Ig +)	Turnover	11.5 ± 1.0	FγG + ANTI-FγG	
			2.3 ± 0.6	4.9
Chronic Lymphocytic Leukemia (Cox)	NP40	HIgM + ANTI-HIgM	FγG + ANTI-FγG	
		16.8 ± 0.7	0.6 ± 0.2	3.5
Chronic Lymphocytic Leukemia (War)	NP40	4.5 ± 0.1	1.3 ± 0.1	1.4
Bursa (Chicken)		ANTI-FγG + GARG	NRS + GARG	
		12.6 ± 0.7	3.6 ± 0.1	1.5

B cells were radioiodinated as follows: to 5×10^6 to 1×10^7 cells suspended in 50 μl PBS containing 20 μg lactoperoxidase were added 100 - 200 μC ^{125}I iodide (carrier-free, The Radio-chemical Centre, Amersham, Bucks, England) followed by 10 μl of 0.03% H_2O_2. The cells were mixed and incubated at 30°C for 5 min. The reaction was stopped with a large excess of chilled PBS and the cells washed twice (at 4°C) prior to further analysis. Turnover was performed as previously described (28). Lysis with the non-ionic detergent NP40 was performed by incubating cells with 0.5% (V/V) NP40 (British Drug Houses, Melbourne) for 10 min. at room temperature. Approximately 1 ml. NP40 solution was added per 5×10^7 cells. Nuclei and debris were removed by centrifugation at 1500 rpm. The supernatants were dialyzed against Tris-NaCl prior to coprecipitation analysis. Data tabulated were obtained on the fourth wash. Each aliquot corresponds to 2 - 3 $\times 10^6$ cells. MIG, mouse immunoglobulin (IgG of normal CBA mice); anti-MIG, rabbit anti-serum to normal mouse IgG immunoglobulin (possesses specificity for κ, λ and γ chains. HIgM, human IgM myeloma protein Frymac; anti-HIgM, rabbit antiserum to human IgM immunoglobulin (possesses activity for κ, λ and μ chains). Anti-FγG, rabbit antiserum to chicken IgG (Y) immunoglobulin (possesses activity for light chains and γ(Y) chain); FγG, chicken IgG (Y). GARG, goat antiserum to rabbit IgG immunoglobulin. NRS, normal rabbit serum. Hcyn, Limulus hemocyanin; Anti-Hcyn, rabbit antiserum to Limulus hemocyanin. Data represent mean and standard errors of at least 4 replicates.

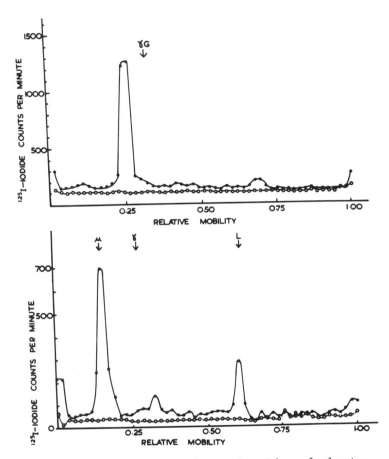

Fig. 3. Analysis by polyacrylamide gel electrophoresis in SDS containing buffers of ^{125}I-labelled surface
immunoglobulin of CLL cells of patient MAT. Upper
figure (1), unreduced samples resolved on 5% polyacrylamide gel. ●-●, specifically precipitated immunoglobulin;
0-0, counts associated with FγG anti FγG precipitate. γG↓,
location of human IgG marker protein (M.W. 150,000).
Lower figure (b), samples reduced with 2-mercaptoethanol
to cleave interchain disulfide bonds and analyzed on 10%
gel under conditions which resolve light chains and heavy
chains. ●-●, specifically precipitated immunoglobulin;
0-0, counts associated with the control precipitate. μ, γ
and L indicate positions at which μ chain, γ chain and light
chain migrate under these conditions. Gels were prepared
as described by Laemmli (81).

for this surface immunoglobulin. When the surface immuno-globulin is reduced to cleave inter-chain disulfide bonds, alkylated to prevent their reformation, and subjected to PAGE analysis (9% gel), polypeptide chains possessing mobilities characteristic of μ chains and light chains are observed (Figure 3b). This result, i. e. the presence of 7S IgM molecules, obtained for B cells of man and mouse. The chicken exhibited light chains and μ chains on bursal lymphocytes. In addition, it also expressed a heavy chain of molecular weight 40,000. A number of laboratories have reported similar conclusions for surface immuno-globulins of murine spleen lymphocytes, presumably B cells (25, 36, 37), human lymphocyte tumor lines (25, 38, 39) and CLL cells (38, 40).

Surface immunoglobulins of T lymphocytes.

Table 2 presents a selection of immunological precipitation data obtained for ^{125}I-surface proteins of T lymphocytes from various sources. Care was taken to use only T lymphocyte populations which showed minimal amounts of cells which were positive for immunoglobulin by either immunofluorescence or short-term autoradiography. Such cells were interpreted as B cells (41). The data shown here illustrate that both thymus and peripheral T cells of CBA mice express surface immunoglobulin which can be detected by the proper use of surface radioiodination, extraction and immunological precipitation. Human thymus lymphocytes also possessed surface immunoglobulin as did those of neonatal chickens. Moreover, the amount of counts specifically precipitated as immunoglobulin is too high to be accounted for by the trace contamination with B cells present in these experiments. The results observed for the Θ+ thymoma lines WEHI 22 and WEHI 7 were especially interesting because both cells represent cloned mouse leukemias which have been adapted to continuous cell culture. There is no possibility of B cell contamina-tion or passive antibody in these situations. Furthermore, I shall present evidence below that these cells synthesize immunoglobulin which mimics that of T cells in certain functional properties. Using the precipitation systems applied to murine T lymphocytes in this table, no significant

TABLE 2

Isolation of ^{125}I-Surface Immunoglobulins of T Cells

Cell source	% Ig + Cells	Extraction	Specific System (cpm x 10^{-3})	Control System (cpm x 10^{-3})	% High M.W. Counts specifically precipitated
Human thymus (5 days old)	<2%	Acid-Urea	HIgM + ANTI-HIgM 9.9 ± 1.6	FγG + ANTI-FγG 1.9 ± 0.5	4.4
CBA Thymus	<1% (>99 Θ+)	Acid-Urea	MIg + ANTI-MIg 4.9 ± 0.9	FγG + ANTI-FγG 1.6 ± 0.4	1.8
CBA Thymus (Cortisone resistant)	<0.2%	Acid-Urea	21.6 ± 1.2	3.4 ± 0.7	3.7
CBA T.TDL (Activated to C57Bl H-2)	<0.2%	Turnover	9.9 ± 0.6	1.2 ± 0.4	4.3
CBA TDL (Cell electrophoresis)	<0.1%	Turnover	9.8 ± 0.4	3.3 ± 0.4	1.7
WEHI 22 (θ + No B thymoma line)	Cells	NP40-Urea	MIgM + ANTI-MIgM 15.1 ± 4.4	FγG + ANTI-FγG 1.5 ± 0.5	1.2

	No B Cells	NP40-Urea	FγG + ANTI-FγG	MIgG + ANTI-FγG	
WEHI 7 (θ + thymoma line)			33.5 ± 3.0	6.9 ± 1.3	0.5
Thymus (newly hatched chicken)	<0.5%	Turnover	8.3 ± 0.7	2.8 ± 0.1	2.4

T cell populations were radioiodinated as described in the legend to Table 1. The thymoma lines were labelled as follows: To 1×10^7 cells in 30 μl PBS containing 10 μg lactoperoxidase were added 4 μl carrier-free ^{125}I-iodide followed by 10 μl 0.03% H_2O_2. The cells were mixed and incubated 4 min. at 37°C. An additional 10 μl of 0.03 H_2O_2 and 10 μl lactoperoxidase in PBS (1 mg 1 ml) were added and the cells mixed. After 4 min., this process was repeated. After another 4 min., 10 μl 0.03% H_2O_2 alone was added with mixing. Following four minutes incubation, the reaction was stopped with a large volume of chilled PBS and the cells washed as above. Turnover was performed as previously described (28). Cells were dissolved in 10M urea, 1.5 M acetic acid (1 ml per 1-2 x 10^7 cells) at 37°C for 1 - 2 hr. The lysate as centrifuged at 1,500 rpm at 4°C for 15 min. and the supernatant retained. It was dialyzed against Tris - NaCl prior to further analysis (see ref. 31 for details). NP40-urea consisted of 1% NP40, 6M urea. Cells were incubated in this solvent, 0.7 ml per 10^7 cells, for 15 min. at room temperature followed by centrifugation. The supernatant was dialyzed against Tris-NaCl prior to further analysis. Data given are counts obtained after 3- 4 washes. Each aliquot corresponds to 2 - 3 x 10^6 cells. Antisera used are as in Table 1 except for MIgM, mouse IgM immunoglobulin from normal CBA mice; Anti-MIgM, rabbit antiserum to this immunoglobulin (possesses activity to λ, λ and μ chains. Means and standard errors of at least four replicates are given.

immunoglobulin was detected in ^{125}I-surface proteins of
fetal liver cells, testis cells or mastocytoma P815 line
cells.
    Table 3 presents data obtained by Haustein, in this
laboratory, which illustrates that particular details of surface radioiodination and extraction are crucial to the attain-
ment of reliable amounts of surface immunoglobulins from
certain lymphocytes.   Harris et al (42) previously showed
that the lymphoma line WEHI 22 synthesizes IgM immunoglobulin and expresses surface immunoglobulin detectable
by immunofluorescence.   We (29, 32) confirmed the latter
result by surface radioiodination.   As shown in Table 3
surface IgM-type immunoglobulin can be isolated from ^{125}I-
labelled WEHI 22 cells by metabolic release and extraction
with acid-urea or urea-NP40, but poorly, if at all, using
NP40 alone under conditions described by Vitetta et al (43).
Furthermore, I would emphasize that optimal conditions
for the radioiodination of lymphocyte tumor lines are markedly different than those previously used for T cells or B
cells (Haustein, D. , in preparation).
    Table 4 presents data obtained in collaboration with
Haustein and Harris (in preparation) which demonstrates
that the Θ+ thymoma lines WEHI 22, WEHI 7 and S49 incorporate significant amounts of H^3-leucine into immunoglobulin.   This result, coupled with previous work of
Harris et al (42), provides unequivocal evidence that Θ+
lymphocytes can synthesize immunoglobulin.   The level of
immunoglobulin synthesis is low compared with plasmacytomas or activated B cells (44).
    Analyses of specifically precipitated surface immuno
globulins of T lymphocytes established that these molecules
resemble the 7S subunits of IgM immunoglobulin.   Figure
4a depicts the PAGE pattern obtained for intact surface
immunoglobulin from thymus lymphocytes of CBA mice.
The predominant component possesses a mobility slightly
retarded relative to the IgG marker (M.W. 150,000).   In
this experiment, special care was taken to remove parathy-
mic lymph nodes which might contribute B cells to the cell
population.   Upon reduction (Figure 4b), the immunoglobulin molecule dissociates into light chains and heavy
chains with a mobility identical to that of μ chains.   Figure

TABLE 3

Isolation of ^{125}I-labeled Surface Immunoglobulin from Thymoma Line WEHI 22

Extraction procedure	Total counts nondialyzable (cpm x 10⁻³)	Precipitation System		Percent of nondialyzable material specifically ppt.
		MIgM + anti-MIgM (cpm x 10⁻³)	FIgG + anti-FIgG (cpm x 10⁻³)	
1% NP40	1,410	2.0 ± 0.2	1.0 ± 0.1	0.07
1% NP40/ 6M Urea	2,025	24.3 ± 4.4	1.5 ± 0.5	1.1
Acid/urea	190	11.4 ± 0.3	3.2 ± 0.1	4.4
Metabolic release	210	6.0 ± 0.3	1.7 ± 0.2	2.0

θ + thymoma line WEHI 22 was labeled as described in legend to Table 2 (D. Haustein, in preparation). Extraction procedures and reagents described above. Data correspond to 2 - 3 x 10⁻⁶ cells and were obtained after 3 or 4 washes. Means and standard errors of at least 4 replicates are given.

TABLE 4

Immunoglobulin Synthesis by Theta Positive Thymoma Lines

	H^3 counts (cpm x 10^{-3}) Released from cells by Lysis with NP40/Urea			
	WEHI 22	WEHI 7	S49	EL 4
Total macromolecular counts (TCA-precipitable)	2,350.0	2,520.0	1,400.0	1,920.0
Counts precipitated by antiglobulin	76.1	3.5	1.4	9.3
Counts precipitated by control system	48.3	1.9	0.4	3.2
Specific counts in Ig	27.8	1.6	1.0	6.1
Per cent Ig	1.2	0.1	0.1	0.3

Cell lines in logarithmic growth phase were incubated for 6 hrs with 50 μc H^3-leucine per ml (10^7 cells per ml) in a medium decreased correspondingly in cold leucine. Cells were washed and lysed with NP40/urea as above. Coprecipitation analysis was performed using

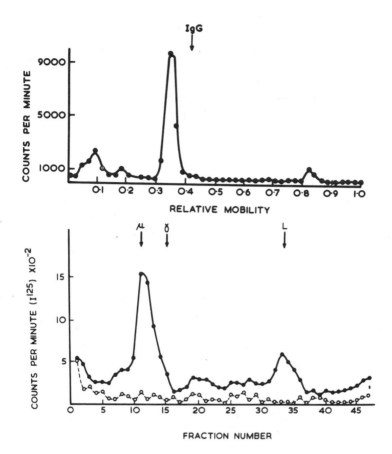

Fig. 4. Analysis by polyacrylamide gel electrophoresis in SDS-containing buffers of ^{125}I-labelled surface immunoglobulin of thymus lymphocytes of CBA mice. Upper figure (a), unreduced ^{125}I-labelled surface immunoglobulin analyzed on 5% gel. ↓ IgG indicates the position at which mouse IgG (M.W. 150,000) migrated under these conditions. The counts associated with the control FγG-anti-FγG system fell within background level values. Lower figure (b), reduced aliquot resolved on 9% gel. ●-●, specifically precipitated immunoglobulin; 0-0, counts associated with the control precipitate. μ, γ and L indicate the migration positions of μ chains, γ chains and light chains, respectively. Gels were prepared according to Laemmli (81).

5 illustrates the polypeptide chain composition of surface immunoglobulin from peripheral CBA T lymphocytes activated in vivo by the method of Sprent and Miller (45) to H2 antigens of C57Bl mice. The lymphocytes were obtained by cannulation of the thoracic ducts of lethally irradiated (CBA x C57Bl)F1 hybrids which were injected with CBA thymus cells. These cells proliferated in response to C57Bl histocompatibility antigens. The coprecipitation data for this cell population are given in Table 2. Because these data were obtained from 3×10^6 cells, only 0.3% or 9×10^3 being B cells (Ig+), the immunoglobulin found could not have resulted from B cell contamination. Approximately 1×10^6 B cells is the minimum number which can be reliably detected (37, 43). In any case, the pattern obtained here typifies all T cell results, with μ-like chains and light chains being resolved. Moroz and Hahn (46) have recently isolated light chains and μ chains from the surfaces of human and C57Bl mouse lymphocytes using techniques similar to those described here.

These data establish that IgM-like immunoglobulin can be isolated from the surfaces of B lymphocytes, T lymphocytes and Θ+ murine leukemia cell lines. Such a demonstration provides an existence proof and adds plausibility to the circumstantial argument that these molecules serve as lymphocyte receptors for antigen. In the remainder of this paper, I shall present evidence that isolated surface immunoglobulins can bind antigen under certain conditions. Moreover I will consider briefly the possible role of T cell IgM in T, B collaboration using immunoglobulin produced by WEHI 22 as a model for T cell IgM.

Antigen-binding properties of isolated surface immunoglobulin.

A number of investigators have now reported that binding of antigen by both B cells and T cells is inhibited by antisera directed against light chains and μ chains (4, 5, 9, 10, 12). Such studies employed method for the enumeration of individual antigen binding cells. The clonal selective nature of antibody formation generally precludes the application of "bulk average" approaches, like the one used here, because the frequency of cells binding a particular

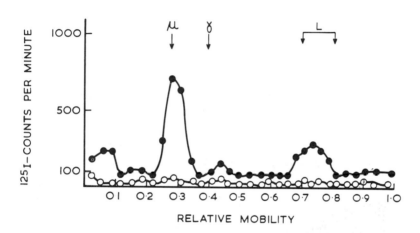

Fig. 5. Analysis by polyacrylamide gel electrophoresis in SDS-containing buffers of ^{125}I-labelled surface
immunoglobulin of CBA T-lymphocytes (from the thoracic
duct) activated to C57 Bl histocompatibility antigens (see
Table 2). ●-●, specifically precipitated mouse immunoglobulin; 0-0, counts associated with FγG, anti-FγG precipitate. μ, γ and L refer to positions corresponding to
μ chains, γ chains and light chains, respectively, 10% gel.
Gels were prepared according to Laemmli (81).

159

antigen is usually low (less than 1 per 1000). However, certain circumstances exist which allow the production of populations of B and T lymphocytes which are enriched in cells of a particular binding specificity.

B. cells. Approximately 1% of lymphocytes from un-immunized congenitally athymic (nu/nu) mice bind DNP specifically (47). This value also holds for thymus lympho-cytes (9, 47) and T and B cells of other mouse strains (9, 11, 47). In all cases the binding is eliminated by incuba-tion of the cells with antisera to immunoglobulins, notably Κ chains and μ chains. If immunoglobulin is the receptor for DNP on these cells, it should be possible to isolate complexes of cell surface immunoglobulin and DNP-antigens. Because approximately 1% of normal B lymphocytes bound this antigen, sufficient radioactivity in DNP-mouse hemo-globin (^{125}I-labelled) was associated with the cell population to allow isolation of these complexes by immunological precipitation (47). It was shown elsewhere (47) that com-plexes of cell surface immunoglobulin and DNP-mouse hemo-globin were released from the surfaces of B cells which had bound the antigen either by metabolic release or limited proteolyses using trypsin.

Activated T cells. I will give two examples illustrating that surface immunoglobulins of T lymphocytes activated to particular antigens demonstrate binding specificity for those antigens. The first example is based upon the system devised by Wagner and Röllinghoff (48) in which cortisone resistant T cells of BALB/c mice are transformed into specific "killer cells" by in vitro incubation with irradiated syngeneic tumor cells. In the experiment reported here (49), T cells were activated to the plasmacytoma line HPC 108. Such activated cells showed cytotoxic activity for HPC 108, but not for the syngeneic plasmacytoma line MOPC 315 which shared H2 antigens with HPC 108 but did not possess the same tumor associated transplantation antigen (TATA). The reaction was abrogated by treatment with anti Θ serum plus complement. Activated T cells were radioiodinated and ^{125}I-labelled cell surface proteins ob-tained by metabolic release. The experimental design out-lined in Figure 1 above was now followed. The activated T cells were found to have IgM-like immunoglobulin on the surfaces. Furthermore, as illustrated in Table 5, a significant proportion of this immunoglobulin bound specifically to the TATA of HPC 108. All binding was abrogated by removal of immunoglobulin.

Antigen specific Ig M-like immunoglobulin was also isolated from the surfaces of CBA T cells activated in vivo as "helper" cells to sheep erythrocytes (50), keyhole limpit hemocyanin (51) and fowl γG immunoglobulin (51). Helper T cells activated to sheep erythrocytes (SRBC) were obtained by reconstituting lethally irradiated (850r) CBA mice with CBA thymus cells plus SRBC plus a synthetic polynucleotide adjuvant consisting of a complex of polyadenylic acid and polyuridylic acid. This complex was previously shown to stimulate T cells (52). Two days after injection of this mixture, spleens were removed as used as a source of helper T cells to SRBC in an in vitro assay consisting of nu/nu spleens and added T cell populations. Specifically activated helper T cells to SRBC produced a plaque-forming cell response >10 times larger than that supported by normal CBA T cells or CBA T cells activated to FγG (52). The response was completely abrogated by treatment of the T cells with anti Θ serum. Using the experimental design of Figure 1 above, we investigated that possibility that helper cells to SRBC might possess surface immunoglobulin showing binding specificity for this antigen. As illustrated in Table 6, such cells express surface immunoglobulin which bound specifically to SRBC. Only IgM-like immunoglobulin was found in these cell preparations. Moreover, treatment of these cells with anti Θ serum plus complement prior to radioiodination completely eliminated detection of immunoglobulin. This result was consistent with the low percentage of B cells (<2%) in the activated populations and the virtual absence of cells forming antibodies to SRBC (<5 PFC/10^6 cells).

T cell immunoglobulin in T, B collaboration.

The preceding data on antigen specific helper cells leads to the possible role of T-cell IgM in collaboration with macrophages and B cells in the generation of an antibody-forming response. Both antigen-specific (13, 14, 18, 53) and nonspecific (53-55) helper functions have been ascribed

TABLE 5

Binding Specificity of HPC 108-activated T-cells for TATA

Treatment of ^{125}I-cell surface proteins	Radioactivity (cpm x 10^{-3}) binding to	
	HPC 108	MOPC 315
Coprecipitated with FγG + rabbit anti-FγG	14.5 ± 1.0	0.6 ± 0.1
Coprecipitated with MIG + rabbit anti MIG	3.0 ± 1.5	1.0 ± 0.1

^{125}I-labelled surface proteins of BALB/c T cells (cortisone-resistant) activated in vitro either with MIG and rabbit anti-MIG (to deplete immunoglobulins) or FγG + rabbit anti-FγG (to serve as a control for adherence of counts to precipitates). The supernatants of these procedures were assayed for binding to either tumor lines HPC 108 or MOPC 315 (2 x 10^5 cells in 100 μl PBS - 5% fetal calf serum per 200 μl ^{125}I-cell surface protein). The mixture was held at 4°C for 3 hr. followed by washes with PBS, 5% fetal calf serum as described elsewhere (49). Data represent mean $\pm$ s. e. from 3 - 4 replicate samples per group. ^{125}I-cell surface proteins were obtained by metabolic release (turnover). See Figure 1 for flow sheet of experimental design. Data of reference 49.

162

TABLE 6

Antigen-Binding by Surface Immunoglobulins of T Cells (CBA)

Activated by Sheep Erythrocytes (SRBC)

Treatment of ^{125}I-Labeled Cell Surface Proteins of ATC-SRBC	Counts ^{125}I (cpm x 10^{-3})		
	Sheep RBC	Horse RBC	Mouse RBC
Coprecipitated with FγG + RAFγG	5.5 ± 0.1	0.2 ± 0.1	0.6 ± 0.3
Coprecipitated with MIg + RAMIg	0.3 ± 0.1	0.2 ± 0.0	0.5 ± 0.1

^{125}I-cell surface proteins were obtained by turnover from CBA T lymphocytes activated to sheep erythrocytes (SRBC). The solution was divided into two aliquots, one was incubated with MIg + RAMIg to deplete mouse immunoglobulin; the other was incubated with FγG + RAFγG to control for nonspecific adherence to immune precipitates. The supernatants of these procedures were tested for binding to sheep, horse or mouse RBC as described elsewhere (50). Results represent the mean ± s. e. of 3 replicates in 2 separate experiments. 200 μl of ^{125}I-labelled surface proteins were incubated 1.5 hrs. at 37°C and 3 hrs. at 4°C with 100 μl of a 1% (V/V) suspension of erythrocytes in Eisen's balanced salt solution containing 10% fetal calf serum. The cells were washed four times and the radioactivity in the pellet determined. Data of reference 50.

163

to T cells and "factors" of both persuasions have been implicated. If specific T cell helper function is mediated via a factor, this collaborative factor is most probably immunoglobulin (56) and various groups have reported evidence consistent with this position (13, 14, 18, 57). In particular, Feldmann and Nossal (18) have proposed that T cell IgM, complexed with antigen, binds to macrophages by means of its F_c piece. These bound complexes are now presented to B cells in such a manner as to initiate differentiation of the specific B cells into antibody-secreting plasma cells. This type of model predicts that T cell immunoglobulin should be cytophilic for macrophages. Cone (this symposium) will describe studies which provide results consistent with this prediction.

I commented above that studies with murine thymoma lines show unequivocally that $\Theta+$ lymphocytes can synthesize immunoglobulin. Stocker, Harris and I (58) performed experiments to determine whether immunoglobulin produced by such cells manifested functional similarity to normal T cell immunoglobulin. If the above model of T, B collaboration is correct and immunoglobulin of thymoma lines possesses the proper F_c piece, it should be possible to inhibit specific cell cooperation in vitro by introducing an excess of thymoma immunoglobulin to compete for receptor sites on the macrophage. This effect should be observed for thymus dependent antigens; but it should not apply to antigens such as DNP-polymerized flagellin which is independent of T cells and macrophages in vitro. Figure 6 illustrates the effect of a concentrated globulin fraction obtained from culture fluid of WEHI 22 upon the in vitro response of CBA spleen cells (T, B and macrophages) to donkey RBC and DNP-POL. The thymus-dependent response is virtually eliminated, whereas the DNP-POL response is unaffected. This suppression was abolished by removal of immunoglobulin from the WEHI 22 concentrate using antiglobulin (anti $\varkappa$, γ) bound to Sepharose 4B. Although other possibilities such as a direct effect of WEHI 22 immunoglobulin or T cells cannot be excluded, we presently favor the hypothesis that this immunoglobulin competes with antigen-specific T cell IgM for the macrophage surface. Similar results have been obtained by Feldmann and Boyleston (59) using the $\Theta+$ thymoma line EL-4.

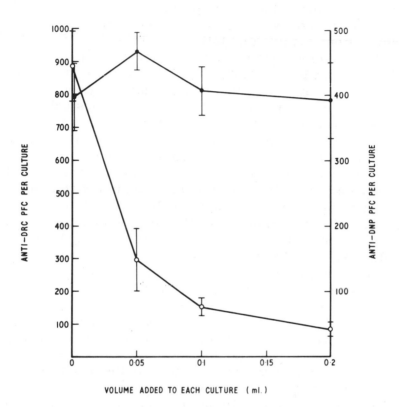

Fig. 6. Effect of different amounts of WEHI-22
culture fluid concentrate on immune responses in vitro.
●-●, plaque forming cells to DNP; 0-0, plaque forming
cells to donkey red blood cells (DRBC). The culture
fluid concentrate was enriched in immunoglobulin. It
was prepared by precipitation with 45% saturated ammonium sulfate. Conditions for tissue culture are described
in reference 58. Taken from reference 58.

DISCUSSION

Experiments described in this paper were designed to provide information on the physico-chemical and biological properties of lymphocyte surface immunoglobulin. Three salient conclusions follow from the data given. Firstly, B lymphocytes and T lymphocytes express IgM-like immunoglobulin (M.W. approx. 200,000) on their outer membranes. Although the surface immunoglobulins of T cells and B cells are generally similar in physical and antigenic properties, the possibility exists that some differences related to their divergent biological functions may exist (51, 60). The amount of immunoglobulin found on T cell populations virtually free of B cells renders it highly unlikely that this IgM-like immunoglobulin arose from contamination by B cells or plasma cells. In addition, "helper function" of such immunoglobulin (51) coupled with the fact that it was not cytophilic for T cells (60) strengthens this conclusion. Moreover, studies with cloned lines derived from murine thymomas establish unequivocally that $\Theta+$ lymphocytes can synthesize immunoglobulin. In the second place, isolated surface immunoglobulin of both normal B cells and activated T cells exhibits binding specificity for antigens. The specificity of activated helper T cell populations militates further against the possibility that B or plasma cell contamination accounts for the observed results because the reactions were susceptible to anti Θ treatment, the contamination was miniscule, and the activation conditions totally unsuitable for production of antibody-forming B cell progeny. Activated T cells are effector cells rather than primary recognition cells, but studies involving inhibition of antigen binding by the latter cells (4-12) indicate that the receptor for antigen here is also IgM-like immunoglobulin. The third major conclusion of the present experiments is that immunoglobulin produced by one $\Theta+$ thymoma line inhibits cooperation among T cells, B cells and macrophages in the induction of antibody formation in vitro. This result is consistent with the proposal that immunoglobulin from such T cell tumors possesses an F_c region structure similar to that of collaborative T cell IgM-like immunoglobulin and can compete with the latter in a nonspecific step such as concentration on the macrophage surface.

The results obtained for B cells are essentially those that would be expected on the basis of a large body of literature directed toward investigation of membrane immunoglobulin of these cells (for review see 15, 16). The demonstration that T cells possess 7S IgM-like immunoglobulin which shows specificity for antigens and serves as a collaborative factor in specific T, B cooperation is consistent with a number of recent studies of antigen binding by T cells (4-12) and specific helper function (13, 14). In this paper, I described the isolation of surface immunoglobulins of T cells and thymus lymphocytes of man, mouse and chicken. Moroz and Hahn (46) have recently isolated light chains and μ chains from thymus lymphocytes of man and C57Bl mouse. Ladolis et al (61) have also used surface radioiodination and membrane isolation to obtain immunoglobulins of rat thymus and spleen lymphocytes.

It is now well documented that IgM-like immunoglobulin plays some role in the binding of foreign antigen by T cells (4-12) and in other T cell activities which show specificity for such antigens including delayed type hypersensitivity (62-64) and "helper" function (13, 14, 57). The present data support the receptor function of immunoglobulin in these T cell reactions. Other T cell reactions, in particular those manifested in allogeneic situations, exist where the role of immunoglobulin is difficult to ascertain (65, 66). Two prime examples of such phenomena are the mixed lymphocyte reaction (MLR) and the graft versus host reaction (GVHR) which might differ from classical immune reactions (67-69). It is interesting that the genes conditioning both the MLR (70) and the GVHR (71) are closely linked, if not identical, and are also closely associated with the Ir-1 locus. The nature of the recognition systems and/or stimuli for proliferation in these responses remain problematic.

An apparent paradox exists because the presence of IgM-like immunoglobulins on T cell membranes can be readily demonstrated by inhibition of antigen binding (4-12), "hot antigen suicide" (2) or delayed type hypersensitivity (62-64), yet direct binding of labelled antiglobulin reagents yields variable results. Some workers claim to be unable to detect binding of fluorescein-labelled (72) or radioiodine-labelled (73) antiglobulins to T cells; whereas others report that the majority of T cells bind anti-Ig, but conditions of special sensitivity are required (41, 74). Others, however, have observed that peripheral T cells possess membrane Ig which is readily detected using virus-labelled (75) or fluorescein-labelled (76) antiglobulins. One possible solution to this dilemma is that surface immunoglobulin of T cells is arranged in such a manner that only its variable regions, containing the combining sites for antigens, are exposed (5, 29). The normally antigenic constant regions would be somehow obstructed. Alternative possibilities are that T cell surface immunoglobulin combined with either antigen or antiglobulin is rapidly shed or internalized. Other systems exist where components are present on plasma membranes, but are somehow masked with respect to binding of antisera directed against them. One such system is the TA_3/HA mouse mammary carcinoma line from which membrane-bound H-2 antigens can be isolated by surface radioiodination and membrane preparation (77), by direct immunological assays. Another such puzzle is the finding that antisera directed against components specified by genes closely linked to the Ir-1 locus, which was proposed to encode a non-immunoglobulin T cell receptor for antigen (78), bind readily to B cells but not to T cells (79, 80). Detailed analysis of the structural and biological properties of lymphocyte membranes are required to resolve these problems of differential expression of membrane components.

ACKNOWLEDGMENTS

This work was supported by grants from the Anna Fuller Fund, the American Heart Association (72 - 1050), the Damon Runyon Memorial Fund (DRG-1215), and the United States Public Health Service (AI-10886). I thank Miss Pat Smith for expert technical assistance. This is paper No. 1990 from the Walter and Eliza Hall Institute of Medical Research.

REFERENCES

1. Ehrlich, P. , Proc. Roy. Soc. B. 65, 424 (1900).
2. Basten, A. , Miller, J. F. A. P. , Warner, N. L. and Pye, J. , Nature New Biol. 231, 104 (1971).
3. Humphrey, J. H. , Roelants, G. and°Willcox, N. , Cell Interactions and Receptor Antibodies in Immune Responses, O. Makela, A. M. Cross and T. V. Kosunen (eds.), Academic Press, New York, 1971, p. 123.
4. Dwyer, J. M. , Warner, N. L. and Mackay, I. R. , J. Immunol. 108, 1439 (1972).
5. Hogg, N. M. and Greaves, M. F. , Immunology 22, 967 (1972).
6. Bach, J. F. , Reyes, F. , Dardenne, M. , Fournier, C. and J. Y. Muller, Cell Interactions and Receptor Antibodies in Immune Responses, O. Makela, A. M. Cross and T. V. Kosunen (eds.), Academic Press, New York, 1971, p. 111.
7. Marchalonis, J. J. , Cone, R. E. and Rolley, R. T. , J. Immunol. 110, 561 (1973).
8. Ashman, R. F. and Raff, M. C. , J. Exp. Med. 137, 69 (1973).
9. Lawrence, D. A. , Spiegelberg, H. L. and Weigle, W. O. , J. Exp. Med. 137, 470 (1973).
10. Roelants, G. E. , Forni, L. and Pernis, B. , J. Exp. Med. 137, 1060 (1973).
11. Rutishauser, U. and Edelman, G. M. , Proc. Nat. Acad. Sci. U. S. 69, 1596 (1972).
12. DeLuca, D. , Decleer, J. , Miller, A. and Sercarz, E. E. , Cell. Immunol. 10, 1 (1974).
13. Lesley, J. F. , Kettman, J. R. and Dutton, R. W. , J. Exp. Med. 134, 618 (1971).
14. Feldmann, M., J. Exp. Med. 136, 737 (1972).
15. Marchalonis, J. J. , J. Medicine, in press (1974).
16. Warner, N. L. , Advances Immunol. , in press (1974).
17. Bretscher, P. and Cohn, M. , Science 169, 1042 (1970).
18. Feldmann, M. and Nossal, G. J. V. , Transplant Rev. 13, 3 (1972).
19. Allan, D. and Crumpton, M. J. , Biochem. J. 123, 967 (1971).
20. Marchalonis, J. J. and Nossal, G. J. V. , Proc. Nat. Acad. Sci. U. S. 61, (1968).

21. Marchalonis, J.J., Biochem. J. 113, 299 (1969).
22. Marchalonis, J.J., Cone, R.E. and Santer, V., Biochem. J. 124, 921 (1971).
23. Phillips, D.R. and Morrison, M., Biochemistry 10, 1766 (1971).
24. Baur, S., Vitetta, E.S., Sherr, C.J., Schenkein, I. and Uhr, J.W., J. Immunol. 106, 1133 (1971).
25. Kennel, S.J. and Lerner, R.A., J. Mol. Biol. 76, 485 (1973).
26. Czech, M.P. and Lynn, W.S., Biochemistry 19, 3597 (1973).
27. Tsai, C.M., Huang, C.C. and Canellakis, E.S., Biochim. Biophys. Acta. 322, 47 (1973).
28. Cone, R.E., Sprent, J. and Marchalonis, J.J., Proc. Nat. Acad. Sci. U.S. 69, 2556 (1972).
29. Marchalonis, J.J., Cone, R.E. and Atwell, J.L., J. Exp. Med. 135, 956 (1972).
30. Atwell, J.L., Cone, R.E. and Marchalonis, J.J., Nature New Biol. 241, 251 (1973).
31. Cone, R.E. and Marchalonis, J.J., Biochem. J. in press (1974).
32. Marchalonis, J.J. and Cone, R.E., Transplant Rev. 14, 3 (1973).
33. Marchalonis, J.J., Atwell, J.L. and Haustein, D., Biochim. Biophys. Acta., in press (1974).
34. Grey, H.M., Rabellino, E. and Pirofsky, B., J. Clin. Invest. 50, 2368 (1971).
35. Wilson, J.D. and Nossal, G.J.V., Lancet 2, 1153 (1971).
36. Grey, H.M., Kubo, R.T. and Cerottini, J.C., J. Exp. Med. 136, 1323
37. Liskowska-Bernstein, B., Rinny, A. and Vassalli, P., Proc. Nat. Acad. Sci. U.S. 70, 2879 (1973).
38. Eskeland, T., Klein, E., Inoue, M. and Johansson, B., J. Exp. Med. 134, 265 (1971).
39. Sherr, C.J., Baur, S., Grundke, I., Zeligs, J., Zeligs, B. and Uhr, J.W., J. Exp. Med. 135, 1392 (1972).
40. Moroz, C., Shalmon, J. and Hahn, J., Eur. J. Immunol. 3, 16 (1973).
41. Nossal, G.J.V., Warner, N.L., Lewis, H. and Sprent, J., J. Exp. Med. 135, 405 (1972).

42. Harris, A. W., Bankhurst, A. D., Mason, S. and Warner, N. L., J. Immunol. 110, 431 (1973).
43. Vitetta, E. S., Bianco, C., Nussenzweig, V. and Uhr, J. W., J. Exp. Med. 136, 81 (1972).
44. Melchers, F. and Andersson, J., Transplant. Rev. 14, 76 (1973).
45. Sprent, J. and Miller, J. F. A. P., Nature New Biol. 234, 195 (1971).
46. Moroz, C. and Hahn, Y., Proc. Nat. Acad. U. S. 70, 3716 (1973).
47. Rolley, R. T. and Marchalonis, J. J., Transplantation 14, 734 (1972).
48. Wagner, H. and Röllinghoff, M., Nature New Biol. 241, 53 (1973)
49. Rollinghoff, M., Wagner, H., Cone, R. E. and Marchalonis, J. J., Nature New Biol. 243, 21 (1973).
50. Cone, R. E. and Marchalonis, J. J., Austral. J. Exp. Biol. Med. Sci. 51, 689 (1973).
51. Feldmann, M., Cone, R. E. and Marchalonis, J. J., Cell. Immunol. 9, 1 (1973).
52. Cone, R. E. and Marchalonis, J. J., Austral. J. Exp. Biol. Med. Sci. 50, 69 (1972).
53. Gorczynski, R. M., Miller, R. G. and Phillips, R. A., J. Immunol. 111, 900 (1973).
54. Dutton, R. W., Falkoff, R., Hirst, J. A., Hoffmann, M., Kappler, J. W., Kettman, J. R., Lesley, J. F. and Vann, D., Progress in Immunology, B. Amos (ed.) Academic Press, New York, 1971, p. 355.
55. Katz, D. H. and Benacerraf, B., Advances Immunol. 15, 1 (1972).
56. Cohn, M., Genetic Control of Immune Responsiveness, H. O. McDevitt and M. Landy (eds.) Academic Press, New York, 1972, p. 370.
57. Rieber, E. P. and Riethmuller, G., submitted for publication.
58. Stocker, J. W., Marchalonis, J. J. and Harris, A. W., J. Exp. Med. in press (1974).
59. Feldmann, M. and Boyleston, A. W., unpublished observations reported by M. Feldmann. The Lymphocyte: Structure and Function. J. J. Marchalonis (ed.) Marcel Dekker, New York, in press.

60. Cone, R. E., Feldmann, M., Marchalonis, J. J. and Nossal, G. J. V., Immunology 26, 49 (1974).

61. Ladoulis, C. T., Gill, T. J. III., Chen, S-H. and Misra, D. N., Progress in Allergy 18, in press (1974).

62. Cooper, M. G. and Ada, G. L., Scand. J. Immunol. 1, 247 (1972).

63. Theis, G. A. and Thorbecke, G. J., J. Immunol. 110, 91 (1973).

64. Rajapakse, D. A., Papamichail, M. and Holborow, E. J., Nature New Biol. 245, 155 (1973).

65. Crone, M., Koch, C. and Simonsen, M., Transplant. Rev. 10, 36 (1972).

66. Mason, S. and Warner, N. L., J. Immunol. 104, 762 (1970).

67. Hildemann, W. H. and Reddy, A. L., Fed. Proc. 32, 2188 (1973).

68. Segall, M., Schendel, D. J. and Zier, K. S., Tissue Antigens 3, 353 (1973).

69. Lafferty, K. J., The Biochemistry of Gene Expression in Higher Organisms, J.K. Pollack and J.W. Lee (eds) Australia and New Zealand Book Co., Sydney, 1973, p. 593.

70. Bach, F. H., Widmer, M. B., Bach, M. L. and Klein, J. J. Exp. Med. 136, 1430 (1972).

71. Klein, J. and Park, J. M., J. Exp. Med. 137, 1213 (197

72. Rabellino, E., Colon, S., Grey, H. M. and Unanue, E. R., J. Exp. Med. 133, 156 (1971).

73. Unanue, E. R., Grey, H. M., Rabellino, E., Campbell, P. and Schmidtke, J., J. Exp. Med. 133, 1188 (1971).

74. Bankhurst, A. D., Warner, N. L. and Sprent, J., J. Exp. Med. 134, 1005 (1971).

75. Hämmerling, U. and Rajewsky, K., Eur. J. Immunol., 1, 147 (1971).

76. Goldschneider, I. and Cogen, R. B., J. Exp. Med. 138, 163 (1973).

77. Molnar, J., Klein, G. and Friberg, Jr., S., Transplantation 16, 93 (1973).

78. Benacerraf, B. and McDevitt, H. O., Science 175, 273 (1972).

79. Hammerling, G., Deak, B. D., Mauve, G,, Hammerling U. and McDevitt, H. O., Immunogenetics, 1, in press (1974).

80. Goding, J. H. , Nossal, G. J. V. , Shreffer, D. and Marchalonis, J. J. submitted.
81. Laemmli, U. K. , Nature (Lond.), 227, 680 (1970).

ALLOANTISERUM INDUCED BLOCKADE OF IR GENE PRODUCT FUNCTION

W.E. Paul, E.M. Shevach, S.Z. Ben-Sasson
F. Finkelman and I. Green

Laboratory of Immunology
National Institute of Allergy and Infectious Diseases
National Institutes of Health
Bethesda, Maryland 20014

ABSTRACT. The activation of guinea pig thymus derived lymphocytes by antigens, the response to which is controlled by histocompatibility-linked immune response (Ir) genes, may be specifically blocked by alloantisera prepared by reciprocal immunization of strain 2 and strain 13 guinea pigs. This blockade is specific in that anti-2 serum blocks the response of $(2 \times 13)F_1$ cells to antigens responsiveness to which is controlled by 2-linked Ir genes while anti-13 serum blocks response dependent on 13-linked Ir genes. The inhibitory antibodies appear to be directed at antigens specified at the 2/13 locus rather than at the Ir gene products themselves. Anti-2 serum blocks responses to the copolymer of glutamic acid and alanine (GA) of cells from $2^{+}GA^{+}$ animals but not of cells from $2^{-}GA^{+}$ animals.
Studies of the 2 alloantigen indicate a molecular weight of ~25,000 Daltons, absence of a low molecular weight polypeptide chain and an expression principally on lymphocytes.
We suggest a model in which the Ir gene product exists as a molecular complex with the 2/13 histocompatibility antigen. In this model, the Ir gene product is responsible for the specific recognition functions of the complex and the alloantigens mediate biologic functions, such as histocompatibility dependent cellular interactions.

INTRODUCTION

The capacity of animals to mount immune responses to many individual antigens or sets of closely related antigens is controlled by specific immune response (Ir) genes, which are linked to the major histocompatibility complex of the species. The precise cellular locus of action of Ir genes is still controversial, but the bulk of evidence suggests that the prime expression of these histocompatibility-linked Ir genes is within thymus-derived (T) lymphocytes (1). Recent studies suggest that these genes, or closely linked

175

genes, are also important in macrophage-T lymphocyte interaction in guinea pigs (2) and in T lymphocyte interaction
with precursors of antibody secreting cells in the mouse (3).

As an approach to the analysis of the function of Ir
gene products, we have studied the effect of alloantisera,
produced by reciprocal immunization of inbred strain 2 and
13 guinea pigs, on in vitro T lymphocyte responses of
(2 x 13)F$_1$ lymphoid cells. In these experiments we have used
a series of antigens, responsiveness to which is controlled
by histocompatibility-linked Ir genes. These antigens are
presented in Table 1, together with the histocompatibility
type with which responsiveness is associated. Our initial
studies involved the 2, 4-dinitrophenyl (DNP) conjugate of
the copolymer of L-glutamic acid and L-lysine (GL) and the
copolymer of L-glutamic acid and L-tyrosine (GT). Responsiveness to DNP-GL is controlled by a 2-linked Ir gene (4) while
responsiveness to GT is a 13-linked trait (5). In addition,
we evaluated the response of (2 x 13)F$_1$ cells to purified
protein derivative of tuberculin (PPD), responsiveness to
which is not limited to either strain 2 or strain 13 guinea
pigs.

F$_1$ guinea pigs were immunized with DNP-GL and GT
emulsified in complete Freund's adjuvant. Two to three
weeks later, sterile mineral oil was infused into the
peritoneal cavity and the resultant exudate was harvested
3-4 days subsequently. From this exudate, an enriched
population of lymphocytes was prepared by passage over rayon
wool columns. The lymphocytes in the resultant cell population are almost exclusively T lymphocytes (6) and are
exquisitely responsive to antigens both in terms of DNA
synthesis and production of migration inhibition factor (MIF)
(7). The antigen-stimulated proliferative response is
primarily a T lymphocyte function in the guinea pig system.
With the cell preparation we have employed, in which the
vast majority of lymphocytes present are T lymphocytes, the
specific proliferative response is almost entirely due to T
cells.

The purified lymphocyte population was exposed to antigen for a limited period of time or, alternatively, peritoneal exudate cells from a non-immunized syngenic animal were
pulsed with antigen and then mixed with the immune lymphocyte
population. Heat-inactivated normal guinea pig serum, anti-2
serum or anti-13 serum was added to the cell culture (final
conc. 10%). The cells were cultured for 72 hours. One µCi
of ^{3}H-thymidine (^{3}H-TdR) was added for the last 4 or 16 hours
of the culture period and the amount of ^{3}H-TdR incorporated
into acid precipitable material was measured.

176

TABLE 1

IR GENES OF INBRED GUINEA PIGS

Strain	Histocompatibility Type	Presence of Ir Genes Controlling Responses to:
2	2	DNP-GL GA
13	13	GT DNP-GPA (low dose)
$(2 \times 13)F_1$	2,13	DNP-GL GA GT DNP-GPA (low dose)

Abbreviations:

DNP - 2,4-dinitrophenyl
GL - copolymer of L-glutamic acid and L-lysine
GA - copolymer of L-glutamic acid and L-alanine
GT - copolymer of L-glutamic acid and L-tyrosine
GPA - guinea pig albumin

This alloantiserum inhibition experiment had a striking outcome, as shown in Table 2. The response to DNP-GL, which is controlled by a 2-linked Ir gene, was completely blocked both by anti-2 serum and an $\overline{Fab_2'}$ fragment of the $\gamma 2$ fraction of anti-2 serum, while anti-13 serum had little or no effect. The response to GT, which is controlled by a 13-linked Ir gene, was not significantly affected by anti-2 serum but was almost completely blocked by anti-13 serum. The PPD response showed no specific blockade by either anti-serum alone. Thus, a 2-linked response of $(2 \times 13)F_1$ cells is blocked by an anti-2 serum while a 13-linked response of the same cell population is blocked by an anti-13 serum (8).

It is highly unlikely that this blockade is due to general inactivation of the responsive cells. Although many pieces of evidence argue against general inactivation the most powerful finding is the specificity of the blockade. Generalized inactivation with specific blockade in this system would require allelic exclusion, with those F_1 cells responsive to DNP-GL expressing only strain 2 alloantigens and those F_1 cells responsive to GT expressing only strain 13 alloantigens. Our studies of F_1 guinea pig lymphocyte populations provide no evidence of such allelic exclusion (9). Indirect immunofluorescenes reveals that more than 95% of peritoneal exudate lymphocytes are stained by anti-2 serum alone, anti-13 serum alone, or anti-2 serum plus anti-13 serum. Similarly, the number of F_1 cells lysed, in the presence of complement, by anti-2 serum plus anti-13 serum is no more than that lysed by either serum alone. These results thus indicate that the blocking activity of the alloantisera must be a localized cell surface phenomenon rather than a generalized inactivation of the cell. This, in turn, strongly suggests that alloantisera inhibit antigen-recognition or specific stimulation by blocking the Ir gene product directly or indirectly.

Before addressing the question of the precise specificity of the inhibitory activity in the alloantisera, we wished to ascertain whether T lymphocyte functions other than antigen-induced thymidine incorporation could be blocked by alloantisera. One classical function of T lymphocytes is antigen-stimulated production of MIF (10). The capacity of anti-2 and anti-13 serum to block stimulation of MIF production by $(2 \times 13)F_1$ cells in response to DNP-GL and to DNP-guinea pig albumin (DNP-GPA) was determined. Responsiveness to the former is, as noted above, a 2-linked trait, while responsiveness to DNP-GPA is principally a function of a 13-linked Ir gene, particularly when guinea pigs are immunized with low doses of DNP-GPA (11). In order to assay the

TABLE 2

ALLOANTISERUM BLOCKADE OF DNA SYNTHESIS RESPONSE
OF $(2 \times 13)F_1$ CELLS TO DNP-GL AND GT

Stimulant	Serum		
	NGPS	Anti-2	Anti-13
--	3,499	1,479	1,484
DNP-GL	68,361	1,231	46,385
GT	17,070	12,147	1,770
PPD	20,049	12,086	15,159
PHA	56,887	44,281	28,094

Response is measured by incorporation of tritiated thymidine
into acid precipitable material and is presented as cpm.
All sera were heat inactivated and are present at a final
concentration of 10%. The duration of the culture is 72
hours.

MIF activity in supernatants of stimulated lymphocytes in the presence of alloantisera, a migrating population of strain 13 macrophages was used when anti-2 serum was employed and strain 2 macrophages were used when the effect of anti-13 serum was under study. This was done to avoid the direct inhibitory activity of alloantisera on macrophage migration. Table 3 demonstrates that anti-2 serum blocks MIF production in response to DNP-GL but not DNP-GPA while anti-13 serum blocks the response to DNP-GPA but not DNP-GL (12). This indicates that specific blockade of T cell activation in Ir gene controlled systems is not limited to a single T cell function. Indeed, as there is suggestive evidence that MIF producing cells may be different from some or all T cells responsible for the proliferative response to antigen (13), our result suggests that alloantisera induced blockade is not limited to a single T cell class.

A major question in the analysis of alloantisera blockade of lymphocyte activation is the specificity of the blocking sera. We envisage two major alternatives:

1. The blocking antibodies within the alloantisera are directed to the product of the Ir gene itself and block through their interaction with this active product.

2. The blocking antibodies within the alloantisera are directed at the histocompatibility antigen coded for at the 2/13 locus and block Ir gene product function indirectly.

The first possibility can be tested in a variety of ways. If the Ir gene product mediates a specific recognition function, as seems likely, then Ir gene products should possess unique antigenic determinants for which the inhibitory alloantibodies might be specific. If the Ir gene product is clonally distributed and clonal expansion occurs as a result of immunization, then cells from appropriately immunized animals should be much more efficient in adsorbing the inhibitory antibodies than cells from control animals. To test this possibility, the relative capacity of lymph node cells from a strain 2 guinea pig immunized to DNP-GL in complete Freund's adjuvant (CFA) and of a strain 2 guinea pig immunized to CFA alone to adsorb the capacity of anti-2 serum to inhibit the response of (2 x 13)F$_1$ cells to DNP-GL was determined. No difference in the adsorptive capacity of these cell populations was observed (Table 4), making it unlikely that the inhibitory antibodies were directed at unique antigenic determinants (idiotypes) of a clonally distributed DNP-GL-Ir gene product. Similarly, cells from strain 2 guinea pigs immunized to DNP-GL were no more effective than control cells in eliciting inhibitory alloantisera in strain 13 animals.

TABLE 3
ALLOANTISERUM BLOCKADE OF MIF PRODUCTION BY
$(2x13)F_1$ CELLS IN RESPONSE TO DNP-GL AND DNP-GPA

Antigen	Strain 13 Macrophages		Strain 2 Macrophages	
	NGPS	ANTI-2	NGPS	ANTI-13
0	100	100	100	100
DNP-GL	40	91	36	42
DNP-GPA	51	51	37	75

Response is measured as percent of migration of macrophages
exposed to supernatants of antigen-stimulated culture compared to migration of macrophages exposed to supernatants of
unstimulated cultures. When the effect of anti-2 serum was
tested, a migrating population of strain 13 macrophages was
employed. When anti-13 serum was being tested, strain 2
macrophages were used.

TABLE 4

ABSORPTION OF BLOCKING ACTIVITY BY CELLS FROM DNP-GL IMMUNE AND CONTROL ANIMALS

		Serum		
		Anti-2 Serum		
			Absorbed with:	
Antigen	NGPS	0	"CFA" Cells	"DNP-GL" Cells
0	1,169	924	677	591
DNP-GL	15,764	1,784	5,840	4,893
GT	5,082	5,673	5,172	4,944

CPM of tritiated thymidine incorporated into acid precipitable material by $(2x13)F_1$ cells. Anti-2 serum was unabsorbed or absorbed with either $2x10^8$ cells from strain 2 guinea pigs immunized to CFA alone ("CFA" cells) or $2x10^8$ cells from strain 2 guinea pigs immunized to DNP-GL in CFA ("DNP-GL" cells).

The most powerful approach to establish whether the inhibitory antibodies are directed against the DNP-GL-Ir gene
product or the 2 histocompatibility (H) antigen would be to
determine the capacity of specific alloantisera to block in
vitro responses to DNP-GL of cells from guinea pigs of a recombinant genotype in which the gene controlling the 2 alloantigens (the 2-gene) and the Ir gene controlling responses
to DNP-GL (the DNP-GL-Ir gene)had become separated. If anti-
2 serum caused blockade of the response to DNP-GL of cells
from a 2⁻ DNP-GL⁺ animal, it would strongly suggest that the
alloantisera functioned through antibody directed at the Ir
gene product. On the other hand, the failure of anti-2 serum
to block the DNP-GL response of 2⁻ DNP-GL⁺ cells would imply
that the blocking antibody was not directed at the Ir gene
product, but rather at the 2 alloantigen and that blockade
was an indirect process.

Unfortunately, such recombinant guinea pigs have not yet
been developed. However, in outbred guinea pig populations,
one encounters animals which have a different arrangement of
H and Ir genes than is observed in inbred animals. Table 5
presents the four principal phenotypes observed in outbred
populations (14). The Ir gene controlling responses to the
copolymer of glutamic acid and alanine (GA), which is associated with the 2 histocompatibility gene in inbred and many
outbred animals (5), frequently occurs in 2⁻ outbred guinea
pigs. These 2⁻GA⁺ guinea pigs allow the performance of the
experiment described above. One important reservation
exists, however. It is possible that the GA-Ir gene found
in 2⁻ guinea pigs is not identical to the GA-Ir gene found
in 2⁺ guinea pigs. If this were the case, then an anti-2
serum might fail to block the response to GA of cells from
2⁻GA⁺ animals not because it lacked antibody to the GA-Ir
gene product, but rather because it lacked antibody to the
unique GA-Ir gene product of 2⁻ animals. Although we regard
this possibility as unlikely for a variety of reasons, it
must be borne in mind in the interpretation of our data.

We have tested the capacity of anti-2 serum to block the
response to GA of cells from GA immunized (2 x 13)F₁ and outbred 2⁺GA⁺ and 2⁻GA⁺ animals. The results were quite clear
(15). In the great majority of experiments, anti-2 serum
blocked the response to GA of (2 x 13)F₁ cells and of outbred 2⁺GA⁺ cells but had no effect on the response of outbred 2⁻GA⁺ cells (Table 6). This result is supported by two
related experiments. Alloantiserum produced by strain 13
guinea pigs immunized with cells from 2⁺GA⁺ animals blocks
the response to GA of lymphocytes from (2 x 13)F₁ guinea
pigs while alloantisera produced by strain 13 guinea pigs

TABLE 5

COMMON PHENOTYPES OF INBRED AND OUTBRED GUINEA PIGS

	Histocompatibility Type	Ir Type
Inbred:		
Strain 2	$2^+, 13^-$	DNP-GL$^+$, GA$^+$, GT$^-$
Strain 13	$2^-, 13^+$	DNP-GL$^-$, GA$^-$, GT$^+$
F_1	$2^+, 13^+$	DNP-GL$^+$, GA$^+$, GT$^+$
Outbred:		
	$2^+, 13^-$	DNP-GL$^+$, GA$^+$, GT$^-$
	$2^-, 13^+$	DNP-GL$^-$, GA$^-$, GT$^+$
	$2^+, 13^+$	DNP-GL$^+$, GA$^+$, GT$^+$
	$2^-, 13^+$	DNP-GL$^-$, GA$^+$, GT$^+$

TABLE 6

FAILURE OF ANTI-2 SERUM TO BLOCK RESPONSES
TO GA OF CELLS FROM A 2^-GA$^+$ GUNIEA PIG

	2^+GA$^+$ Cells		2^-GA$^+$ Cells	
Antigens	NGPS	Anti-2	NGPS	Anti-2
--	2,989	2,250	845	810
	24,258	4,098	40,489	51,740
DNP-PLL	37,218	6,284	1,256	1,040
PPD	29,261	20,118	96,314	147,452

CPM of tritiated thymidine incorporated into acid precipitabl
material by cells from 2^+GA$^+$ and 2^-GA$^+$ animals immunized to G
and DNP-poly-L-lysine (DNP-PLL) in CFA. Cells were stimulate
with nothing, GA, DNP-PLL or PPD. The response to DNP-PLL is
controlled by the GL gene or a gene very closely linked to it
The 2^- animals used here are all GL$^-$ and unresponsive to DNP-
PLL.

immunized with cells from 2^-GA^+ animals does not block the GA
response of cells from F_1 animals. Finally, cells from 2^-GA^+
animals fail to adsorb the capacity of 13 anti-2 serum to
block the response of $(2 \times 13)F_1$ cells to GA, while 2^+GA^+
cells are effective adsorbants of the blocking activity of
these sera (15).

These experiments provide strong evidence that the capacity of anti-2 serum to block the response to GA is due to
the interaction of the antiserum with the 2 histocompatibility antigen rather than with the GA-Ir gene product. Although the reservation discussed above concerning the possible
distinctness of the GA-Ir gene product of 2^- animals remains,
one piece of evidence suggesting it is unlikely may be cited.
If the blocking activity of the anti-2 sera were, in fact,
due to antibody to the GA-Ir gene product and anti-2 serum
failed to block responses to GA of 2^-GA^+ cells because such
cells possessed a different GA-Ir gene product, then a 13
anti-2^-GA^+ serum should contain antibody to this distinct
GA-Ir gene product. Therefore, we tested the capacity of a
13 antiserum raised by immunization with cells of 2^-GA^+ random bred animal to block the response to GA of cells from
2^-GA^+ animals and cells from 2^-GA^+ animals. We found such
sera without blocking activity, although they were very cytotoxic for cells from outbred animals of both phenotypes.
This experiment strengthens the contention that alloantisera
exert their blocking activity by binding to the 2 alloantigen
rather than to the Ir gene product.

The finding that functions of Ir gene products are blocked by sera directed at the products of linked but distinct
genes suggests that an intimate relationship exists between
these molecules on the surface of the cell. In view of current evidence indicating that independent surface proteins are
capable of free diffusion in the plane of the membrane, this
finding is most easily explained if a stable bond exists between the 2 alloantigen and the Ir gene product. If a molecular complex between 2 alloantigens and Ir gene products
exists, a study of the chemical structure of this antigen
might be most illuminating. Consequently, we have initiated
studies of the guinea pig histocompatibility antigens using
lactoperoxidase catalyzed surface iodination. In addition
to studying the structure of the 2 and 13 alloantigens described above, we have also investigated a guinea pig histocompatibility antigen which is specified at a distinct, but
very probably linked, genetic locus. This antigen, B, is a
member of a family of histocompatibility antigens originally
described by Sato and deWeck (16). Three antigens B, C and
D were initially described and evidence now exists that one

or more additional alternatives exists at this locus (17).
Strain 2 and 13 guinea pigs are B$^+$, C$^-$, D$^-$. Anti B sera are
highly cytotoxic but, thus far, have failed to block activation by antigen of lymphocytes from inbred and (2 x 13)F$_1$
guinea pigs under conditions in which anti-2 or anti-13 sera
are potent blocking agents. Thus, it is possible that the B
antigen is not linked to Ir gene products on the cell surface
and the study of this antigen would be an excellent control
in the study of the 2/13 antigens. On the other hand, we may
have simply failed to test the response to an antigen for
which a B linked Ir gene product is present.

In order to study both the B and 2 antigens we have
labelled strain 2 lymph node cells with ^{125}I using catalytic
iodination (18,19). After washing, the cells were lysed with
the nonionic detergent, Nonidet P40 and ultracentrifuged. The
supernatant was dialyzed and then analyzed by sequential
immunoprecipitations followed by SDS-acrylamide gel electrophoresis. An initial non-specific precipitation was performed by adding normal rabbit immunoglobulin (Ig) followed by an
equivalence amount of sheep anti-rabbit Ig. We then added
rabbit anti-guinea pig Ig followed by sheep anti-rabbit Ig to
precipitate surface Ig. This precipitate was extensively
washed, reduced, dissolved in sodium dodecyl sulfate (SDS)
and electrophoresed on an SDS-acrylamide gel. We routinely
observe peaks consistent with μ chain, γ chain and L chain in
such precipitates, as would be anticipated from surface
immunofluorescence studies of guinea pig lymph node cells
(20). To the remaining supernatant, we add a 2 anti-13 antibody and precipitate this with rabbit anti-guinea pig Ig.
Upon analysis as above no radioactive peak is observed (Fig.
1), as expected since the strain 2 lymphocytes lack the 13
antigen and surface immunoglobulin had been completely removed during the first precipitation step. The next precipitation involves the addition of anti-2 antibody to the supernatant followed by precipitation with anti-Ig. When this
precipitate is dissolved and analyzed (Fig. 1), a single
radioactive peak with an apparent molecular weight of approximately 25,000 Daltons is found.

The final treatment of the extract of strain 2 lymph
node cells is the addition of an anti-B serum followed by
anti-Ig. This specific precipitate when run on SDS-acrylamide gel reveals a large peak with a molecular weight of
∿ 45,000 Daltons (Fig. 1). In addition, a second peak of
smaller magnitude with an apparent molecular weight of
∿ 11,000 Daltons is consistently observed. This latter peak
may be the guinea pig analog of the low molecular weight
polypeptide chain found in HL-A antigens of humans (21-23).

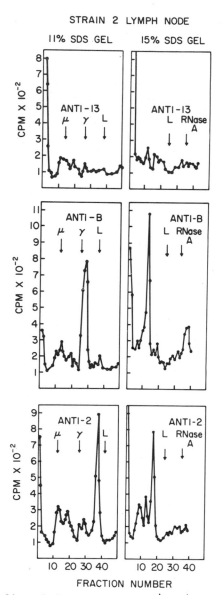

Fig. 1.   Sodium dodecyl sulfate (SDS)-polyacrylamide gel electrophoresis of immune precipitates of NP-40 extracts of ^{125}I-labelled strain 2 lymph node cells.   The direction of migration is from left to right.   The positions of a group of molecular weight markers, μ chain, γ chain, L chain and Rnase A, are indicated by arrows.   The precipitates were analyzed on both 11% and 15% gels using the Laemmli system.   The antiserum used for each analysis is indicated.

187

Evidence has been presented that the low molecular weight
HL-A associated chain of humans is either identical, or very
similar, to β2 microglobulin (21,23,24).

Several interesting points concerning the B and 2 antigens may be noted. Firstly, they appear to be on separate
molecules, as shown by their independent precipitation behavior and by experiments demonstrating independent "capping"
of B and 2 on the cell surface. Secondly, anti-2 serum is a
powerful inhibitor of lymphocyte activation by antigens the
response to which is controlled by 2-linked Ir genes while
anti-B serum, thus far, has not displayed such activity.
Thirdly, the 2 antigen is expressed principally on lymphocytes and macrophages. We are unable to detect it on several
tumor cells including a viral-induced sarcoma and two chemical carcinogen-induced hepatomas. B can be found on these
tumor lines and thus appears to have a wider tissue distribution than 2. Fourthly, the 2 antigen is smaller than B and
than both the D and K series H-2 antigens (25) and the LA and
Four series of HL-A antigens (22,26). In addition, we have
not yet detected a low molecular weight chain in association
with 2, while this is routinely found with both B and HLA
antigens. This data raises the possibility that the B, C, D
series of antigens may be the guinea pig analog of the D
and/or K H-2 antigens of mice and the LA and/or Four antigens
of humans. The 2/13 antigens may prove to be more analogous
to the recently described Ia antigens of mice (27-30). These
antigens are coded for in the Ir region of the H-2 complex,
appear to have a more limited tissue distribution than the D
and K antigens and initial molecular weight studies indicate
a value of ∿ 25,000-30,000 Daltons (31).

The precise function of the Ir gene product is still uncertain. The fact that it confers upon the animal the capacity to respond to individual antigens or limited sets of
antigens implies a specific function in antigen-recognition.
The simplest hypothesis would be that the Ir gene product,
probably acting as a molecular complex with the alloantigens
coded for at the 2/13 locus, functions as the antigen-binding
receptor of the T cell. In this model, the Ir gene product
would, most likely, be the antigen-recognition portion of the
complex and the alloantigen would be a constant portion of
the complex, presumably involved in biologic functions such
as cellular interactions. An interesting analogy to immunoglobulin genetics and structure may be drawn in which the
2/13 genes are comparable to the IgC$_H$ genes and specify constant region structures which may be associated with any of
a large series of the products of linked Ir genes, the latter
analogous to IgV$_H$ genes. Indeed, the analogy may be pushed

somewhat further. One might postulate that both immunoglobulin constant and variable region genes and the genes coding for Ir gene products and 2/13 alloantigens might derive from a primordial recognition gene. This would allow a unified system of antigen recognition and yet account for the apparent distinctness of many aspects of antigen recognition by B and T lymphocytes.

Alternatively, the Ir gene product may play an auxillary role in aiding the binding and/or "processing" of antigen, or in determining the capacity of the antigen to activate the cell. As such it may be expressed exclusively on T cells or on macrophages, T lymphocytes and B lymphocytes. The latter might serve to explain the need for sharing of histocompatibility complex-determined surface structures in both macrophage-T cell (2) and T cell-B cell interactions (3). In either case, Ir gene products play a crucial role in the process of antigen-recognition and cell activation. A complete evaluation of their mode of function and of their structure will provide a major advance in our capacity to manipulate these important phenomena.

REFERENCES

1. H.O. McDevitt and M. Landy (editors). Genetic Control of Immune Responsiveness. Academic Press, New York, 1972, p. 1.
2. E.M. Shevach and A.S. Rosenthal, J. Exp. Med., 138, 1213, (1973).
3. D.H. Katz, T. Hamaoka and B. Benacerraf, J. Exp. Med., 137, 1405 (1973).
4. L. Ellman, I. Green, W.J. Martin and B. Benacerraf, Proc. Natl. Acad. Sci., U.S.A., 66, 322 (1970).
5. H.G. Bluestein, L. Ellman, I. Green and B. Benacerraf, J. Exp. Med. 134, 1259 (1971).
6. A.S. Rosenthal, D.L. Rosenstreich, J.M. Davie and J.T. Blake, Proceedings of the Sixth Leukocyte Culture Conference, Academic Press, N.Y., 1972, p. 433.
7. D.L. Rosenstreich, J.T. Blake and A.S. Rosenthal, J. Exp. Med., 134, 1170 (1971).
8. E.M. Shevach, W.E. Paul and I. Green, J. Exp. Med. 136, 1207 (1972).
9. S.Z. Ben-Sasson, E.M. Shevach, W.E. Paul and I. Green, Manuscript in preparation.
10. T. Yoshida, H. Sonozaki and S. Cohen, J. Exp. Med. 138, 784, (1973).
11. I. Green, W.E. Paul and B. Benacerraf, J. Immunol. 109, 457 (1972).

12. S.Z. Ben-Sasson, E.M. Shevach, I.Green and W.E. Paul, manuscript in preparation.
13. R.E. Rocklin, J. Immunol. 110, 674 (1973).
14. E.M. Shevach, L. Lee, S. Pickeral and I. Green, manuscript in preparation.
15. E.M. Shevach, I. Green and W.E. Paul, J. Exp. Med. 139, 679 (1974).
16. W. Sato and A.L. deWeck, Z. Immunitaetsforsch., Allerg. Klin. Immunol., 144, S.49 (1973).
17. E. M. Shevach, unpublished observations.
18. D.R. Phillips and M. Morrison, Biochem. Biophys. Res. Commun. 40, 284 (1970).
19. E.S. Vitetta, S. Baur and J.W. Uhr, J. Exp. Med. 134, 242 (1971).
20. J.M. Davie, W.E. Paul, R. Asofsky and R.W. Warren, J. Immunol. In press.
21. K. Nakamuro, N. Tanigaki and D. Pressman, Proc. Natl. Acad. Sci., U.S.A., 70, 2863 (1973).
22. P. Cresswell, M.J. Turner and J.L. Strominger, Proc. Natl. Acad. Sci, U.S.A., 70, 1603 (1973).
23. P.A. Peterson, L. Rask and J.B. Lindblom, Proc. Natl. Acad. Sci., U.S.A., 71, 35 (1974).
24. H.M. Grey, R.T. Kubo, S.M. Colon, M.D. Poulik, P. Cresswell, T. Springer, M. Turner and J.L. Strominger, J. Exp. Med. 138, 1608 (1973).
25. B.D. Schwartz, K. Kato, S.E. Cullen and S.G. Nathenson, Biochemistry 12, 2157 (1973).
26. D. Snary, P. Goodfellow, M.J. Hayman, W.F. Bodmer and M.J. Crumpton, Nature, 247, 461 (1974).
27. V.D. Hauptfeld, D. Klein and J. Klein, Science, 181, 167 (1973).
28. D. H. Sachs and J. L. Cone, J. Exp. Med., 138, 1289, (1973).
29. C.S. David, D.C. Shreffler and J.A. Frelinger, Proc. Natl. Acad. Sci., U.S.A., 70, 2509 (1973).
30. G. Hammerling and H.O. McDevitt, Immunogenetics, In press.
31. S.E. Cullen, C.S. David, D.C. Shreffler and S.G. Nathenson, Proc. Natl. Acad. Sci. U.S.A., in press.

FURTHER CHARACTERIZATION OF Ia (IMMUNE RESPONSE REGION ASSOCIATED) ANTIGEN MOLECULES

Susan E. Cullen and Stanley G. Nathenson
Department of Microbiology and Immunology
and Cell Biology
Albert Einstein College of Medicine
Bronx, New York 10461

ABSTRACT. An earlier report (Cullen, S. E., David, C. S., Shreffler, D. C. and Nathenson, S. G., P.N.A.S., 1974, in press) has shown that antisera raised between H-2 identical, I-S region non-identical mouse strain pairs (anti Ia antisera) can be used to isolate Ia (I region associated) antigen molecules from spleen cells solubilized by the non-ionic detergent NP-40. These Ia antigen molecules are probably glycoproteins since they can be radiolabeled with monosaccharide precursors. The evidence for multiple Ia antigen molecules determined by single haplotypes has been strengthened by the finding that haplotype a (strain B10.A) has at least two populations of Ia molecules. Physical and chemical heterogeneity among serologically different Ia molecules is suggested, but not yet adequately proven.

INTRODUCTION

Recombinant mouse strain pairs are now available which differ in the central portion of the major histocompatibility complex (MHC), but are identical in the two H-2 genes (H-2K and H-2D) which map at the outer ends of the MHC region (Table 1). The K and D genes determine antigen molecules which are considered to be the major transplantation antigens. By eliminating differences between the K and D genes, the new recombinant pairs may provide the means of investigating the other functions of the MHC (1).

It has been found by several groups (2,3,4,5,6) that the chromosomal segment between K and D, which includes the I and S regions,[1] determines lymphocyte antigens (Ia; I region associated antigens) which induce the production of cytotoxic antibodies. The function of the Ia antigens is still in the realm of speculation, but they could be related

---

[1]The nomenclature used in this paper follows the recommendations of the Nomenclature Committee, Bar Harbor Workshop 1973, Immunogenetics, in press.

TABLE 1

Description of H-2 Identical, I-S Region Non-identical Strain Pairs

Strain	Haplotypes[a] in F$_1$	Resultant[a] haplotype	F$_1$ MHC[a] with probable crossover site				Resultant MHC[a]			
			K	I	S	D	K	I	S	D
A.TH	a/s	t2(th)	k/s	k/s	d/s ↗	d/s	s	s	s	d
A.TL	a1(aℓ)/s	t1(tℓ)	k/s ↖	k/s	k/s	d/s	s	k	k	d
B10.AQR	a/q	y1(y-Klj)	k/q ↖	k/q	d/q	d/q	q	k	d	d
B10.T(6R)	a/q	y2(y-Sg)	k/q	k/q ↖	d/q	d/q	q	q	q	d

[a]Haplotype designations and MHC region designations according to recommendations of Nomenclature Committee, Bar Harbor Workshop 1973 (Immunogenetics, in press). Old haplotype designations in parentheses.

to a known MHC function such as control of immune response, mixed lymphocyte reactivity, or graft vs host reactivity. The I region has been most strongly implicated in all of these functions. The Ia antigens could also be another in the series of histocompatibility antigens, or could be associated with genetic traits as yet undiscovered.

The purpose of our study has been to use the anti Ia antisera to isolate the Ia antigen molecules as an aid in genetic and serological analysis and ultimately to structurally characterize these important molecules.

MATERIALS AND METHODS

Antisera. Anti Ia antisera were provided by C. S. David and D. C. Shreffler. They include A.TH anti A.TL (I^s anti I^k, (A.TH x B10)F_1 anti A.TL ((I^s x I^b) anti I^k), and A.TH x B10.D2)F_1 anti A.TL ((I^s x I^d) anti I^k).

Antigen. Spleen cells were radiolabeled with radioactive amino acid or monosaccharide precursors by short term incubation in vitro. Conditions for amino acid labeling: 2×10^7 spleen cells/ml incubated for 5 hours at 37°C in 5% CO_2 in leucine deficient, glutamine supplemented modified Eagle's minimum essential medium (MEM) with 50-100 μCi/ml ^{3}H-leucine or 5-10 μCi/ml ^{14}C-leucine (50-100 Ci/mmol and about 250 mCi/mmol respectively, New England Nuclear Corp.).

Conditions for monosaccharide labeling: 2×10^7 spleen cells/ml were incubated for 5 hours at 37°C in 5% CO_2 in glutamine supplemented MEM with 50-100 μCi/ml ^{3}H-fucose, ^{3}H-mannose, ^{3}H-galactose, or ^{3}H-N-acetylglucosamine. (^{3}H-mannose; Amersham, about 2 Ci/mmol, all others; New England Nuclear Corp., about 5 Ci/mmol.

After labeling, the cells were solubilized by the nonionic detergent Non-Idet P-40 (NP-40, Shell Chemical Co., Ltd.) as previously described (7). 2×10^8 cells were suspended in 0.15 M NaCl, 0.01 M Tris-Cl pH 7.4, 0.5% NP-40, and kept on ice for 30 minutes. After this solubilization step, the suspension was centrifuged at 100,000 x g for one hour to remove nuclei, debris and insoluble material. Supernatants could be stored at -80°C.

Assay. Indirect immune precipitation was used as described earlier (7,8) to isolate antigen molecules. Solubilized radiolabeled spleen cell supernatants were

193

pretreated to remove radiolabeled immunoglobulins synthesized during the labeling period in order to prevent interference with subsequent analysis of Ia molecules. Pretreatment consisted of mixing the antigen preparation with normal mouse serum and goat anti mouse IgG. By this procedure, the radiolabeled IgG was precipitated with the carrier IgG in the normal mouse serum. After pretreatment, the antigen preparations were tested for reactivity with anti Ia antiserum by indirect precipitation, again using goat anti mouse IgG. Appropriate controls for non-specific precipitation were included. Anti Ia antiserum was titrated and used in excess when necessary. Goat anti mouse IgG was used at equivalence with each mouse antiserum.

Immune precipitates were further examined by dissolving them in 2% sodium dodecyl sulfate (SDS) and 2% 2-mercapto-ethanol. The dissolved precipitates were subjected to electrophoresis on 10% polyacrylamide-SDS gels using a modified Maizel system (9,7). Gels were sliced and counted using a Protosol-Omnifluor-Toluene cocktail (Protosol and Omnifluor, New England Nuclear Corp.) in a Beckman LS-250 scintillation counter.

RESULTS

Structure and composition. Preliminary results with the antisera A.TH anti A.TL and A.TL anti A.TH have been previously reported (8). Precipitates formed by specific reaction with these antisera and appropriate ^{3}H-leucine labeled antigens were dissolved in 2% SDS and electrophoresed. For example, gel electrophoresis of precipitates made with an $\underline{I}^k$ anti $\underline{I}^s$ antiserum and ^{3}H-leucine labeled B10.S ($\underline{I}^s$) antigen showed the presence of two peaks. When compared to ^{14}C-immunoglobulin H and L chains, these peaks had molecular weights in the range of 60,000 and 30,000. The 60,000 molecular weight species was isolated by gel filtration on BioGel 1.5 m in 0.05 M Tris-Cl pH 7.4, 0.5% SDS, and analyzed by polyacrylamide gel electrophoresis. Electrophoresis in SDS alone showed the expected 60,000 molecular weight peak, but electrophoresis in SDS and 2-mercaptoethanol showed a peak of about 30,000. This suggested that the 60,000 molecular weight material was composed of two polypeptide chains similar in molecular weight joined by disulfide bonding.

The Ia molecules are clearly differentiable from H-2 molecules by several criteria; a) the genetic region determining Ia is separable from the regions determining H-2 antigens by recombination (2,3); b) the tissue distribution of Ia antigens is much narrower than that of H-2 (3); c) the molecular weights of Ia and H-2 in strongly dissociating and reducing conditions (SDS and 2-mercaptoethanol) are different (8); d) when H-2K and H-2D molecules are removed from labeled spleen cell antigen preparations by indirect precipitation, the material remaining unprecipitated contains the Ia antigens (8).

Attempts to label the Ia antigens with radiolabeled monosaccharide precursors did not always meet with success, but we were finally able to show that ^{3}H-fucose, ^{3}H-mannose, ^{3}H-galactose and ^{3}H-glucosamine were all incorporated into specifically precipitable molecules which migrated in the 30,000 molecular weight region of SDS gels under reducing conditions. Figure 1 shows several such results using preparations of NP-40 solubilized B10.D2 spleen cell extracts radiolabeled with ^{3}H-mannose or ^{3}H-fucose and precipitated with the antiserum $\underline{I}^s$ anti $\underline{I}^k$. Precipitates were dissolved in SDS, reduced, and electrophoresed on SDS-polyacrylamide gels. Panels (a) and (b) show that mannose and fucose are incorporated into specific peaks which migrate between the ^{14}C-labeled H and L chain markers in the region of about 30,000 molecular weight.

The reaction of a double labeled (^{3}H-mannose, ^{14}C-leucine) preparation with the specific antiserum (c) shows that both labels peak in the 30,000 molecular weight range. These peaks seem to be partially non-coincident, which could be due to the presence of several different molecular species with different mannose/leucine incorporation ratios. Positions of the ^{14}C-labeled H and L chain markers in this case is inferred from the result shown in panel (a). Panel (d) shows absence of radiolabel when control serum was used to make the precipitate. Results similar to (a) and (b) were seen when ^{3}H-galactose and ^{3}H-N-acetyl glucosamine were used.

Demonstration that several antigen molecules exist in one haplotype. The data obtained by David et al., and David and Shreffler (3,11) on strain specificity of anti Ia sera in cytotoxicity tests were exactly reproduced using the indirect immune precipitation test (8). In the previous paper it was also observed that extracts of strain B10.HTT reacted with both $\underline{I}^s$ anti $\underline{I}^k$ and $\underline{I}^k$ anti $\underline{I}^s$ antisera (8). We were able to show by indirect immune

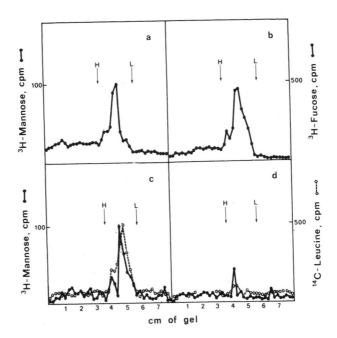

Figure 1. Electrophoresis of reduced immune precipitates made with NP-40 solubilized extracts of B10.D2 spleen
cells labeled with (a) ^{3}H-mannose, (b) ^{3}H-fucose, (c,d) ^{3}H-
mannose and ^{14}C-leucine. The specific anti Ia antiserum $\underline{I}$
anti $\underline{I}^k$ was used to make the precipitates in (a,b,c), and
all three panels show peaks in the 30,000 molecular weight
range. Normal mouse serum was used for the control precipitate shown in panel (d). ^{14}C- labeled H and L chain markers
were coelectrophoresed with precipitates (a) and (b), but
their positions are inferred for panels (c) and (d).

precipitation that the antigenic determinants detected by these two different sera were found on different antigen molecules. Thus it was concluded that there could be more than one Ia molecule determined by a single haplotype.

We decided to examine a further case using the strain B10.A as an antigen source. It had been noted (3) that several antibody populations existed in the antiserum I^s anti I^k. This antiserum reacted with I^k strains, and also with I^b and I^d strains. Absorption of the serum with I^b strain cells left reactivity for I^d and I^k strains. Absorption with I^d strain cells left reactivity with I^b and I^k. The sera $(I^s \times I^b)$ anti I^k and $(I^s \times I^d)$ anti I^k were then raised and showed expected reactivity with respect to I^b, I^d and I^k strains.

We wished to use these sera to determine whether there were a number of separable antigen molecules, or if there was a single antigen molecule bearing multiple determinants. The antigen source, B10.A (I^k), was tested and found to be reactive with these sera. The antigen extract was then divided in 4 aliquots and mixed with normal mouse serum or with amounts of the three anti Ia sera determined to give antibody excess. Precipitates were made, and the supernatants were retained and subdivided in 4 aliquots, each of which was reacted with the normal control serum and the three antisera. These second round precipitates were analyzed on SDS polyacrylamide gels under reducing conditions, and the results are presented in Figure 2. It is clear that the two antisera, $(I^s \times I^b)$ anti I^k and $(I^s \times I^d)$ anti I^k are reactive with different molecules because the removal by precipitation of antigen molecules reactive with one serum does not clear molecules reactive with the other serum. It is also apparent that the serum I^s anti I^k includes antibodies reactive with both of these antigen molecules.

DISCUSSION

Although these studies are still in a very preliminary stage, several facts concerning Ia antigens have emerged. Like the H-2 molecules to which they are so closely linked genetically, at least some of the Ia antigen are glycoprotein molecules, and they have been shown to be associated with the surface membrane (8).

On the other hand, Ia antigens (about 30,000 molecular weight) are smaller than the H-2 antigens (about 45,000

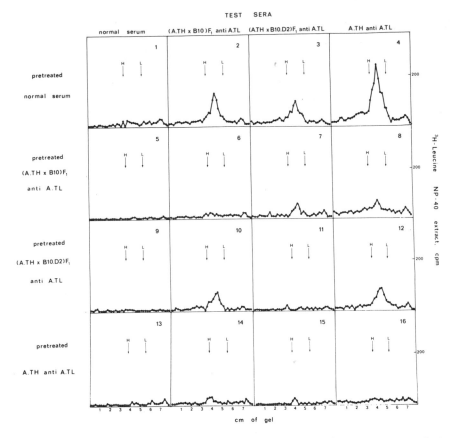

Figure 2. Electrophoresis of reduced immune precipitates from the second round of the sequential precipitation experiment (see text). The first row (1-4) shows the positive reaction patterns for the antisera after a pretreatment step using control normal mouse serum. All test sera are positive. The second row (5-8) shows the reaction pattern after precipitation with $(\underline{I}^s \times \underline{I}^b)$ anti $\underline{I}^k$. Frame 6 shows that the antigen molecule reactive with this serum has been completely removed while the other two sera are still positive (7,8). Row three (9-12) shows that after preprecipitation with $(\underline{I}^s \times \underline{I}^d)$ anti $\underline{I}^k$, all antigen molecules reactive with that serum are removed (11) whereas the other two sera (10,12) remain positive. Row 4 (13-16) shows that the antiserum $(\underline{I}^s$ anti $\underline{I}^k$ removes molecules reactive with all three sera (14,15,16). Thus the antisera $(\underline{I}^s \times \underline{I}^b)$ anti $\underline{I}^k$ and $(\underline{I}^s \times \underline{I}^d)$ anti $\underline{I}^k$ react with different populations of Ia molecules, and the antiserum $\underline{I}^s$ anti $\underline{I}^k$ includes antibodies reacting with both populations.

198

molecular weight). The tissue distribution of H-2 and Ia antigens have also been shown to differ (3) and the two types of antigens are separable genetically and serologically.

Immunization between strains differing in the I region of the MHC can result in the production of sera reacting with several different antigenic determinants (3,11), and these sera have been used to show that at least two Ia molecules are determined by haplotype t3 of the strain B10.HTT (8) and by haplotype a of the strain B10.A. So far no two antigenic determinants have been shown to be present on the same Ia molecule, but this possibility has not been ruled out.

In addition to the serological differences between Ia antigen molecules, there is probably some heterogeneity in size and composition of the molecules bearing the Ia antigenic specificities. This supposition is suggested by two observations: 1) the generally broad character and occasional shoulders of the Ia profile observed in most polyacrylamide-SDS gel patterns suggests multiple molecules of different molecular sizes; 2) the lack of coincidence of monosaccharide and amino acid label (cf. Figure 1) may indicate that some molecules might contain different monosaccharides or different amounts of carbohydrate.

Thus it is clear that an understanding of the molecular complexity which is suggested by these preliminary observations is a major problem to be resolved in order to fully comprehend the genetic and functional properties of the Ia antigen system. Toward this end studies on the physical and immunochemical properties of the entities bearing the Ia antigenic sites are being actively pursued.

ACKNOWLEDGMENTS

This research was supported by Grants AI-07289 and AI-10702 from the United States Public Health Service. S.E.C. is a Fellow of the Leukemia Society of America.

REFERENCES

1. Demant, P., Transpl. Rev. 15, 162-200 (1973).
2. Hauptfeld, V., D. Klein and J. Klein, Science 181, 167-169 (1973).

3. David, C. S., D. C. Shreffler and J. A. Frelinger, Proc. Nat. Acad. Sci. U.S. 70, 2509-2514 (1973).
4. Sachs, D. H. and J. L. Cone, J. Exp. Med. 139, 1289-1304 (1973).
5. Götze, D., R. A. Reisfeld and J. Klein, J. Exp. Med. 138, 1003-1008 (1973).
6. Hämmerling, G. J., B. D. Deak, G. Mauve, U. Hämmerling and H. O. McDevitt, Immunogenetics, in press.
7. Schwartz, B. D. and S. G. Nathenson, J. Immunol. 107, 1363-1367 (1971).
8. Cullen, S. E., C. S. David, D. C. Shreffler and S. G. Nathenson, Proc. Nat. Acad. Sci. U.S., in press.
9. Shapiro, A. L., E. Venuela and J. V. Maizel, Jr., Biochem. Biophys. Res. Commun. 28, 815-820 (1967).
10. Muramatsu, T. and S. G. Nathenson, Biochemistry 9, 4875-4883 (1970).
11. David, C. S. and D. C. Shreffler, Transplantation, in press.

RECEPTORS FOR ANTIGEN ON "B, T, B-T AND NUL" LYMPHOCYTES IN NORMAL AND "NUDE" MICE

by
Francis Loor and Georges E. Roelants
Basel Institute for Immunology, CH-4058 Basel, Switzerland.

List of abbreviations:
α: anti; ABC: antigen-binding cell; BSA: bovine serum albumin FCS: fetal calf serum; FITC: fluoresceine isothiocyanate-conjugated; M: mouse; N: normal; R: rabbit; S: sheep; TIGAL: heavily iodinated (T,G)-A--L; TMV: Tobacco mosaic virus; TRITC: tetramethylrhodamine isothiocyanate-conjugated; θ: Thy 1.1 or Thy 1.2 determined antigen; θB: θ antigen when detected by the R antibody.

ABSTRACT.   A rabbit anti-mouse θ reagent was made specific by absorbtion in nude mice in vivo. When used in double fluorescence with anti-Ig reagent it allows the recognition of 4 lymphocyte types: $Ig^+\theta^-$, $Ig^-\theta^+$, $Ig^-\theta^-$, $Ig^+\theta^+$. In nude mice spleen more than 20% of the lymphocytes are of T lineage. Antigen binding receptors are found among all cell types.

By using combined autoradiography for ^{125}I-antigen and fluorescence for surface Ig and θ it is found that prior anti-Ig treatment induces the polar redistribution of receptors for antigen on both B and T cells followed by their removal from the cell surface. When put in culture for a few hours, both B and T cells are able to bind antigen again and the receptors are again cleared by anti-Ig. These results show that both B and T cells synthesize their Ig receptors for antigen.

INTRODUCTION

Two major types of arguments have frequently been used against the existence of antigen-binding T lymphocytes, (a) the lack of their detection in normal mice (1), and (b) the finding that spleen from congenitally athymic (nude) mice is not deficient in antigen binding cells (ABC) "though they lack T cells" (2).

The first type of argument was controversial since some authors found T-ABC, although usually in lower numbers than B-ABC (3, reviewed in 4). It was recently shown that

201

provided the dose of antigen is high enough, T cells are able to bind, at saturation, as much antigen as B cells, but that the binding was more dependent on the antigen concentration (5).

ABC are not diminished in nude mice but it was recently shown that the peripheral lymphoid organs of these mice have a few T cells (1,6) and also precursors for T cells (7,8). These precursors can repopulate a grafted allogeneic thymus (8), migrate to other lymphoid organs (8) and exert T lymphocyte functions (9).

It is generally admitted that receptors for antigen on B cells are Ig but it has been suggested by some authors that T cell receptors are of different nature (10). This question is still controversial.

We present data showing on the one hand that antigen receptors on T cells are immunoglobulins,most probably synthesized by the T cells themselves, and on the other hand that in nude mice, ABC are also found among cells of the T lineage, i.e. T precursors before their passage through the thymus or T cells following an abnormal differentiation pathway because of lack of thymus.

MATERIALS AND METHODS

Our general procedures are schematised in the following figures: Fig. 1: preparation and absorbtion in vivo of rabbit IgG with anti-mouse brain θ antigen activity (RIgG-α-MθB); Fig. 2: double labelling of the cells for θ and θB; Fig. 3: double labelling of the cells for membrane Ig and θB; Fig. 4: triple labelling of the cells for membrane Ig, θB and radioactive antigen; Fig. 5: the detection of Ag receptors on T and B cells, their polar redistribution by anti-Ig reagents and their resynthesis in culture. The preparation of fluorescent antibodies and the specificity controls, the capping and cell culture procedures, and the fluorescence microscopy techniques, have been described in detail (3,5,8, 11,12).

RESULTS

1. In the nude spleen, TIGAL-binding lymphocytes are also of T lineage

When stained with fluorescent anti-mouse Ig reagents, as many as 40% nude mouse spleen lymphocytes appear to lack easily detectable membrane immunoglobulins. When stained with fluorescent anti-θ alloantibodies only 1-2% show clear membrane fluorescence, but up to 20% show a vague membrane fluorescence which suggests that these cells are of T lineage though they express only a low density of θ antigen.

The rabbit anti-mouse brain θ reagent (RIgG-α-MθB), prepared as described in Fig. 1, allows a better identification of the latter cells. First, the RIgG-α-MθB can be used in conjunction with α-MIg reagent for double staining for T and B markers (see Fig. 3). Second, it can be used in indirect immunofluorescence, which amplifies the detection of the θ antigen. Being themselves mouse Ig, α-θ alloantibodies cannot of course be used in similar ways.

Our main specificity controls for the detection of cells of T lineage by the RIgG-α-MθB are as follows: this antibody binds to the same cells as α-θ alloantibodies when double staining for θ and θB is performed (see Fig. 2); preincubation of the cells, both from normal and from nude mice with α-θ alloantibodies can virtually block further binding of RIgG-α-MθB; when double staining for Ig and θB markers is performed on spleen or lymph node cells from normal mice (Fig. 3), Ig and θB markers are found mostly on different cell populations (Table I).

Table I shows the distribution of cells having the Ig and/or θB markers in spleen and lymph nodes from normal and nude mice. Results are presented as mean (range) from 7 individual normal mice (5 BALB/c, 2 NMRI) and from 7 individual nude mice (5 BALB/c-nu, 2 NMRI-nu). Controls performed with NRIgG (also absorbed in vivo) instead of RIgG-α-MθB did not show any significant binding of NRIgG (less than 0.1%) except in the case of one NMRI and of one NMRI nude. These values are incorporated in the table.

Lymph node and spleen from normal and nude mice have also

been exposed to ^{125}I-TIGAL prior to double staining for Ig and θB (see Fig. 4). TIGAL binding cells can be found in each of the four cell types: typical B cells (positive for Ig only) typical T cells (positive for θB only), as well as double positive and double negative cells, though no data are yet available to quantitate their frequency.

2. T cell receptors for TIGAL are T cell made immunoglob-ulins

The experimental design is as described in Fig. 5. Our findings are schematically represented in Fig. 6 and a sample is given in Table II.

Lymph node lymphocytes from non-immunized mice which bind ^{125}I-TIGAL were classified as T ($θ^+$ or Ig$^-$) and B ($θ^-$ or Ig$^+$) cells, by use of specific fluorochrome-conjugated reagents. Pretreatment of the lymphocytes with non-inhibitory doses (3) of fluorescent anti-Ig prior to TIGAL induces a redistribution of the TIGAL binding as caps, which follows the capping of the detectable membrane Ig on B cells, but leaves unaffected the distribution of θ antigen on T cells. After 1 hr, B- or T-TIGAL binding cells were no longer detected. Antigen binding by both B and T cells and detectable membrane Ig on B cells simultaneously reappear as early as 3 hours only after capping, though sometimes complete resynthesis requires 12-18 hours. If these cells are again treated by the anti-mouse Ig reagent, the Ag receptors are again redistributed as caps, on both B and T cells, and later disappear, with again the same kinetics as the capping and endocytosis of detectable membrane Ig on B cells.

DISCUSSION

The data presented here show that cells of the T lineage exist in large numbers in nude mice and already express receptors for antigen without thymic influence. Moreover, they strongly argue for the immunoglobulin nature of the receptors on B and T cells.

Nude mouse lymphocytes can no longer be used as a source of pure B cells. Indeed, by use of the in vivo absorbed RIgG-α-MθB which binds to the same cells and probably to the same determinant as α-θ alloantibodies, one can demonstrate that a large fraction of nude spleen lymphocytes are of T lineage. Some other cells lack detectable amounts of both Ig and θ markers, some others have both. The former cells could be immature lymphocytes which have not yet differentiated, i.e. are not yet committed to follow a B or T pathway, or that have not yet expressed their differentiation antigens in detectable amounts. Their higher proportion in nudes than in normal mice is not necessarily an argument for them pertaining to the T lineage. The maturation of all lymphocytes in nude mice, both T and B, might be retarded and their migration patterns altered. Double negative cells have already been described (13), but their belonging to the T lineage was rejected because it was assumed that the only cells of T lineage homing in the spleen were coming from the thymus. It was not at all considered that the spleen might be the usual transit pathway of the T precursors coming from the bone marrow, which would then result in their accumulation in the spleen of thymectomized animals.

The significance of the latter cells, the double positive, is difficult to evaluate: they could be cells of T lineage with passively adsorbed membrane Ig, cells of B lineage with Fc receptors picking up our RIgG-α-MθB (though this could be excluded as a major cause as NRIgG is usually not picked up), or cells actually synthesizing both θB and Ig markers. These double positive cells are also more frequent in nudes than in normal mice. Among various interpretations, one could suggest they are cells of T lineage following an abnormal differentiation pathway because of lack of a thymus (turning back to a B function?) , or actual precursor cells with still both pathways of differentiation open.

Finally, other likely candidates for the T cell precursors are the cells identified as T cells by the RIgG-α-MθB but not or very hardly by α-θ alloantibodies (though they seem to bind to the same determinant). When analysed by free flow electrophoresis, these cells band at a position different from typical mature T cells (G.E. Roelants, F. Loor, H. von Boehmer, unpublished). These cells, which can probably be characterized as having a low density of θ antigen, were also present in larger amounts in nudes.

All these 4 cell types were found to bind TIGAL, which shows that the lack of thymus does not impede the expression of receptors for antigen by cells of the T lineage, even not

fully differentiated. In the normal mouse, and though no pre
-cise quantitation has been made so far, the majority of the
TIGAL binding cells was found among the single positive cells,
i.e. the typical B and typical T cells. Thus, the finding of
the Ag binding by some double positive or double negative
cells does not significantly affect the interpretation of results obtained previously by classifying B cells as Ig^+ or
θ^- and T cells as Ig^- or θ^+. Both the Ig and θ classification were routinely done and gave identical results.

In normal, unprimed mice, TIGAL-binding lymphocytes are
rare cells: in the study presented here, 0.10% of the lymph
node lymphocytes examined. In the whole cell population,
there were 17% B cells (Ig^+ or θ^-) and 83% T cells (Ig^- or θ^-
). About 2/3 of the TIGAL binding cells were B cells and
1/3 were T cells, which represents 0.41% of the total B cells
and 0.03% of the total T cells. These percentages of ABC fit
well with the plateau levels found for TIGAL binding B and
T cells by Roelants and Rydén in an independent study (5).

Pretreatment of the cell suspension by non-blocking doses
of α-MIg antibody first redistributes the antigen receptors as
caps, which later disappear from the cell surface. When the
cells are put in culture, the antigen binding capacity starts
to reappear as ea_ly as 3 hours only after the capping,
though maximal recovery is usually completed by 12-18 hours
only. At this point, a new treatment with α-MIg antibody
will again induce the Ag receptors to cap and disappear.
Ag receptor capping, disappearance, reappearance and recapping on B and T cells follow the same general kinetics as the
capping, endocytosis, resynthesis, recapping of detectable
membrane Ig on B cells. This strongly suggests that membrane
Ig are responsible for Ag binding on both B and T cells.

Since only rare T cells can bind TIGAL, some of them
binding as many as 50,000 molecules (5), it is rather unlikely that the binding occurs via cytophilic antibody of B
cell origin; indeed one should not expect the concentration
of such antibody on rare T cells only. Moreover, the data
presented here show recovery of Ag binding capacity by the T
cells after capping, and it is still less likely that the
few TIGAL binding B cells present in this population of
normal lymph node cells would have synthesised or shed, during the time of culture anti-TIGAL Ig that would stick again

to very rare T cells and just the same number than before capping. One would then have to postulate that B cell-derived α-TIGAL Ig would be selectively taken up by those rare T cells only. In this respect, it is essential to remember that in our experimental design, the cells can see TIGAL, only after all the steps of α-Ig antibody treatment and never before. Thus, it cannot be argued that TIGAL-specific T cells were triggered by antigen, expressed Fc receptors and bound α-TIGAL antibody secreted by or shed from B cells. This also eliminates the possibility of triggering of TIGAL specific B cells during the culture period, and binding the secreted antibody to TIGAL, itself attached to non-Ig T cell receptors.

We cannot exclude that some T cells recognize an idiotype on α-TIGAL antibody of B cell origin and selectively pick them up from the culture medium. This would be expected to inhibit the antigen binding capacity and also would suppose a very high affinity for the idiotype-α-idiotype system, given the very low concentration of α-TIGAL antibodies in the culture medium. Anyhow, as far as we know, anti-idiotype recognition structures are immunoglobulin themselves.

The speculation remains that in T cell membrane cytophilic Ig of B cell origin are associated with other components including a non-Ig TIGAL receptor. This is more difficult to rule out since one could actually mount a whole set of speculations on that first one! However, we think that one can disregard these possibilities for a number of reasons. Since α-Ig antibody can remove all the T cell receptors for Ag, one would have to postulate that all T cell non-Ig receptors for Ag are associated with Ig, and all lymphocyte membrane biology known so far is against this, as no cocapping of individual membrane components has been found until now. But still, if there was nevertheless a one to one association of cytophilic Ig of B cell origin and of T cell Ag receptors, one should find some T cells with up to a few thousand molecules of adsorbed Ig, which would be easy to detect by fluorescence as for instance in the case of the macrophage membrane (14). The possibility remains that there are very few cytophilic Ig of B cell origin per cluster of T cell Ag receptors. If such a clustering exists as a native distribution of Ag receptors in the T cell membrane, then those clusters would be very selective with regard to the membrane components they include: receptors for antigen and receptors for Fc, but no θ, and no H2. Indeed α-Ig capping does not affect at all the distribution of θ or H2. If they were in the clusters, they would also constitute polymeric antigen and some capping should be induced by α-θ or α-H2, which is again not the case. Moreover, α-θ, α-H2 or a very polyspecific ALS pretreatment of the lymphocytes did not affect Ag binding (3).

These last hypotheses are highly speculative and what remains is that Ag receptors on T cells can be blocked or redistributed by α-Ig reagents, either polyspecific α-Ig, or specific α-μ and α-L chain and that this activity is lost if the α-Ig antibodies are removed from the serum by absorbtion with solid Ig (3).

It is of course intriguing that these T cell membrane Ig cannot be detected by immunofluorescence, since they can be as numerous as on some B cells, and that attempts to isolate them from the cell membrane gave such controversial results (15,16). One should keep in mind that not all T cells have to express Ig receptors. Actually there are 10 times less T cells than B cells binding TIGAL, and may be only 10% of T cells might have membrane Ig, which would decrease very much the efficiency of their biochemical isolation. Moreover, those T cells with membrane Ig might show only the useful part of it, i.e. their active sites. The absence of detection of these receptors by fluorescent reagents which can block or cap them is irrelevant to the problem of the Ig nature of those receptors. Indeed the same puzzling fact remains whether the activity of the fluorescent anti-Ig preparation is due to anti-Ig or to contaminating antibody which would also be tagged with fluorochrome. We believe that the absence of staining must be due to a peculiarity of the T cell membrane. That T cells have a different membrane from B cells is getting increasingly evident. It has been suggested that T cell Ig receptors might be partially buried due, for instance, to a more hydrophobic Fc or to a thicker, denser glycocalix. Antibodies raised in phylogenically distant species might be a tool for detecting those T cell Ig active sites as they might recognize their invariable segments as foreign (Loor, F., du Pasquier, L., Pink, J.R.L., and Roelants, G.E., manuscript in preparation).

In conclusion, T cells can bind soluble antigen, via self-made immunoglobulin receptors, but it is not excluded that other mechanisms of self-not-self recognition exist.

ACKNOWLEDGEMENTS

We thank Dr. E. Mozes for the generous gift of TGAL. This work was realized with the outstanding technical assistance of Miss Lena-Britt Hägg and Miss Aina Rydén. Francis Loor is Chercheur Qualifié Honoraire from the Belgian National Funds for Scientific Research, from which he got travel funds to attend this meeting.

REFERENCES

1. Lamelin, J.P., Lisowska-Bernstein, B., Matter, A., Ryser, J.E., and Vassali, P., J. Exp. Med. 136,984 (1972).

2. Dwyer, J.M., Mason, S., Warner, N.L., and Mackay, J.R., Nature (London) New Biol. 234,252 (1971).

3. Roelants, G.E., Forni, L., and Pernis, B., J. Exp. Med. 137,1060 (1973).

4. Roelants, G.E., C.T. Microbiol. Immun. 59,135 (1972).

5. Roelants, G.E., and Rydén, A., Nature (London) 247,104 (1974).

6. Raff, M.C., Nature (London) 246,350 (1973).

7. Pritchard, H., and Micklem, H.S., Clin. exp. Immunol. 14,597 (1973).

8. Loor, F., and Kindred, B., J. Exp. Med. 138,1044 (1973).

9. Kindred, B., and Loor, F., J. Exp. Med. in press (1974).

10. Genetic Control of Immune Responsiveness. H.O. McDevitt and M. Landy, editors. Academic Press, New York and London. pp. 205-272 (1972).

11. Loor, F., Forni, L., and Pernis, B., Eur. J. Immunol. 2, 203 (1972).

12. Roelants, G.E., Rydén, A., Hägg, L-B., and Loor, F., Nature (London) 247,106 (1974).

13. Stobo, J.D., Rosenthal, A.S., and Paul, W.E., J. Exp. Med. 138,71 (1973).

14. Loor, F., and Roelants, G.E., Submitted for publication.

15. Marchalonis, J.J., and Cone, R.E., Transplant. Rev. 14,3 (1973).

16. Vitetta, E.S. and Uhr, J.W., Transplant. Rev. 14,50 (1973).

Figure 1: Preparation of RIgG-α-MθB

1. Immunisation of rabbits with CBA/J mouse brain: 2 I.M. injections of 3 CBA/J mice brain homogenized in complete Freund's adjuvant, at 1 week interval, boost 5 months later. Bleed 2 weeks after boost.

2. Preparation of the IgG from the immune serum (and from preimmune serum as control) by repeated $(NH_4)_2SO_4$ precipitation (1.6 M, 0°C) followed by purification on DEAE-cellulose (pH 6.3, 0.0175M phosphate buffer).

3. In vivo absorption of the non-α-θ antibodies in nude mice: IP injection of 10 mg IgG/1 ml/nude mouse. Bleed out the mice 8 to 10 hours later.

4. Isolation of the filtered RIgG from the mouse serum, by the same procedure as above (step 2): most of the mouse Ig gets stuck to the DEAE, while the RIgG passes through.

5. Concentration of the RIgG-α-MθB (Diaflo membrane UM2) up to 10-20 mg/ml. Keep at $^+4$°C, in PBS + 0.5% BSA + 10 mM NaN$_3$. To be used on the cells at final concentration 250 μg/ml. NRIgG similarly prepared and absorbed as control.

Figure 2: Double labelling for θ and θB

1. $2.5.10^6$ cells in 0.1 ml medium (RPMI 1640 + 0.5% BSA + 10mM NaN$_3$ buffered with 0.03M HEPES and NaOH to pH 7.2) + 50 μg (0.1 ml) TRITC-C3H IgG-α-Thy 1.1 (or TRITC-AKR IgG-α-Thy 1.2)

1. /cont.

    15 min. at 0°C.

2. No wash
    + 50 µg (0.1 ml) RIgG-α-MθB
    15 min. at 0ºC.

3. Wash 3x. Pellet.
    + 50 µg (0.1 ml) FITC-SIgG-α-RIg.
    15 min. at 0°C.

4. Wash 3x. Pellet.
    Microscopic observation of cells in suspension and of
    smeared fixed cells.

Figure 3: Double labelling for membrane Ig and θB

1. $2.5.10^{6}$ cells in 0.1 ml (RPMI 1640 + 0.5% BSA + 10 mM
    NaN_3 buffered with 0.03M HEPES and NaOH to pH 7.2).
    + 50 µg (0.1 ml) RIgG-α-MθB (or NRIgG as control)
    30 min. at 0ºC.

2. Wash 3x. Pellet.
    + in 0.2 ml $\begin{cases} 50 \text{ µg TRITC-SIgG-α-RIg} \\ 50 \text{ µg FITC-SIgG-α-MIg.} \end{cases}$

3. Wash 3x. Pellet.
    Microscopic observation of cells in suspension and of
    smeared, fixed cells.

Figure 4: Triple labelling for membrane Ig, θB and antigen

1. Incubation of cells with ^{125}I-TIGAL (82-109 µCi/µg) at
    saturating doses for detection of antigen binding cells
    (5):
    2.5 µg TIGAL/25.10^{6} cells/ml, for 30 min, at 0°C.

2. Wash through FCS gradients.
    Resuspend in RPMI 1640 + 0.5% BSA + 10mM NaN_3, buffered
    with 0.03M HEPES and NaOH to pH 7.2.

3. Proceed for double labelling of membrane Ig and θB: as
    for Fig.3 , but smear on gelatine coated slides, fix

3. /cont.

in absolute ethanol (5 min.). Process for auotoradiography.

Figure 5: Detection, capping and resynthesis of Ag receptors

1. 50.10^6 normal lymph node cells/ml medium (RPMI 1640, 10% FCS, 2mM glutamin, 100 I.U./ml penicillin-streptomycin, buffered with 0.03M HEPES and NaOH to pH 7.2). and FITC-RIgG-α-MIg (500 μg/ml, FITC-RIgG-α-TMV as control).
Mix equal volume of cell suspension and fluorescent conjugates for 10 min at 0°C, then for 50 min at 37°C.

2. (Optional) wash 3x. Pellet.
+ Sser-α-RL 1/40 final dilution.
15 min. at 37°C.

3. Wash 3x. Pellet. Resuspend at $0.5.10^6$ cells/ml.
Samples of 4 ml are cultured at 37°C for variable lengths of time in Falcon Tissue Culture Flasks 3012.

4. Wash 2x with medium containing 1.5 mM NaN$_3$, 0°C.
+ ^{125}I-TIGAL (200-468 μCi/μg).
2.5 μg Ag/25.10^6 cells/ml.
30 min., 0°C, 1.5 mM NaN$_3$.

5. Wash through FCS gradients (0°C, 1.5 mM NaN$_3$).
Resuspend at 50.10^6 cells/ml. Divide cell samples into 2 parts A and B.
A = + TRITC-RIgG-α-MIg (500 μg/ml).
B = + TRITC-AKR IgG-α-Thy 1.2 (500 μg/ml).
Mix equal volume of cell suspension and fluorescent conjugates 30 min., 0°C. 1.5 mM NaN$_3$.

6. Wash 3x. Pellet. Smear on gelatine coated slides, fix in absolute ethanol (5 min.), process for autoradiography (Ilford K5 emulsion).

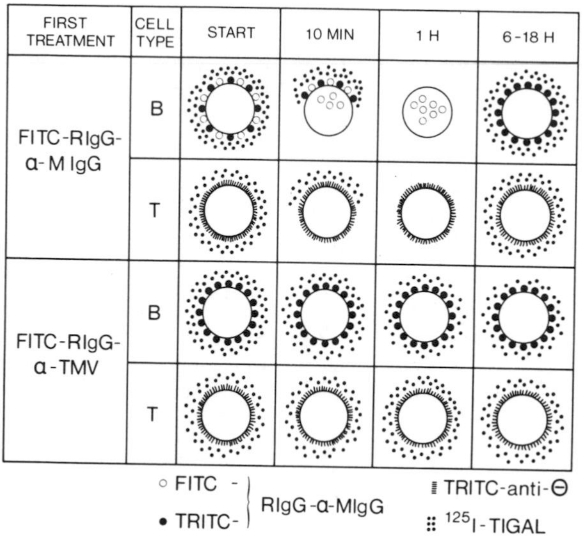

FIRST TREATMENT	CELL TYPE	START	10 MIN	1 H	6-18 H
FITC-RIgG-α-M IgG	B				
	T				
FITC-RIgG-α-TMV	B				
	T				

○ FITC -
● TRITC- } RIgG -α-MIgG

▦ TRITC-anti-Θ
⸬ ^{125}I-TIGAL

Figure 6:
Capping and resynthesis of immunologlobulin receptors for antigen on T and B lymphocytes for experimental protocol see Figure 5 and text (12).

213

TABLE I: PROPORTION OF LYMPHOCYTES WITH SURFACE IG AND/OR MθB MARKERS IN SPLEEN AND LYMPH NODES OF NORMAL AND NUDE MICE [1]

MARKERS [2]		SPLEEN		LYMPH NODES	
Ig	θB	Normal mice	Nude mice	Normal mice	Nude mice
-	-	11.9 (6.4-18.0)	23.3 (19.4-26.2)	5.6 (3.0- 9.8)	9.5 (3.1-16.9)
+	-	4.9 (3.0- 8.4)	5.8 (3.4- 9.4)	6.8 (4.0-11.3)	19.5 (11.1-31.5)
++	-	37.3 (30.2-41.4)	37.3 (29.2-42.4)	30.4 (18.9-45.5)	58.5 (48.5-73.9)
-	+	5.3 (2.6-10.0)	6.2 (4.2-10.4) 0.1	5.0 (3.6- 7.0) 0.1	0.9 (0 - 1.9) 0.1
-	++	36.7 (28.4-44.6)	15.5 (13.2-18.4)	48.8 (29.1-65.8) 0.1	4.1 (1.5- 7.3)
+	++	0.3 (0 - 0.6) 0.2	2.1 (0 - 4.4) 0.9	0.3 (0 - 0.5)	0.8 (0.3- 1.8)
+	+	1.0 (0.2- 1.8) 0.1	2.2 (0.4- 3.2) 0.3	0.3 (0 - 1.0) 0.1	1.1 (0.2- 2.6) 0.1
++	+	1.8 (0.8- 2.8) 0.3	2.9 (2.0- 3.8) 0.4	2.4 (0.3- 6.2) 0.1	4.5 (1.3- 9.3) 0.2
++	++	1.3 (0.6- 1.8) 0.7	5.1 (3.4- 9.2) 1.6	0.3 (0 - 0.6) 0.1	1.3 (0.5- 2.2) 0.2

[1]mean of 7 mice (range). Under the range is indicated the proportion of cells picking up NRIg absorbed in nude mice, when higher than 0.1% (see text).
[2]- : no detectable fluorescence; + faint fluorescence; ++ strong fluorescence.

214

TABLE 2: ACTIVE SYNTHESIS OF Ig RECEPTORS FOR ANTIGEN BY B AND T LYMPHOCYTES (ref.12)

	Proportion of B cells in total population	ABC frequency $\times 10^{-5}$ *		Groups compared	Statistical analysis P value†	
		B	T		B	T
1 Untreated population	17%	69	28			
2 1 h after first capping with RIgG–α–MIgG	17%	0	0‡	1 : 2	<0.0005	<0.01
3 18 h after first capping with RIgG–α–MIgG	9%	25	21	2 : 3	<0.001	<0.005
4 1 h after second capping with RIgG–α–MIgG	7%	0	0	3 : 4	<0.001	<0.005
				1 : 3	<0.025 >0.40§	>0.60
5 1 h after RIgG–α–TMV	17%	84	47	1 : 5	>0.50	>0.30
6 18 h after RIgG–α–TMV	10%	23	21	1 : 6	<0.025 >0.50§	>0.50

* 50,000 to 75,000 lymphocytes were examined per group.

† Based on χ^2 test.

‡ One cell was found with ~ thirty grains still in a small cap.

§ When corrections were made for the decrease in the overall proportion of B cells, which was found in two experiments out of five.

CYTOPHILIC PROPERTIES OF T LYMPHOCYTE MEMBRANE ASSOCIATED IMMUNOGLOBULINS

Robert E. Cone

Basel Institute for Immunology, Basel, Switzerland.

ABSTRACT. Lactoperoxidase catalyzed radioiodination of membrane proteins was used to incorporate ^{125}I (iodide) into membrane immunoglobulins of thymus influenced (T) and bone marrow derived (B) lymphocytes. Surface immunoglobulins were isolated by incubation of radiolabelled cells in cell culture medium for several hours. Released immunoglobulins were incubated with peritoneal exudate cells or lymphocytes. Serological and autoradiographic techniques were employed to assess the association of the released surface immunoglobulins with the various cell types. Immunoglobulins obtained from normal thymocytes or antigen-activated T lymphocytes were found to be cytophilic for a non-lymphoid macrophage-like cell in peritoneal exudate but showed no capacity to bind to either thymus or B lymphocytes. Under the experimental conditions employed surface immunoglobulins from B lymphocytes did not bind to either peritoneal exudate cells or lymphocytes. These results indicate that there may be structural differences between T and B lymphocytes surface immunoglobulins, at least in their heavy polypeptide chains.

INTRODUCTION

Immunoglobulins which resemble the monomeric subunit of pentameric IgM have been isolated from the cell membrane of murine thymus-influenced (T) lymphocytes by a combination of biochemical and serological techniques (1). These studies corroborate a number of reports in which immunoglobulin determinants have been demonstrated at the T cell surface by cyto-serological techniques (2-7). Similar approaches have been employed to demonstrate that one function of T cell surface immunoglobulin may be to serve as the cellular recognition site for antigen (3-6,8,9).

An additional role for T cell immunoglobulins has been suggested by experiments designed to elucidate the mechanism of collaboration between T and B lymphocytes during the humoral immune response in vitro (10,11). In these studies collaboration between T and B cells was shown to occur when the cells were separated by a membrane which would permit the passage of macromolecules only. The soluble "collaborative factor" was shown to consist of a complex of antigen

and membrane immunoglobulin shed from the surface of antigen
activated T cells (11). Moreover, admixture of the T cell
antigen specific collaborative factor with a non lymphoid,
glass-adherent cell population in peritoneal exudate con-
ferred on these cells the ability to induce B cells to produce specific antibody (11,12). Thus, T cell membrane
immunoglobulins may also serve as a soluble mediator of collaboration between T and B lymphocytes and a non-lymphoid,
macrophage-like cell. Since B cell surface immunoglobulin
cannot replace T cell immunoglobulin in this function, these
observations suggest that these molecules may differ in their
cytophilic properties, implying some fundamental structural
differences between T and B cell surface immunoglobulins.
Consequently, the experiments described below were designed
to compare directly the cytophilic properties of T and B
lymphocyte surface immunoglobulins for various cell types.
The results indicate that immunoglobulins obtained from normal and antigen-activated T lymphocytes bind to a macrophage-
like cell in peritoneal exudate whereas, under the conditions
employed, B cell surface immunoglobulins bind neither to
peritoneal exudate cells nor lymphocytes. The results
suggest that although both T and B cell surface immunoglobulins resemble the monomeric subunit of pentameric IgM,
they are structurally distinct molecules.

EXPERIMENTAL RESULTS

Assessment of cytophilicity by direct binding assays. The
cell surface of splenic T lymphocytes which had been activated by keyhole limpet hemocyanin (ATC_{KLH}) or sheep erythrocytes (ATC_{SRBC}), normal thymus cells and spleen cells from
congenitally athymic (nu/nu) mice (B lymphocytes) were radioiodinated with ^{125}I (iodide) using lactoperoxidase (13).
Radiolabelled cell surface proteins were obtained by incubating the labelled cells in cell culture medium for several
hours at 37°C. During this period the cells release ^{125}I-
labelled membrane proteins including immunoglobulin into the
culture fluid (14). The cytophilic properties of the

Abbreviations used:
ATC_{KLH}, ATC_{SRBC} — Splenic T cells enriched for cells
                          specific for the given antigen.
PEC   — Peritoneal exudate cells.
KLH   — Keyhole limpet hemocyanin.
SRBC   — Sheep erythrocytes

released surface proteins were assessed initially by incubation of appropriate "target" cells with the ^{125}I-labelled proteins, followed by washing the cells and a) counting radioactivity associated with the cell, and b) autoradiography at the light microscope level (Fig. 1).

As shown in Fig. 2, when ^{125}I-labelled surface proteins obtained from ATC$_{KLH}$ cells were incubated with peritoneal exudate cells (PEC) or thymus lymphocytes, labelled material remained associated with PEC only (12). Examination of PEC by light microscopic autoradiography (15) revealed that radioactivity was associated with macrophage-like cells but not lymphocytes (Table 1). Moreover, when ^{125}I-labelled surface proteins which had been absorbed with PEC, were added to fresh PEC, the number of labelled cells was reduced by 80-90%. These results indicated that a small proportion of ^{125}I-labelled T cell surface proteins could bind specifically to the macrophage-like cells. The immunoglobulin nature of these binding proteins was suggested by the observation that cell surface protein mixtures depleted of immunoglobulin were deficient in the PEC-binding proteins (Fig. 2). The ability of cell surface immunoglobulins obtained from various lymphoid cell types to bind to PEC and lymphocytes in such direct binding assays is summarized in Table 2. Cell surface immunoglobulins from normal thymocytes, ATC and a lymphoma possessing a T cell antigenic marker, θ (Thy-1) (16) exhibited the capacity to bind to PEC. B lymphocyte surface immunoglobulin was also bound by PEC but to a much less extent.

Assessment of cytophilicity by supernatant depletion assays. To quantitate the binding of cell surface immunoglob -ulins to other cells further, an assay system was developed in which ^{125}I-labelled lymphocyte surface proteins were mixed with PEC or lymphocytes, the cells removed by centrifugat -ion,and the amount of ^{125}I-labelled immunoglobulin in the supernatant was then determined by coprecipitation with mouse γ globulin and a polyvalent rabbit anti mouse immunoglobulin antiserum (15). Thus, absorption of surface immunoglobulins would be indicated by depletion of immunoglobulin from the mixture of cell surface proteins. Incubation of cell surface proteins from thymus lymphocytes or ATC with thymus lymphocytes did not remove any ^{125}I-labelled material specif -ically precipitable with anti-immunoglobulin antisera (15). However, as shown in Fig. 3, $5 \times 10^5 - 1 \times 10^6$ PEC absorbed completely the amount of labelled immunoglobulin released

Fig. 1

ASSAY FOR CYTOPHILIC PROPERTIES OF LYMPHOCYTE
SURFACE IMMUNOGLOBULINS

lymphocytes
thymus
activated T cell
nu/nu splenic (B) lymphocytes

lactoperoxidase catalyzed
incorporation of ^{125}I (iodide)
into membrane proteins

^{125}I-labelled cell surface proteins
obtained by incubation of radiolabelled cells in cell culture medium.

"shed" ^{125}I-labelled surface proteins are dialyzed and centrifuged
at 20,000 xg for 1 hr.

cell surface proteins incubated
at 4°C with peritoneal exudate
cells or lymphocytes

washing   autoradiography   quantitation of
direct counting   immunoglobulin
                                                 absorbed

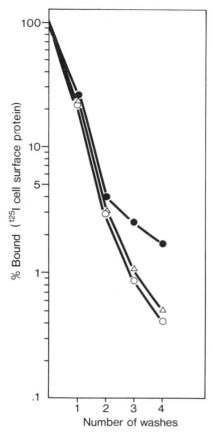

Fig. 2: Binding of ^{125}I-labelled T cell surface proteins
to various cell types as a function of washing. Antigen
activated T cells were prepared by injecting 1 x 10^8 thymus
cells intravenously into mice which had received 900 r
whole body X-irradiation. The mice then received keyhole
limpet hemocyanin emulsified in Freund's complete adjuvant.
Spleens enriched for ATC$_{KLH}$ were removed after seven days,
a single cell suspension was prepared and dead cells were
removed by centrifugation through a BSA gradient (details
in ref. 12). ATC were radiolabelled with ^{125}I and cell
surface proteins were obtained by incubation for 3-4 hrs
at 37°C of 1 x 10^8 ^{125}I-labelled ATC$_{KLH}$ in 2 ml minimal
essential medium (MEM) buffered with 20 mM HEPES. 100 μl
of cell surface proteins were incubated for 2 hr with 1 x
10^7 normal thymus lymphocytes (CBA/H/wehi) or peritoneal
exudate cells (PEC) obtained by saline lavage from mice injected 4 days previously with protease peptone.
(•————•) ^{125}I cell surface proteins + PEC;
(o————o) ^{125}I cell surface proteins + thymocytes;
(△————△) ^{125}I cell surface proteins depleted of immuno-
        globulin + PEC.

Table 1

BINDING OF ^{125}I-LABELLED T CELL SURFACE PROTEINS TO PERIT-
ONEAL EXUDATE CELLS SHOWN BY AUTORADIOGRAPHY

Cell surface proteins	Cell examined	Per cent labelled cells	
		8 days exposure	92 days exposure
ATC_{KLH}	macrophages	2.5	63.0
	lymphocytes	0	0
ATC_{KLH} pre-absorbed with macrophages	macrophages	0.25	15.0
	lymphocytes	0	0

1×10^8 ATC_{KLH} were labelled with ^{125}I. Radiolabelled surface proteins were obtained by incubation of the ^{125}I-
labelled lymphocytes in 2 ml minimal essential medium (MEM)
buffered with 20 mM HEPES. ^{125}I-labelled cell surface proteins (100-200 μl) were incubated at 4°C with peritoneal
exudate cells (10^6 cells) for 1-2 hr. The supernatant from
this incubation was held with a second population of PEC
under identical conditions (15).

Table 2

CYTOPHILIC PROPERTIES OF SURFACE IMMUNOGLOBULINS DETERMINED BY DIRECT BINDING ASSAYS

Cell surface immunoglobulins	Peritoneal exudate cells	Thymus lymphocytes	nu/nu splenic lymphocytes	% Immunoglobulin bound by 2×10^6 cells [a]
Antigen activated T cells	+	-	-	70 - 100
nu/nu spleen (B) lymphocytes	±	-	-	10 - 20
thymus lymphocytes	+	-	-	65 - 92
θ positive cell line (WEHI-22)	+	-	-	100

a) Figure obtained by comparing the percent of cell surface protein counts (^{125}I) bound to the percent specifically precipitable with anti-immunoglobulin antisera.

by 5 x 10[6] thymus or ATC lymphocytes in 3 hours. In similar
experiments (Table 3), PEC absorbed little or no surface
immunoglobulins obtained from nu/nu spleen cells. The specificity of PEC receptors for T cell surface immunoglobulins is
underscored by the finding that excess non-radioactive T cell
proteins blocked the binding of T cell immunoglobulin to PEC
whereas excess B lymphocyte protein was without appreciable
effect (Table 4).

Biochemical nature of T and B lymphocyte surface proteins
binding to PEC. Cell surface proteins obtained from T and
B lymphocytes which were specifically precipitated with
anti-immunoglobulin antisera were analyzed by disc polyacrylamide gel electrophoresis (1,9,12,15). The results
were consistent with previous observations that T cell immuno
-globulins (1) and B cell surface immunoglobulins (1,17) resemble a monomeric subunit of pentameric IgM. Accordingly,
to characterize further the nature of the ^{125}I-lymphocyte
surface proteins bound by PEC, cells which had bound T or B
cell surface proteins were dissolved in sodium dodecyl sulfate (SDS), reduced and alkylated and the solubilized [125]I-
labelled lymphocyte surface proteins which had been absorbed
by the PEC were resolved by disc gel electrophoresis. As
shown in Fig. 4, ^{125}I-labelled T cell surface proteins absorbed by PEC were resolved into two major components. One component penetrated the gel to the same extent as murine immuno
-globulin μ chains and the other resembled murine immunoglobulin L chains in its mobility in the gel. A component
with a mobility slightly retarded relative to that of murine
immunoglobulin γ chain as well as a component with a mobility
similar to light chains was observed when ^{125}I-labelled B
cell surface proteins absorbed by PEC were analyzed. These
results were consistent with the fact that PEC removed T cell
surface immunoglobulin from a mixture of T cell surface proteins. B cell surface proteins which were absorbed by PEC
were found to be significantly different from the cytophilic
T cell material and, if immunoglobulins, they resemble molecules of the IgG-class.

DISCUSSION

The experiments described above demonstrate that a fraction of cell surface proteins obtained from T lymphocytes are
strongly cytophilic for a macrophage-like cell in peritoneal

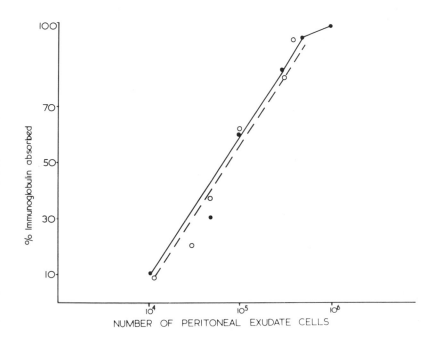

Fig. 3: Absorption of T cell surface immunoglobulin by PEC.
PEC or thymus cells were suspended in 100 µl PBS and incubated with 200 µl ^{125}I-labelled cell surface proteins
obtained from (●) ATC$_{KLH}$, (o) normal thymus cells. The
cells were incubated for 2 hr at 0°C, centrifuged and the
supernatants coprecipitated with mouse gamma globulin and a
polyvalent rabbit anti mouse immunoglobulin antiserum, or,
as controls, fowl gamma globulin and rabbit and fowl gamma
globulin antiserum. Percent immunoglobulin absorbed is
computed by:

$$\frac{\text{cpm specifically precipitated}}{\text{from absorbed cell surface proteins}} \times 100$$
$$\frac{}{\text{cpm specifically precipitated}}$$
from non-absorbed cell surface proteins

225

Table 3

ABSORBTION OF T AND B CELL SURFACE IMMUNOGLOBULINS BY PERITONEAL EXUDATE CELLS

125_I- Cell Surface Proteins	Cells used for absorption		Counts (cpm) specifically precipitated by RAMIg [a]	Per cent absorption
	Number	Origin		
ATC$_{KLH}$	4×10^5	Thymus	2606+201	-
	4×10^5	PEC	392+ 58	85
Thymus	4×10^5	Thymus	2489+120	-
	4×10^5	PEC	240+ 72	95
nu/nu spleen	4×10^5	Thymus	3256+261	-
	2×10^4	PEC	2780+421	15
	5×10^4	PEC	2500+126	20
	1×10^5	PEC	2700+158	15
	4×10^5	PEC	3109+300	2

Absorbing cells were suspended in 100 μl PBS and were incubated for 2 hrs with 200 μl 125_I-labelled cell surface proteins. The cells were centrifuged and the supernatants retained for coprecipitation. Results represent the arithmetic mean + SE of results obtained in 3 separate experiments with 3 replicates/group.

a - RAMIg = Rabbit anti mouse immunoglobulin antisera (from 15).

Table 4

INHIBITION OF BINDING OF LABELLED T CELL IMMUNOGLOBULIN BY NON-RADIOACTIVE T CELL SUPERNATANTS

Radioactive surface proteins	Absorbing cells	Unlabelled supernatant	cpm precipitated specifically by anti-immunoglobulin	Per cent abosrption
ATC SRBC (4×10^6 cell-equivalent)	10^6 thymus	-	1902 ± 23	-
	4×10^5 PEC	-	870 ± 15	55
	10^6 PEC	thymus (1×10^8 cell equivalent)	1605 ± 41	15
thymus cells (6×10^6 equivalent)	4×10^5 PEC	-	100 ± 41	95
	4×10^5 thymus	-	2895 ± 162	-
	4×10^5 PEC	B cell supernatant (1×10^8 cell equivalent)	420 ± 36	80

1×10^6 lymphocytes or PEC suspended in 100 µl PBS were incubated with 200 µl 125I-labelled cell surface protein $\pm$ 100 µl labelled thymus or B cell supernatants obtained from cells incubated for 3 hr at 37°C. Results represent the arithmetic mean $\pm$ SE of quadruplicate samples. From (15).

227

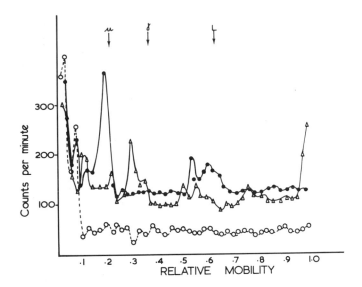

Fig. 4: Polyacrylamide gel electrophoresis in sodium dodecyl sulfate-acrylamide of ^{125}I-labelled T and B cell surface proteins binding to PEC. Cells which had absorbed ^{125}I-
labelled cell surface proteins were dissolved in 3% SDS + 5%
2-β mercaptoethanol. The samples were boiled for 5 min and
iodoacetamide was added to alkylate reduced polypeptides.
(●) ^{125}I-labelled T cell surface proteins extracted from PEC
(Δ) ^{125}I-labelled B cell surface proteins extracted from PEC
(o) ^{125}I-labelled T cell surface proteins extracted from
thymus cells. μ,γ, L refer to mobilities of standard mouse
immunoglobulin μ or γ heavy chains and light chains. 10%
acrylamide, 0.125% bisacrylamide . (From 15).

exudate. The immunoglobulin nature of these cytophilic proteins is indicated by the observations that: a) removal of
immunoglobulin from a mixture of T cell surface proteins elim
-inates cytophilic activity, b) PEC can be used to deplete
immunoglobulin from a mixture of T cell surface proteins, c)
reduced and alkylated T cell proteins which can be recovered
from PEC resemble immunoglobulin μ and light chains when
analyzed by disc electrophoresis in polyacrylamide gels.
These observations are consistent with those of Feldmann (11)
in which the cytophilic properties of T cell immunoglobulin
were demonstrated in a functional assay. Similar observations
(18) have been made for immunoglobulins derived from a T-
lymphoma (19). Rieber and Riethmüller (20) have also reported
that a T cell membrane protein possessing κ-chain determinants and having a molecular weight of approximately 200,000
is cytophilic for PEC.

Since, under the conditions chosen nearly 100% of the ^{125}I-
labelled surface immunoglobulins of normal or activated T
cells were absorbed by PEC, it is likely that the cytophilic
nature of T cell immunoglobulin is a general property of all
T cell antibodies. Neither T nor B cell surface proteins were
absorbed by normal lymphocytes suggesting that these molecules
detected by surface iodination are not adventitiously bound
to the T cell surface. However, the possibility that lymphocytes are saturated by passively absorbed immunoglobulins
while PEC are not, cannot be ruled out in the present experiments. If this were the case, these immunoglobulins would
be uniquely associated with T cells in that a) 8 S IgM is
not normally found in serum, indeed, most serum cytophilic
antibodies belong to the IgG class (21-24), b) B cell surface immunoglobulin is not cytophilic for PEC. Since serum
cytophilic antibodies bind to macrophages via the Fc portion
of the molecule (25,26) differences between T and B cell
surface immunoglobulin are likely to be found in the heavy
polypeptide chain. This raises the question of whether T
cell surface immunoglobulins are a subclass of IgM or another
antigenic class which cross-reacts with μ determinants. The
latter possibility is not inconceivable in that IgD cross-
reacts strongly with anti-μ chain antisera (27) and in fact
resembles an 8 S IgM molecule when analyzed by disc electrophoresis (28). The exact degree of relatedness of T and B
cell surface immunoglobulins will have to be determined by
primary sequence analyses.

The distinctive properties of T cell membranes and membrane immunoglobulin relative to their B cell counterparts, suggest that conditions developed for the isolation of B cell surface immunoglobulin may not apply to T cell surface immunoglobulin (39). This may explain, in fact, the inconsistencies reported in the isolation and detection of T cell immunoglobulins (1,17,30).

The cytophilic properties of T cell immunoglobulins support the feasibility of models of T and B cell collaboration which involve a soluble antigen-specific collaborative factor (10,11) and suggest that T cell immunoglobulin may well be the "associative antibody" of the Bretscher and Cohn Associative Recognition theory (31). In addition to its putative role as a specific collaborative factor, T cell immunoglobulin might also endow non-lymphoid phagocytic cells with antigen specificity in cell-mediated immune reactions. Thus, in addition to its function as the cellular recognition site for antigen, T cell immunoglobulins may play a pivotal role as a regulating factor in humoral and cell mediated immunity.

ACKNOWLEDGEMENTS

This work was supported by grants from the American Heart Association (72-1050), The Anna Fuller Fund, the United States Public Health Service (AI-10886 and AI-6-3958) and the National Health and Medical Research Council of Australia. The work was done primarily at the Walter and Eliza Hall Institute for Medical Research, Melbourne, Australia during the author's tenure as a post-doctoral fellow of the Damon Runyon Memorial Fund.

REFERENCES

1. Marchalonis, J.J., and Cone, R.E. Transplant. Rev. 14:3 (1973)

2. Bankhurst, A.D., Warner, N.L., and Sprent, J.J. Exp. Med. 134:1005 (1971)

3. Basten, A., Miller, J.F.A.P., Warner, N.L., and Pye, J. Nature (Lond.) 231:104 (1971)

4. Greaves, M.F. Transplant. Rev. 5:45 (1970)

5. Hogg, N.M., and Greaves, M.F. Immunology 22:969 (1972)

6. Roelants, G., Forni, L., and Pernis, B. J. Exp. Med. 137:1060 (1973)

7. Warner, N.L., Byrt, P., and Ada, G.L. Nature (Lond.) 226:942 (1970)

8. Cone, R.E., Sprent, J., and Marchalonis, J.J., Proc. Nat. Acad. Sci. (USA) 69:2556 (1972)

9. Cone, R.E., and Marchalonis, J.J. Austr. J. Exp. Biol. Med. Sci. 51:689 (1973) 137:1060 (1973)

10. Feldmann, M., and Basten, A. J. Exp. Med. 136:49 (1972)

11. Feldmann, M., J. Exp. Med. 136:737 (1972)

12. Feldmann, M., Cone, R.E., and Marchalonis, J.J. Cell. Immunol. 9:1 (1973)

13. Marchalonis, J.J., Cone, R.E., and Santer, V. Biochem. J. 124:921 (1971)

14. Cone, R.E., Marchalonis, J.J., and Rolley, R.T. J. Exp. Med. 134:1373

15. Cone, R.E., Feldmann, M., Marchalonis, J.J., and Nossal, G.J.V. Immunology 26:49 (1974)

16. Harris A.W., Bankhurst, A.D., Mason, S., and Warner, N.L. J. Immunol. 108:1126 (1972)

17. Vitetta, E.S., and Uhr, J.W. Transplant. Rev. 14:50 (1973)

18. Feldmann, M., personal communication.

19. Boylston, A., and Nowbray, A. Immunology (In press)

20. Rieber, E.P., and Riethmüller, G. European J. Immunol. (In press)

21. Tizard, I.R. Int. Arch. Allergy 36:332 (1969)

22. Berken, A., and Benacerraf, B.J. Immunol. 100:1219 (1968)

23. Hay, W., and Nelson, D.S. Aust. J. Exp. Biol. Med. 47:525 (1969)

24. Parish, W.E. Nature (Lond.) 268:594 (1965)

25. Tizard, I.R. Bact. Rev. 35:365 (1971)

26. Thrasher, S.T., and Cohnen, S. J. Immunol. 107:672 (1971)

27. Pernis, B., personal communication.

28. Spiegelberg, H. Contemp. Topics in Immunochem. $\underline{1}$:165 (1972).

29. Cone, R.E., and Marchalonis, J.J. Biochem. J. (in press)

30. Crone, M., Koch, C., Simonsen, M. Transplant. Rev. $\underline{10}$:36 (1972).

31. Bretscher, P.A., and Cohn, M. Nature (Lond.) $\underline{220}$:444 (1968).

IN-VITRO BIOSYNTHESIS AND MOLECULAR ARRANGEMENT OF
SURFACE IMMUNOGLOBULIN OF MOUSE THYMUS CELLS

Chaya Moroz and Nitza Lahat

Rogoff-Wellcome Medical Research Institute and
Tel-Aviv University Medical School
Beilinson Hospital, Petah Tikva, Israel

ABSTRACT. Surface immunoglobulin (Ig) was demonstrated on thymocytes from BALB/c and C57BL mice by lactoperoxidase radioiodination of the cells. Active synthesis of Ig in these cells was demonstrated in short-term tissue culture using ^{14}C-amino acids. The demonstration of intracellular and surface Ig required procedures that minimize proteolytic degradation.

IgA was found in the cytoplasm and on the surface of BALB/c thymocytes, whereas IgM was found in the cytoplasm and on the surface of C57BL thymocytes. The surface Ig is of a distinctive structure consisting of non-associated heavy and light chains.

INTRODUCTION

Efforts to demonstrate membrane Igs on T cells have led to conflicting conclusions (1-6). In a previous study (7) we have demonstrated the presence of surface IgM on human thymus cells and its active synthesis in these cells. We suggested that variable proteolysis during the solubilization of membrane components may account for the controversy regarding the presence of surface Igs on T cell membrane.

In the present communication we report on the detection of Ig on the surface of thymus cells from BALB/c and C57BL mice, and bring evidence for the active synthesis of Ig in thymocytes bearing θ antigen. The detection of surface and nascent intracellular Ig as well as the study of their immunochemical nature was made possible by the use of isolation procedures which minimize proteolytic degradation.

MATERIALS AND METHODS

Mice. 6 weeks old BALB/c, C57BL and F_1 hybrids of BALB/c and C57BL mice were used.

Antisera. R III anti-thymocyte C57BL serum, directed against the thymic antigen θ-C3H, was prepared and assayed as described previously (8) and is referred to in the text as anti-θ-C3H.

Goat anti-mouse IgA (α chain specific), goat anti-mouse IgM (u chain specific) and goat anti IgG (γ_2 chain specific) antisera were obtained from Melpar, USA. The potency and specificity of the antisera were determined by hemagglutination and hemagglutination inhibition tests.

In-vitro biosynthesis. Thymus cells were teased and suspended in Eagle's medium containing 1:100 the standard amount of amino acids. Cell suspensions (5×10^7 cells/ml) were preincubated for 15 min at 37° and then 5 uc of ^{14}C-amino acids mixture (uniformly labeled 45 mCi/milliatom of carbon, Amersham, England) were added to each ml of cell suspension. The suspensions were incubated at 37° for 180 min before chilling to 4°. The cells were spun at 500xg for 6 min and the pellet was washed twice with cold Eagle's medium or PBS.

For cytotoxic tests 2×10^7 BALB/c thymus cells were suspended in 1 ml of Eagle's medium, incubated for 45 min at 37° with 1 ml of anti-θ-C3H serum and 1.2 ml of guinea pig serum (C'), both of which had been previously absorbed with 2×10^8 BALB/c spleen cells per ml. The treated cells were washed twice at 500xg for 6 min, resuspended in Eagle's medium to the original concentration and labeled with ^{14}C-amino acids as above. Plasma cells from BALB/c plasmacytoma treated with anti-θ-C3H serum and C', and thymus cells from BALB/c mice treated with C' only served as controls.

Preparation of iodinated thymus cells. Thymuses were teased into 0.15 M NaCl in 0.01 M phosphate buffer, pH 7.2 (PBS), washed 3 times and iodinated according to Marchalonis (9) as modified by Moroz and Hahn (7).

Preparation of cell lysate. The labeled cells were
resuspended for 15 min at 4° either in 9M-urea or Nonidet
P_{40} (NP_{40}), both containing Trasylol (Bayer), as described
previously (7).
The amount of radioactivity incorporated into proteins
was determined following precipitation with 5% trichloro-
acetic acid (TCA).

Immunoprecipitation and electrophoresis. Immune precipitation from urea treated cells was carried out after
exhaustive dialysis (24 h) against PBS-Trasylol at 4°. Radio
active Igs were isolated from cell lysates by coprecipitation
with nonlabeled mouse myeloma protein added to the cell cytoplasm and the above described monoscpecific antisera, according to the procedure described before (7). As control for
non-specific coprecipitation an equal amount of precipitate
was formed with human Bence-Jones λ protein and goat anti-
human λ chain serum (Melpar). Radioactivity in the non-
specific precipitate amounted to about 25% of that in specific precipitates. The dissolved precipitates were characterized by acrylamide gel electrophoresis according to Shapiro
et al (10), as modified by Moroz and Hahn (7).
Standards for the mobility of u, α and light chains
were obtained from reduced and alkylated mouse myeloma IgM
(MOPC-104E) and IgA (MOPC-47A), secreted by the respective
plasma cells labeled with ^{14}C-amino acids for 180 min in
short term tissue culture.

RESULTS

Ig synthesis in mouse thymocytes. The presence of
nascent IgA in the cytoplasm of BALB/c thymocytes and nascent
IgM in the cytoplasm of C57BL mice was established with
appropriate antisera. As shown in table I, 13.4% of the
total radioactive proteins in the cytoplasmic fraction of
BALB/c thymocytes were precipitated with anti- α serum and
only 1.0% with anti-u serum, whereas in the cytoplasmic
fraction of C57BL thymocytes 13.1% of the total radioactive
protein were precipitated with anti-u serum and 4.3% with
anti- α serum. Studies in thymus cells of F_1 hybrids of
BALB/c and C57BL mice revealed that 7.6% of the total radioactivity was precipitated with anti- α serum and 5.2% with
anti-u serum (Table 1).
The possibility that the nascent Ig was synthesized
by a population of B cells (θ^-) in the thymus, as suggested
by Vitteta et al (6), was investigated in BALB/c thymocytes

TABLE 1

^{14}C amino acids incorporated into Ig in the cytoplasm of mouse thymus cells.

Strain	Fraction	Radioactivity cpm	Radioactivity (%)
BALB/c	Total protein*	2.8×10^4	
	α-chain$^+$	3.7×10^3	13.4
	u-chain$^+$	0.3×10^3	1.0
C57BL	Total protein*	2.4×10^4	
	α-chain$^+$	1.0×10^3	4.3
	u-chain$^+$	3.15×10^3	13.1
F_1 (BALB/c x C57BL)	Total protein*	2.5×10^4	
	α-chain$^+$	1.9×10^3	7.6
	u-chain$^+$	1.3×10^3	5.2

* Precipitated with 5% cold TCA.

$^+$ Corrected for non-specific cpm (25%) in immunoprecipitate.

(θ-C3H) pretreated with anti-θ-C3H serum and C'. This treatment killed 95% of the cells as judged by trypan blue staining, whereas in control experiments treatment of thymocytes with C' alone or treatment of plasma cells from BALB/c plasmacytoma with anti-θ-C3H serum and C' killed only 5% of the cells. Protein synthesis in the residual viable thymocytes (θ⁻) was 3% (Table 2).

Igs on the surface of mouse thymus cells. The presence and nature of Igs on the surface of BALB/c and C57BL mice thymus cells were studied by a modification of the radioiodination procedure described in Materials and Methods; the cells were treated with iodoacetamide prior to iodination in order to preclude formation of interchain disulfide linkages which may result from use of H_2O_2 in the labeling procedure.

When the cytoplasmic fraction of iodinated BALB/c thymocytes was reacted with anti-mouse IgA, IgM and IgG_2 antisera, 13.7% of the TCA-precipitable radioactivity was precipitated with anti- α serum and only 1.1% with anti-u serum. On the other hand, in C57BL cytoplasm 18% of the total radioactivity was precipitated with anti-u serum and only 1.4% with anti- α serum (Table 3).

On acrylamide gel electrophoresis the iodinated proteins from BALB/c mice thymocytes exhibited mainly 2 peaks, a slow moving peak corresponding to α or γ chains, and a fast moving peak corresponding to light chain. The iodinated proteins from C57BL thymus cells resolved into 3 peaks: 2 slow moving peaks, a major one corresponding to u chain and a minor one corresponding to α or γ chain, and a fast moving peak corresponding to light chains (Fig. 1A). The mobility of the light chain peaks obtained from BALB/c and C57BL is within the range of the mobility of light chains obtained from the mouse myeloma proteins used as standards. The iodinated Igs isolated from BALB/c thymocytes with anti- α serum and subjected to electrophoresis on acrylamide, exhibited a major peak corresponding to monomeric α-chains with no peak corresponding to light chain; anti-u serum precipitated only minute amounts of monomeric u-chains (Fig. 1B). On the other hand, the iodinated Igs isolated from C57BL cells with anti-u serum exhibited a major peak corresponding to monomeric u-chains (Fig. 1C). The slow moving peaks (Fig. 1B) and the spreading of the monomeric u-chain peak (Fig. 1C) observed in the electrophoretic pattern of the precipitated heavy chains was resolved into a single peak corresponding to α chain and u-chain monomers, respectively, following

TABLE 2

Effect of treatment with anti-θ serum on protein
synthesis in BALB/c mouse thymus cells.

Treatment	% cells stained with Trypan blue	Radioactivity cpm	Loss of biosynthetic activity (%)
Medium + C'	5	3×10^6	
Medium + anti-θ-C3H	5		
Anti-θ-C3H + C'	95	9×10^4	97

TABLE 3

^{125}I incorporated into Ig on the surface of mouse thymus cells.

Strain	Fraction	Radioactivity cpm	Radioactivity (%)
BALB/c	Total protein*	3.25×10^4	
	α-chain$^+$	4.5×10^3	13.7
	u-chain$^+$	0.35×10^3	1.1
C57BL	Total protein*	2.05×10^4	
	α-chain$^+$	0.3×10^3	1.4
	u-chain$^+$	3.7×10^3	18

* Precipitated with 5% cold TCA.

+ Corrected for non-specific cpm (25%) in immunoprecipitate.

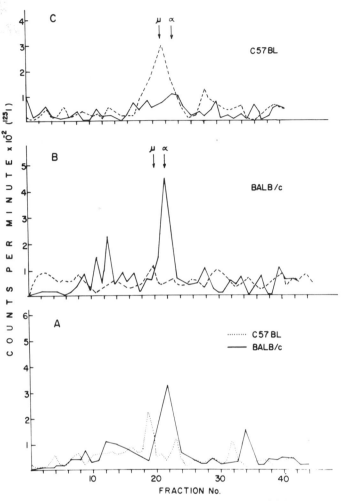

Fig. 1. Acrylamide gel electrophoresis of ^{125}I-labeled surface proteins and isolated Igs from thymus cells of BALB/c and C57BL mice. Iodinated cells were solubilized with 9M urea-Trasylol-0.2M iodoacetamide at 4° followed by exhaustive dialysis against PBS-Trasylol for 16 hr at 4°. For electrophoresis, the dialyzed proteins were treated with 1% SDS for 1 min at 100° and dialyzed against 0.1% SDS in 0.01M sodium phosphate buffer, pH 7.1 and Trasylol for 120 min at 4°. Immunoprecipitates were dissolved in 1% SDS - 0.01M sodium phosphate buffer, pH 7.1 - Trasylol for 1 min at 100° and dialyzed as above. (A) ^{125}I-labeled proteins from thymocytes of BALB/c and C57BL mice. (B) ^{125}I-labeled Igs obtained from thymocytes of BALB/c mice by reaction with ——— anti-α serum and ------- anti-u-serum. (C) ^{125}I-labeled Igs obtained from thymocytes of C57BL mice by reaction with ——— anti-α serum and ------- anti-u serum.

240

complete reduction and alkylation. The minor peaks moving
faster than u chain may represent u chains which were
digested to various degrees by proteolysis in spite of the
precautions taken, as has been previously described (7).
A minor peak corresponding to monomeric α-chains was consistently obtained after reaction of C57BL cytoplasm with
anti-α serum (Fig. 1C).

The molecular arrangement of IgA on the surface of
BALB/c thymocytes. Demonstration of non-covalently linked
monomeric α and light chains on the surface of BALB/c thymocytes raised the possibility that the Ig peptide chains are
separately distributed in the cell membrane rather than in
a non-covalently linked tetrapeptide structure. This possibility was investigated by lactoperoxidase radioiodination
of BALB/c thymocytes pretreated at 4° and 37° with goat
anti-mouse α chain serum. As controls served thymocytes
treated as above with goat anti-human IgM.

On acrylamide gel electrophoresis the iodinated surface proteins of thymocytes treated with goat anti-α chain
antibodies at 4° and iodinated in the cold exhibited a slow
moving peak corresponding to 7S Ig and a fast moving peak
corresponding to light chains (Fig. 2A). The peak corresponding to α chains evident in the pattern of iodinated
surface proteins of cells treated with a non-specific antiserum (Fig. 2C) was absent. The light chain peak of the
cells treated with anti-mouse α chain antibodies was quantitatively similar to that of the control cells (Fig. 2C).

In contrast, thymocytes treated with anti-mouse α
chain serum at 37° prior to iodination in the cold (Fig. 2B),
exhibited on acrylamide gel a single peak identical to the
light chain peak of the cells treated with a non-specific
antibody at 37° (Fig. 2C). The iodinated α chain peak of
the control cells as well as the peak corresponding to 7S
Ig present on the surface of thymocytes pretreated with
anti-mouse α chain serum at 4° were absent (Fig. 2B).

The iodinated surface proteins of the different cell
preparations were reacted with rabbit anti-goat IgG or with
goat anti mouse-α chain serum. As seen in Table 4, in
control cells pretreated with goat anti human IgM at 4° or
37° I^{125} labeled α chains were precipitated. Minute
amounts of labeled goat 7S IgG were also precipitated and
may represent non specific absorption of goat IgG to the
cell surface. In contrast, in cells treated with goat anti-
mouse α chain serum 3-4 times more I^{125} labeled goat IgG
was precipitated from the cell with no labeled α chains.

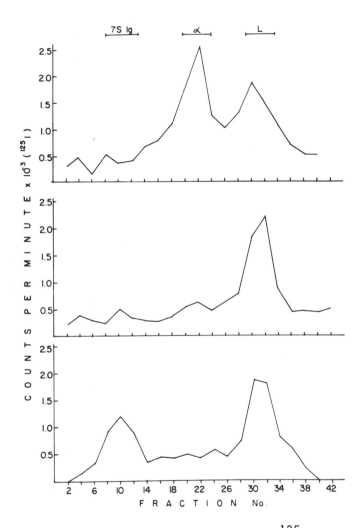

Fig. 2. Acrylamide gel electrophoresis of ^{125}I-labeled surface proteins of BALB/c thymocytes pretreated with goat anti-mouse α chain serum. Thymocytes were preincubated for 60 min at 4° with goat anti-mouse α chain serum or in control experiment with goat anti-human IgM serum. Half of the cells were further incubated for 15 min at 37°. All cell preparations were iodinated for 30 min at 4°. Iodinated cells were solubilized with 0.5% NP$_{40}$-Trasylol at 4°. For electrophoresis samples were treated as in Fig. 1. (A) ^{125}I-labeled proteins from thymocytes pretreated with anti-mouse α chain serum at 4°. (B) at 37°. (C) thymocytes pretreated with anti-human IgM at 4° or 37°.

TABLE 4

^{125}I incorporated into Ig on the surface of BALB/c thymocytes pretreated with anti-mouse α chain serum.

Treatment of cells prior to iodination	Radioactivity cpm x 10^{-3*}	
	Goat IgG**	mouse α chains**
Goat anti-human IgM at 4°	3.8	6.3
Goat anti-human IgM at 37°	2.2	5.3
Goat anti-mouse α chain at 4°	12.1	0
Goat anti-mouse α chain at 37°	2.7	0.8

* Numbers in columns have been multiplied by 10^{-3}.

** Isolated by immune precipitation and corrected for non-specific cpm in immunoprecipitate.

In cells treated with the latter antiserum at 37° minute amounts of I^{125} labeled goat IgG and almost no radiolabeled α chains were precipitated. We conclude that goat anti-mouse α chain antibodies had associated to the surface chains at 4° rendering the chains inaccessible to iodination by lactoperoxidase. The antibodies however did not cover by steric hindrance the surface light chains which were iodinated by the enzyme. Moreover, upon heating to 37° the goat-antiα-αchain complexes were removed from the surface resulting in thymocytes carrying on the surface the free light chains only.

DISCUSSION

In a recent study on Ig of human thymus cells we provided evidence for varying proteolysis during the solubilization of membrane components and the isolation of surface and intracellular Ig (7). Preliminary observations on mouse thymus cells suggested that in the absence of special precautions used to minimize proteolysis, various degrees of protein degradation occur in the cells. Indeed, in the present study on thymus cells from BALB/c and C57BL mice, employing various conditions to minimize protein degradation including low temperature, short time for the entire preparative process, and the use of Trasylol as a general protease inhibitor, surface Ig was detected by enzymic iodination of the cells. u was the major heavy chain class found on thymocytes from C57BL mice whereas α was the major heavy chain class on thymocytes from BALB/c mice.

The latter finding is of particular interest because of the high proportion of induced plasmacytomas in BALB/c mice producing γA myeloma protein (11). It has been suggested (12) that large numbers of immunocytes in the peritoneum where the induced plasmacytoma arise, are differentiated to produce γA type immunoglobulin. Our finding on BALB/c mice thymocytes raises the question of a relationship between the thymus and the synthesis of IgA in B cells.

The detection of noncovalently linked monomeric heavy and light chains on thymocytes from BALB/c and C57BL mice was made possible by a procedure that minimizes formation of interchain disulphide bridges, and is compatible with our previous finding in human thymus cells (7). Although the light chains were not isolated from the mouse thymus cells, their existence is suggested by the radioactive peak corresponding to the mobility of light chain marker observed on acrylamide gel electrophoresis of all iodinated cell preparations. It seems therefore that, as in human thymocytes, the Ig on the surface of mouse thymus cells consists of noncovalently linked heavy and light chains. Since precipitation of the heavy chains did not bring down light chains it is suggested that the Ig peptide chains in the surface membrane are only noncovalently linked but also not associated. Indeed, anti-α antibodies complexed at 4° to α chains on the cell surface of BALB/c thymocytes prior to radioiodination, covered the surface α chain leaving the membranal light chains accessible to lactoperoxidase iodination. The association of goat anti-mouse α chain antibodies to surface α chains was not due to non-specific absorbtion of cytophilic antibodies, since non-specific goat antibodies absorbed very little to the cells at 4° or 37° and did not cover the surface α chinas which were fully iodinated by lactoperoxidase. Moreover, the membranal α chain-anti-α complexes were rapidly removed from the surface upon heating to 37°, rendering thymocytes with surface light chains only.

The possibility that the surface Ig was passively absorbed to the cells is unlikely since the active synthesis of IgA and IgM was demonstrated in BALB/c and C57BL mice, respectively. The killing of 95% of BALB/c thymocytes with anti-θ-serum and complement resulted in 97% decrease in the ^{14}C amino acid incorporation into intracellular proteins. This decrease undoubtedly includes inhibition of Ig synthesis by thymocytes bearing θ antigen, in which cells 14.5% of the total radioactivity was precipitated as Ig heavy chains.

We conclude that mouse T cells possess surface Ig of a distinctive structure consisting of noncovalently linked and non-associated heavy and light chains, and that the type of heavy chain class expressed may vary in different inbred strains of mice. The genetic regulation of the expressed heavy chain class in the thymus may be studied in BALB/c x C57BL hybrids. These studies are currently under investigation in our laboratory. A preliminary observation (Table 2) suggests that in BALB/c x C57BL F_1 hybrid the thymocytes express either one of the parental CH genes in about the same frequency.

ACKNOWLEDGMENTS

We are grateful to Prof. F. Karush and Prof. A de Vries for helpful discussions. The project was supported by a grant from the Chief Scientist of the Ministry of Health, Israel.

REFERENCES

1. Bankhurst, A.D., Warner, N.L. and Sprent, J., J. Exp. Med. 134, 1005 (1971).

2. Nossal, G.J.V., Warner, N.L., Lewis, H. and Sprent, J., J. Exp. Med. 135, 405 (1972).

3. Marchalonis, J.J., Cone, R.E. and Atwell, J.L., J. Exp. Med. 135, 956 (1972).

4. Marchalonis, J.J., Atwell, J.L. and Cone, R.E., Nature New Biol. 235, 240 (1972).

5. Dwyer, M.M., Warner, N.L. and Mackey, I.R., J. Immunol. 108, 1439 (1972).

6. Vitteta, E.S., Uhr, J.W. and Boyse, E.A., Proc. Nat. Acad. Sci. 70, 834 (1973).

7. Moroz, C. and Hahn, J., Proc. Nat. Acad. Sci. 70, 3716 (1973).

8. Witz, I.P., Kaliss, N. and Samuel, T., Cellular Immun. 2, 362 (1971).

9. Marchalonis, J.J., Cone, R.E. and Santer, V., Bioch. J. 124, 921 (1971).

10, Shapiro, A.L., Scharff, M.D., Maizel, J.V., Jr. and Uhr, J.W., Proc. Nat. Acad. Sci. 56, 216 (1966).

11. Potter, M. and Lieberman, R., Cold Spring Harbor Symp. Quant. Biol. 32, 187 (1967).

12. Potter, M. and Lieberman, R., Advances in Immunol. 7, 91 (1967).

THE LYMPHOCYTE PLASMA MEMBRANE

Martin C. Raff and Stefanello de Petris

MRC Neuroimmunology Project
Department of Zoology, University College London
London WC1E 6BT   and
Basel Institute of Immunology
Basel, Switzerland

ABSTRACT. In the unperturbed state, the lymphocyte plasma membrane is fluid with most constituent proteins and lipids randomly distributed and free to move relative to one another in the plane of the membrane. However, under certain conditions, contractile actinomyosin-like cytoplasmic components appear to be able to interact with membrane molecules and influence their distribution and mobility. This microfilament network may also interact with microtubules. Multivalent ligands which bind to and cross-link membrane proteins or lipids can induce them to passively cluster into patches, following which they are actively carried to one pole of the lymphocyte. In some cases, ligand binding induces the pinocytosis of the ligand-receptor complex. Some functional implications of the fluid nature of the lymphocyte plasma membrane are discussed.

INTRODUCTION

It is probable that more is known about the plasma membrane of lymphocytes than any other nucleated mammalian cell. This is largely due to the ease of preparing relatively homogenous suspensions of lymphocytes and to their being the focal point of immunological research. Yet, despite the fact that much has been learned in recent years about the general organisation of the plasma membrane, we know remarkably little about the structure or function of its various components. The technical difficulties of obtaining workable quantities of intact membrane proteins in soluble form and of crystallizing them, taken together with the dangers of extrapolating from studies on solubilized proteins to their properties in the membrane, suggest that we are a long way from solving the structure of any of these molecules. Even in the case of immunoglobulin (Ig) in the membrane of B lymphocytes, which is known to function as receptor for antigen, its complete structure, the way it is inserted in the membrane and the mechanism by which its interaction with antigen triggers the cell, have yet to be established. Although it

247

has been shown that most, and perhaps all, lymphocyte membrane components are turning over (see below), it is still
unclear how they are assembled and how they are lost. In
addition, very little is known about their interaction with
cytoplasmic components. In the case of the lipids, although
a basic bilayer structure seems established (1,2,3), there
is little information on possible assymetry between the
inner and outer leaflets (4), compositional and conformational heterogeneity in the plane of the bilayer (5), or the
nature and extent of lipid-protein interactions.

In this paper, we review some of the things that have
been learned and several of the important questions that have
been raised about lymphocyte membranes from studies using
labelled antibodies and lectins.

THE ORGANISATION OF THE LYMPHOCYTE PLASMA MEMBRANE

Although lymphocytes can pick up certain proteins or
protein-protein complexes from their environment, the majority of membrane proteins are made by the cell that bears
them, and most of these are probably held in the membrane by
hydrophobic interactions in the interior of the lipid bilayer (6). It is unlikely that any protein is entirely
buried in the bilayer, and although little is known of
lymphocyte membrane proteins which are exposed to the cytoplasm but not to the exterior of the cell, by analogy with
the erythrocyte membrane (7), it is probable that many
exist. If they do, nothing is known of their nature,
distribution or behaviour. For technical reasons, the only
lymphocyte membrane proteins that have been studied are those
exposed on the cell surface. In the erythrocyte membrane,
all of the surface exposed proteins appear to penetrate
through the membrane and to be exposed on the cytoplasmic
surface as well (7), whether this will prove to be the case
for all or any of the lymphocyte proteins remains to be seen.
As seems to be true of the great majority of cell membranes,
the carbohydrate side chains of the glycoproteins and glycolipids are probably all on the exterior side of the membrane
(8,9). Most of the lymphocyte proteins which have been
studied zppear to be 'turning over' with a half-life of 4-30
hours (10,11,12,13). Some of the conflicting data on the
rates for Ig (12, and F. Melchers, personal communication)
and H-2 (11,14) turnover on mouse lymphocytes may be related
to differences in the cells studied and in the methods used.
Whether loss of membrane protein under normal conditions
involves pinocytosis, shedding of lipid and protein
containing vessicles, or proteolysis is not clear. The

pathway of membrane protein synthesis and insertion is also unknown. It is still debated whether they are made on membrane-bound polyribosomes like secreted proteins or on free ribosomes like cytoplasmic proteins (7). It is likely that following insertion into the endoplasmic reticulum membrane, they are carried to the Golgi apparatus, during the course of which they may be glycosylated, and finally pinch off in vessicles which fuse with the plasma membrane (15).

In a resting lymphocyte, most (or all) of the membrane proteins exposed at the cell surface are diffusely and randomly distributed and able to move laterally in the plane of the membrane. This has been demonstrated for Ig (16), Concanavalin A (ConA) receptors on lymphocytes (17) and a variety of alloantigens on mouse thymocytes (17). The lateral mobility of membrane lipids is also well established (18). Before it was recognized that membranes were fluid and that multivalent ligands binding to surface molecules could cross-link and redistribute them, the non-uniform distributions seen in mapping experiments with multivalent ligands were misinterpreted as indicating a highly ordered arrangement of membrane macromolecules (20,21). An apparent exception to the rule of randomness recently has been reported, suggesting that Ig molecules are distributed in a non-random manner on human B lymphocytes, even where efforts were made to avoid the labelled anti-Ig antibody redistributing the membrane Ig (22). We have not been able to confirm these findings and have found a random distribution of Ig on human blood and tonsil B lymphocytes when labelled with fluorscein or ferritin-conjugated monovalent Fab anti-Ig (D. Lawson, C. Evans and M. Raff, unpublished observations). Although membrane proteins and lipids can move laterally and rotate in the plane of the membrane, their movement across plasma membranes (i.e. flip-flop) occurs only very slowly, if at all (23). Immunoferritin electron microscopic mapping studies of Ig on mouse B lymphocytes (16,24) suggest that Ig molecules are in the membrane as single molecules or small aggregates of two or three like or unlike molecules, rather than as large 'islands' of protein. It is difficult to reconcile these findings with antibody blocking studies (25), which have indicated that various alloantigens on mouse thymocytes (TL, θ, H-2) are distributed in a constant relationship to one another, although it is possible that membrane proteins form loose associations with one another, which are broken when antibodies react with them.

We have recently observed an interesting exception to the general rule of random distribution of lymphocyte membrane molecules (27). When mouse thymocytes were treated with anti-θ antibody and then fixed with gluteraldehyde at 22 °C and finally labelled with ferritin-conjugated anti-mouse Ig antibody, about 10% of the cells were elongated with pronounced uropods. In such cells, the ferritin was concentrated over the anterior part of the cell with little labelling on the uropod and virtually no labelling on the constricted 'waist' of the cell, which marked the beginning of the uropod and appeared to be the site of a 'constriction ring'. Theta thus appears to be preferentially localized to the fluid parts of the membrane and excluded from those parts which are presumably immobilized by interaction with contractile cytoplasmic structures (see below). Since θ-bearing molecules may be glycolipids (26), it will be important to establish whether any membrane proteins are also excluded from these constricted regions.

When multivalent ligands, such as antibodies, lectins or antigens bind to molecules on the surface of living lymphocytes, they can induce three distinct types of redistribution of the molecules in the plane of the membrane:

1) patch formation (13,16), which is the clustering of the molecules into aggregates, probably in a passive manner similar to an agglutination or precipitation reaction, only occurring in two dimensions;

2) cap formation (13,19,24,27,28,29), which is the active movement of the patches to one pole (that containing the cell organelles) of the cell, and

3) pinocytosis (19,24,30) of the complexes. Since only those molecules to which the ligand binds are redistributed (19,27) one can make use of these phenomena to map the lymphocyte membrane by studying which determinants co-cap and which cap independently. In this way it has been shown the two ends of the major histocompatibility loci in man (LA and Four) (31) and mouse (H-2K and H-2D) (32) code for two distinct proteins, and that β_2-microglobulin and HLA are associated (i.e. they co-cap) on the membrane of human lymphocytes (B. Bernocco and R. Ceppellini, personal communication). This approach should be useful for establishing the relationship between T cell receptors, Immune Response (IR) gene products and lymphocyte-defined (LD) antigens.

RELATIONSHIP OF SURFACE RECEPTORS AND ANTIGENS TO INTRAMEMBRANOUS PARTICLES

When cells are frozen and their plasma membranes fractured through the middle of the lipid bilayer, both halves of the membrane can be viewed, as replicas, by electron microscopy (33,34). Such freeze fracture microscopic studies demonstrate numerous small bumps on both fracture faces (although more numerous on the inner face) whih are referred to as intramembranous particles (IMP) (35). In the erythrocyte membrane, the IMP are of uniform size (80A°), densely packed (4200 particles/μ^2) and randomly distributed (35), and although their nature has not been established, there is indirect evidence that they are associated with one or two types of membrane protein (7,35) which are exposed on the cell surface. Experiments combining freeze fracture, freeze etch and ligand binding have suggested that the IMP of erythrocytes are associated with surface ABO antigens (37) and receptors for viruses and lectins (38), although these studies are not entirely convincing as yet. In lymphocytes, and other nucleated mammalian cells, IMP are less uniform in size and far fewer in number (39,40 and S de Petris, unpublished observations). Although they were reported to be distributed in a clustered fashion in mouse T lymphocytes and in a random manner in B lymphocytes (40), the clustered distribution, subsequently has been shown t o be an artifact induced by the glycerol which is used as a cryoprotectant (41). If lymphocytes are prefixed with gluteraldehyde prior to freezing, the IMP are always randomly distributed (41). All attempts to demonstrate a relationship between IMP and lymphocyte surface antigens or receptors have so far failed. Thus, after capping H-2 Ig, PHA (42) or ConA receptors (42 and S. de Petris, unpublished observations) on mouse lymphocytes, the density and distribution of IMP were found to be unchanged. These experiments suggest that most of the molecules so far studied are not associated with IMP, or that if they are, the association is weak and can be broken by the interaction with ligand. The most convincing evidence for the protein nature of at least some IMP is their appearance in artificial lipid bilayers when purified rhodopsin molecules are inserted (W. Hubbel, personal communication). On the other hand, recent studies of the Semlike Forest virus have shown that viral envelope proteins which penetrate through the viral lipid bilayer are not associated with particles visible by freeze fracture microscopy (K. Simons, personal communication). Thus the freeze-fracture studies on lymphocytes discussed above, in no way exclude the possibility that the IMP are protein in nature or that the antigens and receptors so far studied penetrate through the membrane.

INTERACTIONS BETWEEN MEMBRANE MOLECULES AND CYTOPLASMIC COMPONENTS

The fact that lymphocytes can move, cap, form constriction rings, and put our microvilli, implies that their plasma membranes cannot be entirely fluid all of the time. These localized and directed membrane movements must mean that contractile cytoplasmic components can interact directly or indirectly with membrane molecules and control their movement. The nature of the cytoplasmic components and how they interact with the membrane is still unknown. Two possible candidates are microtubules and actin-like microfilaments, and there is increasing evidence that both somehow may play a role.

The possible role of microtubules is suggested by the experiments of Edelman and his colleagues who have shown that ConA can inhibit the antibody-induced capping of Ig and other surface molecules on lymphocytes, and that this inhibition can be released by microtubule-deaggregating drugs, such as colchicine and vinblastine (43). The interpretation of these experiments is made difficult by the high concentration of the drugs (10^{-4}M) required to demonstrate the release phenomenon, which raises the possibility of a direct membrane effect. The studies of Ukena and Berlin on rabbit polymorphonuclear leucocytes, however, also tend to support a role for microtubules in controlling membrane proteins (44). They have shown that during phagocytosis of latex particles, large amounts of membrane are internalized, but that certain transport enzymes appear to be spared. If cells are first treated with colchicine or vinblastine at relatively low concentrations (10^{-6}M) then the transport sites are internalized along with other membrane components. Since, in morphological studies, microtubules do not appear to interact with the plasma membrane, if they do play a role in controlling membrane protein movement, it is likely that they do so indirectly, perhaps via microfilaments.

There is increasing evidence that all motile cells contain actin and myosin-like molecules (45,46,47) and that the actin can be visualized as microfilaments (48), some of which appear to be associated with the cytoplasmic side of the plasma membrane (46). In glycerol extracted lymphocytes, microfilaments which decorate with heavy meromyosin, can be seen under the membrane, and morphologically similar filaments are seen concentrated at the tail of lymphocytes capped with anti-Ig (S. de Petris, unpublished observations). In addition, while colchicine or vinblastine do not inhibit Ig capping induced by anti-Ig, cytochalasin B, which appears to interfere with the contractile function of microfilaments, does inhibit, although even at very high concentrations (50μgm/ml) the inhibition is only partial. More recently it has been shown that cytochalasin B completely inhibits capping of ConA, and when colchicine or vinblastine (at 10^{-6}M) are combined with cytochalasin B (10μgm/ml) the inhibition of Ig capping is also complete (S. de Petris, in preparation) Moreover, cytochalasin can reverse preformed ConA caps, indicating that cytochalasin B-sensitive structures (presumably microfilaments) also play a role in holding the ConA-ConA-receptor complexes together. These intriguing results suggest that while both microtubules and microfilaments can act synergistically to control membrane protein movement, microfilaments appear to play a more direct role, although it is difficult to exclude the possibility that these drug effects reflect non-filament and/or non-tubule effects.

Thus far, all of the ConA preparations that we have used have caused much less inhibition of Ig capping that has been reported by others (13,29). Even at concentrations as high as 100μgm/ml, affinity chromatographically-purified ConA or ConA-fluorescein caps ConA receptors on approximately 50% of mouse spleen cells, but only on approximately 5% of thymocytes. In addition, when used at concentrations of 20μgm/ml or higher, ConA caps all of the Ig on mouse spleen B cells, and under these circumstances both the Ig and ConA receptor capping is completed, inhibited and reversed by cytochalasin B (S. de Petris, in preparation). Since ConA appears to bind to membrane Ig, it is simpler to visualize its inhibiting effects in terms of its cross-linking Ig to other non-cappable membrane proteins, rather than in terms of Ig molecules existing in anchored and non-anchored states, as has been proposed (43). Why some ConA receptors can be capped while others cannot, remains unexplained.

It is difficult to put all of these findings together into a working model. On morphological and pharmacological grounds, it seems likely to us, that under certain conditions, actin-like microfilaments (presumably associated with myosin-like molecules in contractile complex) can interact directly with the cytoplasmic side of membrane molecules and directly or indirectly be responsible for holding them in a fixed location or moving them about relative to other membrane components. An actinomyosin system would be well suited for this role of intermittently controlling membrane molecules, either by polymerization-depolymerization of some of its components, or by a rapidly reversible interaction with the membrane. It is conceivable that these microfilaments also interact with microtubules and possibly with other types of filaments, which provide anchorage within the cell. It is probably unwise to speculate much further until more information is in hand.

FUNCTIONAL IMPLICATIONS OF A FLUID PLASMA MEMBRANE

In teleological terms, it is not difficult to think of good reasons why plasma membranes should be fluid. It provides a simple means of dividing the membrane components evenly between daughter cells at the time of cell division, of distributing proteins and lipids all around the membrane after they are inserted from inside the cell, and of allowing appropriate membrane components (such as enzymes and their appropriate substrates) to readily come together (49). The advantages of having protein and lipid molecules able to move relative to one another in the plane of the membrane are also apparent in considering cell-cell or cell-ligand interactions, where having the relevant membrane molecules able to move, assures a better and more adaptable fit with the interacting ligands. It also makes it easier to understand how cells move, phagocytose and pinocytose. In addition, where a variety of hormones, each binding to their specific receptors, can stimulate the same cell via a cyclic AMP pathway, one could imagine it being particularly economical to have all the receptors share a common pool of membrane adenyl-cyclase, perhaps by having the receptor-ligand complexes finding the adenyl-cyclase by diffusion (50).

In the case of lymphocytes, the specific binding of antigen to membrane receptors can trigger a chain of events leading to the cell dividing and differentiating into an effector cell. Remarkably little is known about the events that follow antigen binding, but it has been shown that antigens can redistribute receptors on both T and B cells and it is reasonable to think that this may play an important role in signalling the cell. Antigen-induced clustering of receptors could operate in various ways, such as forming ion channels or allowing a second membrane molecule to bind in a manner analogous to complement binding to aggreggated Ig in solution. It is not difficult to imagine how pinocytosis, or excessive redistribution, or the blocking of redistribution (e.g. by antigen excess) of receptors could play a role in tolerance induction. These are difficult theories to test experimentally and thus far there is no experimental evidence that strongly supports or refutes the notion that receptor redistribution (rather

than, or together with, antigen-induced conformational
changes in the receptor) is important in lymphocyte
signalling.
The recognition that antibody can redistribute lymphocyte
surface antigens has provided an explanation for the
previously mysterious phenomenon of 'antigenic modulation',
where antibody-coated cells gradually lose their sensitivity
to complement-mediated lysis (51). In the case of Ig on B
cells, it has been shown that anti-Ig can induce the disappearance of the surface Ig by pinocytosis (19,24,30) while
in the case of the TL (our unpublished observations), and
HLA alloantigens (31), there is evidence that redistribution
of the antibody-antigen complexes on the cell surface may be
sufficient in itself to prevent complement-induced lysis.
Although the biological significance of antigenic modulation
is uncertain, it seems to be one way that tumour cells can
protect themselves from immunological attack (52).

REFERENCES

1. Gorter, E. and Grendel, F., J.Exp.Med. 41, 439 (1925).
2. Dahlelli, J.F. and Davson, H., J.Cell Physiol. 5, 495
   (1956).
3. Wilkins, M.H.F., Blaurock, A.E. and Engelman, D.M.,
   Nature New Biology 230, 72 (1971).
4. Bretscher, M.S., Nature New Biology 236, 11 (1972).
5. Stier, A. and Sackman, E., Biochim,Biophys,Acta
   311,400 (1973).
6. Singer, S.J. Structure and Function of Biological
   Membranes, L.I. Rothfield (Ed.), Academic Press, New
   York, p. 145 (1971).
7. Bretscher, M.S., Science 181, 622 (1973).
8. Eylar, E.H., Madoff, M.A., Brody, O.V. and Oncley, J.L.,
   J.Biol.Chem. 237, 1962 (1962).
9. Nicolson, G.L. and Singer, S.J., J.Cell Biol. 60,
   236 (1974).
10. Turner, M.J., Strominger, J.L. and Sanderson, R.A.
    Proc.Nat.Acad.Sci.USA 69, 200 (1972).
11. Schwartz, B.D. and Nathenson, S.G., Transplant.Proc.
    3, 180 (1971).
12. Vitetta, E.S. and Uhr, J.W., J.Immunol. 108, 577 (1972).
13. Loor, F., Forni, L. and Pernis, B., Eur.J.Immunol.
    2, 203 (1972).
14. Vitetta, E.S. and Uhr, J.W., J.Exp.Med. 136, 676 (1972).
15. Palade, G. Subcellular Particles, T. Hayashi (Ed.),
    Ronald Press, New York, p. 64 (1959).
16. de Petris, S. and Raff, M.C., Nature New Biol. 241,257(73)

17. de Petris, S. and Raff, M.C., Eur.J.Immunol. (in press).
18. Kornberg, R.D. and McConnell, H.M., Proc.Nat.Acad.Sci. USA 68, 2564 (1971).
19. Taylor, R.B., Duffus, W.P.H., Raff, M.C. and de Petris, S., Nature New Biology 233, 225 (1971).
20. Aoki, T., Hämmerling, U., de Harven, E., Boyse, E.A. and Old, L.J., J.Exp.Med. 130, 979 (1969).
21. Stackpole, C.W., Aoki, T., Boyse, E.A., Old, L.J., Lumley-Frank, J. and de Harven, E., Science 172, 472 (1971).
22. Ault, K.A., Karnovsky, M.J. and Unanue, E.R., J.Clin. Invest. 52, 2507 (1973).
23. Kornberg, R.D. and McConnell, H.M., Biochemistry 10, 1111 (1971).
24. de Petris, S. and Raff, M.C., Eur.J.Immunol. 2, 523 (1972).
25. Boyse, E.A., Old, L.J. and Stockert, E., Proc.Nat.Acad. Sci.USA 60, 886 (1968).
26. Vitetta, E.S., Boyse, E.A. and Uhr, J.W., Eur.J.Immunol. 3, 446 (1973).
27. Kourilsky, F.M., Silvestre, D., Neauport-Santes, C., Loosfelt, Y. and Dausset, J., Eur.J.Immunol. 2, 249 (1972).
28. Unanue, E.R., Perkins, W.D. and Karnovsky, M.J., J. Exp.Med. 136, 885 (1972).
29. Yahara, I. and Edelman, G.M., Proc.Nat.Acad.Sci.USA 69, 608 (1972).
30. Unanue, E.R., Perkins, W.D. and Karnovsky, M.J. J. Immunol. 108, 569 (1972).
31. Bernocco, B.S., Cullen, S., Scudeller, G., Trinchieri, G. and Ceppellini, R., Histocompatibility Testing, Munksgaard, Copenhagen (in press).
32. Neauport-Santes, C., Lilly, F., Silvestre, D. and Kourilsky, F.M., J.Exp.Med. 137, 511 (1973).
33. Moor, H., Muhlethaler, K., Waldner, H. and Frey-Wyssling, A., J.Biophys.Biochem.Cytol. 10, 1 (1961).
34. Branton, D., Proc.Nat.Acad.Sci.USA 55, 1048 (1966).
35. Pinto da Silva, P. and Branton, D., J.Cell Biol. 45, 598 (1970).
36. Marchesi, V.T., Tillack, T.W., Jackson, R.L., Segrest, J.P. and Scott, R.E., Proc.Nat.Acad.Sci.USA 69, 1445 (72)

37. Pinto da Silva, P., Branton, D. and Douglas, S.A.,
    Nature 232, 194 (1971).
38. Tillack, T.W., Scott, R.E. and Marchesi, V.T., J.Exp.Med.
    135, 1209 (1972).
39. Scott, R.E. and Marchesi, V.T., Cell.Immunol. 3, 301
    (1972).
40. Mandel, J.E., Nature New Biology 239, 112 (1972).
41. McIntyre, J.A., Gillula, N.B. and Karnovsky, M.J.,
    J.Cell.Biol. 60, 192 (1974).
42. Karnovsky, M.J. and Unanue, E.R., Fed.Proc. 32, 55
    (1973).
43. Edelman, G.M., Yahara, I., and Wang, J.L., Proc.Nat.
    Acad.Sci.USA 70, 1442 (1973).
44. Ukena, T.A. and Berlin, R.D., J.Exp.Med. 136, 1 (1972).
45. Bray, D., Cold Spring Harbor Symposium Quant.Biol. 37,
    567 (1973).
46. Ellard, T.D. and Weihing, R.R., Crit.Rev.Biochem. 2,
    1 (1974).
47. Huxley, H.E., Nature 243, 445 (1973).
48. Wessells, N.K., Spooner, B.S., Ash, J.F., Bradley, M.O.,
    Ludena, M.A., Taylor, E.L., Wrenn, J.T. and Yamada, K.M.,
    Science 171, 135 (1971).
49. Singer, S.J., Perspectives in Membrane Biology, S.
    Estrado-O and C. Gitler (Eds.) Academic Press, New
    York (in press).
50. Cuadrecasas, P., Perspectives in Membrane Biology, S.
    Estrado-O and C. Gitler (Eds.) Academic Press, New
    York (in press).
51. Old, L.J., Stockert, E., Boyse, E.A. and Kim, J.H.
    J.Exp.Med. 127, 523 (1968).
52. Boyse, E.A., Old, L.J. and Luell, S., J.Nat.Cancer Inst.
    31, 987 (1963).

PROBING LYMPHOCYTE MEMBRANE ORGANIZATION

Leon Wofsy

Department of Bacteriology and Immunology
University of California
Berkeley, California 94720

ABSTRACT. We discuss here approaches to some problems of lymphocyte membrane organization. By randomly modifying lymphocyte surfaces with a hapten, we have been able to demonstrate that all exposed membrane protein can be capped without effecting an equivalent aggregation of intramembranous particles (IMP). A versatile and highly specific method is described for simultaneous labeling of multiple cell surface antigens for fluorescence and for transmission and scanning electron microscopy.

INTRODUCTION

The mobility of antigens on lymphocyte membranes has been demonstrated repeatedly (1,2). Under appropriate conditions, each specific surface antigen that has been examined can be capped by direct or indirect antibody binding procedures.

It is not yet possible to relate the significance of this observed surface mobility to a mechanism for lymphocyte activation. In fact, very little is understood about the structure and dynamics of lymphocyte membrane organization, and about the mechanisms that may modulate or be affected by the aggregation of surface receptors. One question which is actively being explored, but which cannot yet be answered, is: What influence does the redistribution of surface antigens by multivalent ligands have on internal membrane structures, and, in particular, on the organization of the IMP observed with freeze-fracture electron microscopy (3)? Another question, raised by recent observations that cell interactions in the immune response require a relationship between multiple surface antigens (4), is: Are antigen binding receptors associated structurally on lymphocyte membranes with certain other gene products?

In this talk, we will describe approaches which our laboratory is developing to these two questions. On the first, we have some relevant findings; on the second, we have a method which we hope will prove useful.

I. SURFACE MOBILITY AND IMP
OF LYMPHOCYTES

A number of laboratories have shown that capping by antibody of Ig, H-2, or Θ surface antigens of lymphocytes does not result in redistribution of IMP (5). Contradictory or ambiguous findings have been reported on the effect of lectin binding (PHA or Con-A) on IMP (6,7). Some very elementary questions remain unanswered: Are there protein portions of IMP and, if so, are any exposed at the cell surface? Are the particles freely mobile in the plane of the membrane, or are they restricted, as in the case of the mature erythrocyte, by a spectrin-like membrane network?

The experiments we will describe here show that no sizeable fraction of IMP protrudes as protein moeities at the surface of the lymphocyte membrane. We have been able to cap simultaneously virtually all surface protein, while demonstrating by freeze-fracture electron microscopy that there is no corresponding capping, or large-scale aggregation, of IMP.

Janis Mower has developed an experimental system which permits the covalent coupling of hapten groups randomly to cell surface proteins. With a sandwich of anti-hapten antibody followed by fluorescent anti-Ig from another species, one can determine whether all lymphocyte surface proteins are mobile and can be capped, as shown schematically in Fig. 1. Freeze-fracture of the membranes may then reveal whether any hapten-modified surface antigens are actually covalent extensions of IMP, so that the aggregation of surface protein is necessarily accompanied by a corresponding movement of IMP.

To establish the validity of our experimental system, we examined the effects of hapten-modification on lymphocyte populations and determined that all detectable surface protein was indeed modified. Mouse spleen cells were reacted with 10^{-3}M diazoniumphenyl β-lactoside for 1 hour at 4°C. Modified cells were indistinguishable from unmodified cells in the in vitro response to sheep erythrocyte antigen and in the incorporation of tritiated thymidine when stimulated by PHA or by lipopolysaccharide. The high viability of modified cells was indicated not only by trypan blue exclusion, but by the fact that > 90% underwent

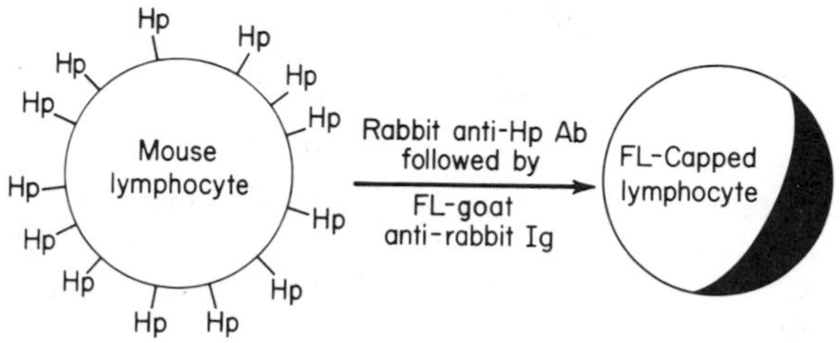

Fig. 1.   HAPTEN-SANDWICH CAPPING OF MODIFIED LYMPHOCYTES

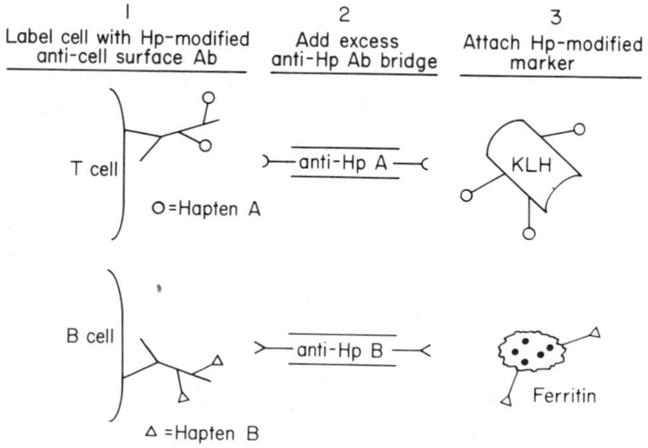

Fig. 2.   HAPTEN-SANDWICH LABELING

261

capping, a metabolically dependent process (2), when treated successively at 37°C with rabbit anti-azophenyl β-lactoside antibody (anti-lac) and fluorescent goat anti-rabbit Ig.

The extent of surface protein modification of mouse splenic lymphocytes was demonstrated in the following experiment: hapten-sandwich capping was achieved with anti-lac and fluorescein (Fl) goat anti-rabbit Ig: then, under non-capping conditions at 4°C, the cells were treated with rhodamine (Rh) goat anti-mouse Ig. Coincident capping of Fl- and Rh-antigens was observed, with no residual diffuse staining of mouse Ig. If any substantial fraction of mouse Ig had not been modified with the lac hapten, it would have been detected readily outside the cap region by the anti-mouse Ig fluorescent reagent.

The same experiment was performed, yielding the same results, with respect to Con-A binding sites. Hapten-sandwich capping, this time with anti-lac and Rh-goat anti-rabbit Ig, was followed by treatment with Fl- Con-A under non-capping conditions. All caps and most large patches were again coincident; no residual diffuse Fl- Con-A staining was observed. Thus, the Con-A binding sites were modified with the lac hapten and could be mobilized into caps by the hapten-sandwich procedure. The results of two-fluorochrome experiments with Con-A binding sites are summarized in Table 1.

Freeze-fracture studies on the capped lymphocytes are now in progress. The most obvious result, already indicated, is that massive aggregation of IMP has not occurred. We are examining some points of interest and possible differences of a less obvious nature in the appearance of fracture faces from capped and uncapped cells.

So, a question has been answered, but we are left with riddles. The vast majority of IMP do not present protein (or free amino saccharide) groups at the lymphocyte surface; if they interact with any class(es) of surface receptors, it must be on the basis of non-covalent association.

In view of reports of the inhibition of surface capping and patching by high concentrations of Con-A (2,8), we have explored the effect of Con-A on the capping of hapten-modified lymphocytes. Table 2 shows that Con-A, 100 µg/ml, partially inhibits capping of these cells with Fl- goat anti-mouse Ig: about 40% less capped cells are seen after Con-A

TABLE 1

HAPTEN-SANDWICH CAPPING OF MODIFIED LYMPHOCYTES

Rabbit anti-Lac + Rh-Goat anti-Rabbit Ig	F1-Con-A	Rh	F1	Coincident Caps
+	−	all caps or large patches	−	−
−	+	−	all diffuse	−
+	+	all caps or large patches	all caps or large patches	100%
+	+ with α-me-mannoside	all caps or large patches	unstained	−

TABLE 2

EFFECT OF HIGH DOSE CON-A ON SURFACE MOVEMENT

Con-A (100 μg/ml	Rabbit anti-Lac + Rh-Goat anti-Rabbit Ig	Fl-Goat anti-Mouse Ig	Percent Cells Stained	Staining Pattern
−	+	−	100%	all caps or large patches
+	+	−	100%	all caps or large patches
−	−	+	60%	all caps or large patches
+	−	+	60%	60% caps or large patches, 40% diffuse

264

treatment. We also observed, as shown in Table 1, that Con-A can inhibit the capping of its own binding sites (8) on the hapten-modified cells. However, the results in Table 2 show no inhibition by Con-A of hapten-sandwich capping (anti-lac, followed by Fl-goat anti-rabbit Ig).

Whatever Con-A may be doing, the notion that it inhibits the aggregation of surface antigens by somehow "freezing" the membrane may not present an accurate picture. Andrew Raubitschek in our laboratory has looked, with unmodified lymphocytes, at the effect of high concentrations of Con-A on membrane lipid fluidity as indicated by a hydrocarbon (2N19) electron spin resonance (ESR) probe. An Arrhenius plot of the ESR signal in the presence of Con-A, at temperatures from 15-37°C, suggests an increase rather than a decrease in lipid fluidity.

II. SIMULTANEOUS LABELING OF DIFFERENT CELL SURFACE ANTIGENS FOR FLUORESCENCE AND ELECTRON MICROSCOPY

The discovery of many allo- and differentiation antigens allows definition of lymphocyte sub-populations and may permit elucidation of any critical associative relationship between receptors and other antigens on a lymphocyte membrane. Considering the large and growing number of alloantigens detected, a simple and versatile procedure for specific labeling of more than one cell surface antigen at a time is sorely needed. An approach suggested by Lamm et al. (9) had also occurred to us: a hapten may be coupled to anti-cell surface antibodies and to markers suitable for electron microscopy; after labeling cells with the hapten-modified antibody, the corresponding anti-hapten antibody may be used to form a bridge to the hapten-modified marker. This hapten-sandwich labeling scheme, as we have used it to label thymus associated antigens with hemocyanin (KLH) and membrane-bound Ig with ferritin (fer), is illustrated in Fig. 2.

In our procedure, a hapten is coupled to antibody by reacting the Ig fraction of any specific antiserum under mild conditions with a diazonium reagent. An average of over 5 hapten groups per mole can be attached, while less than 30% of the antibody loses its capacity to be bound by an immunoadsorbent. As haptens, we have used p-azobenzene β-D lactoside (lac), p-azobenzene arsonate (ars), and o-azobenzene β-D galactoside (o-gal) with equal effectiveness.

There is a wide choice of anti-hapten bridging antibodies, since azoconjugated immunogens are readily prepared and anti-hapten antibodies are easily purified by affinity chromatography (10).

Double-labeling by the anti-hapten bridge method had previously been prevented by the fact that hapten-modification of desired high molecular weight markers, such as hemocyanin and virus particles, frequently results in their dissociation (9). We found that markers could be protected before hapten-modification by a mild cross-linking treatment that stabilized the association of sub-units without significant intermolecular aggregation. As a result, hapten-modified KLH, ferritin, and tobacco mosaic virus (TMV) served as excellent markers in our electron microscopy studies.

The specificity of the hapten-sandwich labeling procedure was verified with fluorescence and electron microscopy. We used lac-modified anti-mouse brain antibody (lac-anti-MBr) to label thymus associated antigens (11), and ars-modified anti-mouse Ig (ars-anti-MIg) to label membrane-bound immunoglobulin. In double-labeling fluorescence experiments with Fl-anti-lac (for MBr) and Rh-anti-ars (for MIg) we could readily distinguish thymocytes and T cells from B cells, as shown in Table 3. In double-labeling experiments for electron microscopy, lymphoid cells were treated sequentially with lac-anti-MBr, anti-lac, and lac-KLH; and with ars-anti-MIg, anti-ars, and ars-fer. The lac-KLH (MBr) and ars-fer (MIg) labels segregated dramatically on different lymphocytes. Cells which labeled strongly with ars-fer (MIg) exhibited no lac-KLH (MBr); cells which labeled with lac-KLH (MBr) also showed about one-tenth or less as much of the ars-fer (MIg) marker; some lymphocytes and all reticulocytes were completely free of either marker. (We do not yet know whether the inclusion of the small amount of ars-fer marker on the lac-KLH (MBr) labeled cells was specific.)

We have also applied the hapten-sandwich labeling procedure to scanning electron microscopy (SEM). Despite rapid developments in SEM, there has been no generally applicable method for immunospecific labeling of antigens with markers that can be visualized with SEM. David Carter and Michael Nemanic have used hapten-sandwich labeling to specifically attach SEM markers to human erythrocytes, mouse mammary tumor cells, and mouse lymphocytes. To establish specificity of labeling, human erythrocytes modified with the lac hapten were treated with anti-lac antibody and then with

TABLE 3

FLUORESCENT LABELING OF CELLS
THAT BIND Hp-COUPLED ANTIBODIES

Lymphocytes	% Rh ars-anti-MIg, Rh-anti-ars	% Fl lac-anti-MBr, Fl-anti-lac
Spleen	60	30
Thymus	< 2	> 95

either lac-TMV or lac-KLH. Both markers were easily visualized. When anti-o-gal antibody was substituted for the anti-lac bridge, no labeling occurred. Splenic lymphocytes were labeled with lac-anti-MIg, anti-lac, and lac-TMV. The lac-TMV marker was exhibited by about the same fraction of the cells as were stained in fluorescence labeling with Fl-anti-MIg.

Despite reports that, in some circumstances, human B cells can be distinguished morphologically from human T cells on the basis of more and longer microvilli (12,13), we found that cells labeled for MIg were not different in appearance from other unlabeled lymphocytes. Under our conditions, less than 10% of the lymphocytes were characterized by many microvilli, and these cells were found to be unlabeled. We have found, as have others (14), that the extent of microvilli formation is highly dependent on the conditions to which cells are subjected, so that the phenomenon does not provide a generally reliable means of discriminating lymphocyte subpopulations.

Detailed procedures for hapten-sandwich labeling, and electron micrographs which cannot be reproduced here for technical reasons, will be published elsewhere.*

ACKNOWLEDGEMENTS

I am indebted to the collaborators mentioned in the text, as well as to the following who have shared in developing the hapten-sandwich labeling procedure: K. Thompson, P. C. Baker, J. Goodman, J. Kimura, C. Henry, and S. Bartalsky. This work was supported by U. S. Public Health Service grant AI-06610 and National Science Foundation grant GB-34328.

---

*Two companion papers have been submitted for publication: Hapten-sandwich labeling. I. A general procedure for simultaneous labeling of multiple cell surface antigens for fluorescence and electron microscopy. By L. Wofsy, P. C. Baker, K. Thompson, J. Goodman, J. Kimura, and C. Henry. Hapten-sandwich labeling. II. Immunospecific attachment of cell surface markers suitable for scanning electron microscopy. By M. K. Nemanic, D. P. Carter, D. R. Pitelka, and L. Wofsy.

REFERENCES

1. Taylor, R. B., Duffus, W. P. H., Raff, M. C., and dePetris, S., Nature New Biol. 233, 225 (1971).

2. Loor, F., Forni, L., and Pernis, B., Eur. J. Immunol. 2, 203 (1972).

3. Pinto da Silva, P., and Branton, D., J. Cell Biol. 45, 598 (1970).

4. Katz, D. H., Hamaoka, T., and Benacerraf, B., J. Exp. Med. 137, 1405 (1973).

5. Karnovsky, M. J., and Unanue, E. R., Fed. Proc. 32, 55 (1973).

6. Loor, F., Eur. J. Immunol. 3, 112 (1973).

7. McIntyre, J. A., Gillula, N. B., and Karnovsky, M. J., J. Cell. Biol. 60, 192 (1974).

8. Yahara, I., and Edelman, G. M., Proc. Nat. Acad. Sci. U.S.A. 69, 608 (1972).

9. Lamm, M. E., Koo, G. C., Stackpole, C. W., and Hämmerling, U., Proc. Nat. Acad. Sci. U.S.A. 69, 3732 (1972).

10. Cuatrecasas, P., J. Biol. Chem. 245, 3059 (1970).

11. Golub, E. S., Cell. Immunol. 2, 353 (1971).

12. Lin, P. S., Cooper, A. G., and Wortis, H. H., New England J. Med. 289, 548 (1973).

13. Polliack, A., Lampen, N., Clarkson, B. D., DeHarven, E., Bentwich, Z., Siegel, F. P., and Kunkel, H. G., J. Exp. Med. 138, 607 (1973).

14. Lin, P. S., Wallach, D. F. H., and Tsai, S., Proc. Nat. Acad. Sci. U.S.A. 70, 2492 (1973).

POLYCLONAL MITOGENS AND THE NATURE OF
B LYMPHOCYTE ACTIVATION MECHANISMS

Melvyn Greaves, George Janossy, Marc Feldmann
and Michael Doenhoff

ICRF Tumour Immunology Unit, University College London,
Department of Immunology, Clinical Research Centre,
Harrow, Middlesex, and
The Chester Beatty Institute, London

ABSTRACT. Three current competitive models of B lymphocyte
activation involving either single or double signals are
discussed. Experiments with polyclonal, mouse B cell mitogens have been designed to further investigate the validity
of these hypotheses. Evidence is presented to suggest that
direct activation of B lymphocytes via either surface immunoglobulins (using insolubilized haptens) or non-specific sites
(lipopolysaccharide and pokeweed mitogen) can occur. The
mitogenicity of thymus-independent antigens was confirmed
but found to be quantitatively unimpressive; its biological
relevance is therefore questioned. No evidence could be
obtained to support the view that activated complement or
cyclic GMP are necessarily involved with the '2nd' signal
level. Evidence for B lymphocyte heterogeneity is presented
in terms of proliferative responsiveness of spleen versus
lymph node B cells. It is suggested that although some
(principally IgM programmed) B cells can be directly activated with minimal second signal involvement, other (particularly IgG programmed) B lymphocytes have additional requirements which either operate during the early induction phase
or post-inductively as potentiation mechanisms.

INTRODUCTION

The term 'polyclonal mitogens' has been used to denote
ligands that activate a large proportion of T or B lymphocyte populations into mitotic cycle in vitro (1,2). The
responses elicited are qualitatively similar to those induced by conventional immunogens which usually activate far
fewer cells. B lymphocytes activated by Pokeweed or Lipopolysaccharide, for example, differentiate into plasmablasts
or plasma cells (3) and concommittantly synthesize and
secrete considerable quantities of IgM (4,5). The latter

271

has been shown to include multiple antibody specificities
that are immunologically unrelated to the initiating ligand
(6). T lymphocytes similarly 'do their thing' when stimulated by lectins such as Concanavalin A and Phytohaemagglutinin;
they release soluble factors that interact with macrophages
(7) and possibly B lymphocytes (8) and under appropriate
circumstances lectin activated T cells are aggressive for
juxtapositioned 'target' cells (9,10). These observations
have been interpreted (1) to suggest that a large proportion
of lymphocytes can be triggered by a process that does not
readily discriminate between antigens and polyclonal mitogens
and that the 'message' to the cell from its surface is likely
therefore to be a non-specific signal, or 'second messenger'.
The quantity of the latter then regulates the expression of
the cells pre-programmed response. This is of course a
simplistic view and there are currently several widely divergent opinions as to what polyclonal mitogens can really tell
us about lymphocyte triggering by antigens. If we accept
that the 'final common pathway' of antigens and polyclonal
mitogens may be the same, we must consider the following
propositions relating to trigger sites and signals.

    1. Do polyclonal mitogens and immunogens act on separate
cell surface sites to generate equivalent (and possibly
identical) signals at those sites (i.e. parallel responses)?

    2. Do polyclonal mitogens and immunogens trigger lympho-
cytes via common sites? (11,12) The idea here is that
immunogens are concentrated on the lymphocyte surface by
antigen receptors (immunoglobulins in the case of B lymphocytes) and that a secondary interaction with 'non-specific'
mitogen sites then occurs either as a direct result of the
immunogens intrinsic mitogenicity (-thymus independent
antigens, e.g. LPS) or following mitogen generation initiated
by the immunogen in other T cells and/or macrophages
(-thymus dependent antigens, e.g. DNP-HGG). Interactions
with the non-specific sites provide the only signal to the
cell. This original concept presents a challenge to a prime
dogma of immunology that has been accepted almost without
question - namely that cell surface immunoglobulins can in
fact initiate the activation sequence. (It is relevant to
recall that attempts to detect conformational changes in
immunoglobulin molecules following antigen binding provide
one of the most commendable failures in immunology (see-13).)

    This single, non-specific signal concept proposed by
Coutinho and Möller should be distinguished from currently
popular 2 signal models for B lymphocyte activation which
are considered to involve non-specific second signals but
where signal one (generated via antigen bound surface

immunoglobulin) interacts in some way with signal two to activate the cell (14,15).
3. Polyclonal mitogens are considered by proponents of
two signal hypotheses (14) to be potent inducers of second
signals. The corollary is that polyclonal mitogens do not
exist as such but function synergistically by 'completing'
or modifying an undetected first signal. Candidates for
first signal generators in this case would be antigens
interacting with surface immunoglobulins and might derive
from foreign serum in cultures, auto-antigens or foreign
antigens interacting with lymphocytes in vivo prior to the
donors' demise. If this view is correct then polyclonal
mitogens mimic 'normal' second signal generators the candid-
ature for which currently includes soluble products of
activated macrophages and T lymphocytes. Activated complement components (16) and cyclic GMP (17) are also candidates
in a sense, although the 'level' of operation in the activation sequence is ill-defined.
These three propositions correspond to three widely
discussed models of B lymphocyte activation (Table1).
They offer three different explanations not only for activation processes but also for tolerance and the relative T
cell dependency of different antigens.
We report here a series of experiments designed to
analyse the validity of these hypotheses.

METHODS

Our methods for inducing and assaying proliferative
(18,19) and antibody secreting (20,21) responses of mouse
lymphocytes have been fully described in the given
references.

RESULTS AND DISCUSSION

1. Experiments with insoluble ligands
    Model 1 (Table1) implies that interaction with immuno-
globulins only is sufficient to trigger or 'tolerize' B
cells, with specificity for determinants 'normally' associated with 'thymus independent' (TI), or 'thymus dependent'
(TD) antigens, provided some particular demands of determinant presentation are met (evidence reviewed in 22). The
hapten DNP on polymerized flagellin provides the most widely
studied immunogen. Since POL is now claimed to be a polyclonal mitogen (12) the above view is now under challenge
(see Model 2). It ought however to be clear that, theoretically at least, this model does not in fact exclude

273

Table 1

COMPARATIVE MODELS OF B LYMPHOCYTE ACTIVATION

Principle Features	Model 1 (ref.22)	Model 2 (ref.11)	Model 3 (ref. 14)
Activation	Single signal via Ig	Single signal via non-specific (mitogen) site(s)	Double signal via (1) Ig and (2) non-specific site
T-dependent antigens	Small, low epitope density	non- mitogenic	Qualitative distinction denied (TI may be
T-independent antigens	Large, high epitope density	mitogenic	more efficient 2nd signal generators)
Tolerance	Excessive binding or monovalent binding (block) No signal assumed	Excess of single activating signal	Signal 1 only
Polyclonal B cell mitogens	Act independently on different (non-Ig) site to antigens	Act independently on same site(s) as antigens	Exist only as 2nd signal generators

activation via other non-immunoglobulin sites. Neither does it exclude polyclonal responses induced by thymus-independent immunogens since these relatively large molecules with repeating identical determinants might be expected at high concentrations to interact with high avidity with cells having relatively low affinity binding sites.

We suggested previously (1) that experiments with insolubilized lectins lent some support to Model 1 since they provided a parallel example in which B cells appeared to ignore the binding of a soluble ligand (of restricted size and valency) yet responded well when confronted with the same ligand on Sepharose (23) or plastic (24). We have now performed the parallel experiment of putting haptens covalently onto a solid surface. Some representative results are given in Fig. 1 and Table 2. Our results are given in full elsewhere (25). These experiments demonstrated that totally insoluble antigens can trigger IgM antibody responses in B cells in vitro. We presume minimal leakage of soluble antigen to be irrelevant since it would not be expected to be immunogenic for purified B lymphocytes. TNP-KLH-Sepharose and TNP-Polyacrylamide were both capable of activating B cells in cultures, containing less than 1% macrophages and T cells, that were incapable of supporting a response to sheep red blood cells (SRBC) or soluble TNP-KLH. It is therefore likely that the insolubilized antigens directly stimulated B cells via surface contact only and without facilitating influences from other cells. The implication of this interpretation is that antigen bound cell surface immunoglobulins initiated the activation sequence (Model 1). The predictions of Models 2 and 3 however demand that we exclude (a) that these insoluble ligands are not highly effective at generating a second signal via a very small number of residual macrophages and/or T cells (Model 3), or (b) that these ligands are not polyclonal mitogens (Model 2). Unfortunately both these points are virtually impossible to refute completely. If one macrophage is enough then the experimental system will have to be radically changed! TNP-KLH sepharose could be a polyclonal mitogen with cross-linked KLH (cf. 26) or sepharose itself (cf. 27) providing the ultimate signal. If this is the case it is not easy for us to see why the optimal substitution should be intermediate rather than high. It seems even less likely that TNP-polyacrylamide carries a potential to interact secondarily with non-specific mitogenic sites. Furthermore both of these types of antigen preparations were not in fact demonstrably polyclonal activators at least in terms of proliferative responses and antibody production to an irrelevant

Figure 1. ACTIVATION OF MOUSE SPLEEN CELLS BY TNP-KLH
SEPHAROSE

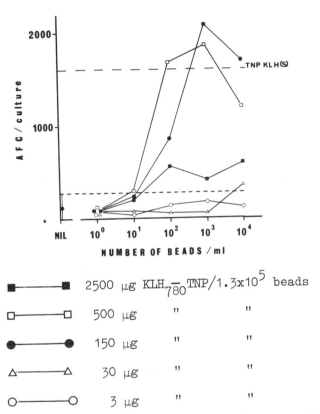

$$\begin{array}{l}\blacksquare\!-\!\!\!-\!\!\!-\!\!\!\blacksquare \quad 2500 \ \mu g \ KLH_{\frac{780}{}}TNP/1.3x10^5 \ beads\end{array}$$

■——■	2500 μg KLH$_{780}$TNP/1.3x10^5 beads	
□——□	500 μg " "	
●——●	150 μg " "	
△——△	30 μg " "	
○——○	3 μg " "	

High dotted line : Mean response of primed spleen cells to
soluble TNP-KLH
Low dotted line : Background anti-DNP response
Day 4 culture direct (IgM) plaque forming cells assayed
against DNP coated SRBC
Each value the arithmetic mean of three cultures. Day 4
direct (IgM) antibody forming cell (AFC) response assayed
against DNP coated red cells.

Table 2

RESPONSE OF NORMAL CBA SPLEEN CELLS TO
INSOLUBILIZED HAPTENS

ANTIGEN	Response AFC/Culture	
	- DNP	- SRBC
NONE	17	163
Soluble TNP-KLH	17	92
DNP-POL $(1\mu g/ml)$	430	180
10^3 TNP-KLH Seph. beads	476	141
10^3 TNP-PolyA beads	983	190
3×10^6 SRBC	-	1622

1.5×10^7 spleen cells per culture day 4 assay. Direct (IgM)
plaque priming cells assayed. Data pooled from a series of
individual experiments in which hapten-beads were titrated.
Optimal response given. Similar responses to TNP-KLH
Sepharose were obtained with spleen cells from nude mice and
with normal spleen cells depleted on T lymphocytes and
macrophages (data in ref 25).
PolyA: Polyacrylamide; aminoethylated for hapten conjugation.
No free amino group left after conjugation.

antigen (SRBC). Even if they were this would be open to at least two different interpretations (vide supra), one of which does not contradict Model 1. More experiments with haptens on various inert surfaces are however necessary to consolidate this point. If no overt polyclonality is demonstrable then Model 2 can only be correct if one postulates that the intrinsic mitogenicity is too weak to be detected as a polyclonal response and that only cells with high affinity anti-hapten binding sites are therefore subject to the essential mitogenic influence. At present this possibility cannot be (a) denied, or (b) tested. These comments should not be taken to suggest that an apparently antigen-specific antibody response cannot result <u>either partly or solely</u> from a non-specific mitogenic influence (11). The existence of such responses does not deny that direct cross-linkage <u>solely</u> of immunoglobulins also generates a B cell response. These experiments with 'insolubilized' haptens parallel earlier experiments with haptens on polymerized flagellin (22). There is however an important reservation to be placed on conclusions based on the use of these polymeric stimulants. The response to both DNP-POL and TNP-Sepharose or Polyacrylamine is <u>restricted to IgM</u> secreting B cells regardless of whether pre-sensitized or 'normal' mice are used as spleen cell donors. The same culture systems supports an IgG response of primed cells to DNP as a soluble T dependent immunogen. It is therefore quite possible that while <u>some</u> IgM programmed B lymphocytes can respond <u>directly</u> to insolubilized haptens, other B cells, particularly those programmed for IgG synthesis have <u>additional</u> requirements for activation that are not satisfied by these polymeric ligands. The same reservations, relating to possible B lymphocyte subsets, are applicable to responses to polyclonal B lymphocyte mitogens such as LPS and pokeweed which stimulate almost exclusively IgM responses (4,5).

2. <u>Mitogenicity of thymus-independent (TI) antigens</u>

The starting point for Model 2 was the observation by Coutinho and Möller (28) that all TI antigens they tested were found to be polyclonal B cell activators in terms of (3H)-thymidine uptake and antibody responses. Human gamma globulin (HGG) as an example of a thymus-dependent (TD) antigen was reported not to have this property. We have repeated these experiments, following the reported methods and in some cases using aliquots of the same TI antigen. The results are summarized in Table 3. They indicate the following points:

1) The results reported by Coutinho and Möller were

Table 3

STIMULATION OF DNA SYNTHESIS IN MOUSE SPLEEN
CELLS BY THYMUS INDEPENDENT ANTIGENS
CONJUGATED WITH HAPTENS

Stimulants	A	B	C
Control	4640	800	6.660
ConA (3µg/ml)	30.200	26.500	156.500
PWM (15 µg/ml)	21.000	n.t.	123.600
LPS. S.marc. (50µg/ml)	15.200	13.950	n.t.
Lipid-A (50µg/ml)	17.650	13.050	104.560
Levan 1 (150µg/ml)	5.350	1.800	57.110
(DNP-) levan 2.(50µg/ml)	6.870	1.970	50.180
−100µg/ml			
(DNP-)levan 3.(60µg/ml)	8.170	4.150	78.000
−100µg/ml			
(DNP-)levan 4.(100µg/ml)	6.245	1.560	47.680
(Stearoyl-)levan 5.(150µg/ml)	5.360	n.t.	n.t.
SIII 1. (500µg/ml)	9.420	3.450	76.860
(DNP-) SIII 2. (100µg/ml)	6.000	2.050	54.570
(DNP-) SIII 3. (100µg/ml)	5.110	1.850	41.580
(DNP-) SIII 4. (100µg/ml)	6.600	2.030	35.240
red cell stroma	1.400	n.t.	7.020

A, B: 5×10^5 spleen cells were cultured in microplate wells
in 0.25ml RPM1-1640 medium supplemented with 10% FCS. In
experiment A FCS 42141 had a relatively high control background and supported mitogenic responses extremely well. In

Legend to Table 3 continued:

experiment B FCS 42070 had low background and supported mitogenic responses moderately well. Cultures were incubated for 64 hours. 1μCi of ^{3}H-thymidine (low specific activity, 50mCi/mmol) was added 16 hours prior to harvesting. Results are expressed as c.p.m. per 0.25ml culture
C: 2.5×10^6 spleen cells were cultured for 2 days in round bottomed plastic tubes in 1 ml serum free medium. 2μCi ^{3}H-thymidine (high specific activity, 5 Ci/mmol) were added 24 hours prior to harvesting. Results show c.p.m. per 1 ml culture. In all cases different doses of antigens were added in duplicates and the observed high stimulation values are shown.
DNP-levan and DNP-SIII 2-4 increasing levels of substitution. Assayed for immunogencity (anti-DNP IgM response) over a wide concentration range in vitro, DNP-levan 3 and DNP-SIII 3 were the only strong immunogens (Desaymard and Feldmann, unpublished observations).
DNP-levan 5 is tolerogenic and has no demonstrable immunogenicity down to 1ng/ml level. Optimal concentrations for mitogenicity are given in parenthesis. In all cases these values were at least 100x the optimal immunogenic dose.
n.t.-not tested.

found to be reproduceable.

2) Conjugates with widely differing immunogenicity in vitro had broadly comparable mitogenicity, and

3) The apparent mitogenicity hinges on certain technical parameters of the test; particularly the amount of thymidine in the culture. We (19) and others (30,31) have discussed this point at considerable length elsewhere. Suffice to point out (see Table 3) that if thymidine is limiting, as it is by a factor of up to 50 in Group C conditions, then the responses are no longer quantitative and good and very weak responses can become less distinguishable. Statistically significant proliferative responses to levan, SIII and Dextran Sulphate certainly do exist but under quantitative assay conditions they are small in magnitude compared to the more conventional B cell mitogens such as LPS (Lipid-A) and PWM. We have not yet assayed these responses for antibody secreting cells so the possibility still remains of a polyclonal activation independent of DNA synthesis. Indeed positive evidence for such a response has been presented (32). We conclude from these experiments that the mitogenicity of TI antigens does not appear to be of sufficient magnitude to provide a strong indication of biological relevance. This in no way denies Model 2 if some TI antigens are considered as polyclonal activators rather than polyclonal mitogens.

3. Mechanisms of activation by polyclonal B lymphocyte mitogens

How such diverse stimulants as Lipid-A, pokeweed, polynucleotides and polyanions activate B lymphocytes is unknown. There is no compelling reason to suppose that a 'common' receptor for these ligands exists or that their mode of action is identical.

One potential explanation for the mechanism of action of polyclonal B lymphocyte mitogens such as LPS is that they actually interact directly or indirectly with immunoglobulins which then initiatethe response! This possibility is raised by the report by Andersson and Melchers (33) that B lymphocyte cell surface IgM appears to become aggregated following the binding of LPS. This conclusion was based on molecular weight estimations of solubilized membrane preparations. We have looked for such an effect by immunofluorescence on intact cells (Greaves and Andersson, unpublished observations) Binding of LPS and Lipid-A, the mitogenic component of LPS, had no discernable influence on either the binding or distribution of rhodamine labelled fab monomers of rabbit antibodies to mouse immunoglobulins (i.e. binding was

diffuse), or on redistribution into patches and 'caps' of
'whole' anti-immunoglobulin antibodies. Similar results were
obtained with Pokeweed mitogen. Thus while indirect effects
on cell surface associated immunoglobulins could exist there
is no direct evidence that polyclonal mitogens activate B
lymphocytes via immunoglobulin molecules.

Do B lymphocyte responses to LPS and PWM involve other
non-B cells? Watson et al (17), proponents of the two
signal (model 3) hypothesis, deny the existence of both true TI
antigens and polyclonal B cell mitogens that directly
activate B lymphocytes since their model consists of obligatory two-signal synergy. While this strict interpretation is
probably not widely shared by all those who subscribe to two
signal hypotheses, it invites challenge since it appears to
contradict available data. We will not discuss the reality
of TI antigens here (see ref 34) but will restrict ourselves
to reporting one relatively straight forward result (Table 4);
which is that cotton filtered spleen cells from nu/nu mice
(with thymic hypoplasia) that have been treated with anti-θ
serum plus complement, responded well to both LPS and pokeweed mitogen although the LPS response was somewhat reduced.
Therefore the suggestion that these B cell responses are T
cell dependent (35) is unlikely to be correct. Non-B, non-T
cells (e.g. monocyte-macrophages ?) may however be important
since most, if not all, TI antigens and B cell mitogens are
pyrogens (36) and supernatants of activated macrophages can
facilitate B cell response to TD antigens (15). They may
also contain polyclonal B cell mitogens (Möller, personal
communication).

It could also be argued that our observations and those
of others reflect two signal synergy dependent upon LPS (or
PWM) and a silent antigen (first signal initiator) in the
culture system. Since responses are quite impressive in
mouse serum supplemented medium, and to a lesser extent in
serum free medium (Table 3 and ref. 32), the most obvious
candidates are lost and the alternatives are not readily
amenable to test.

4. Cyclic nucleotides as first and second signals (Model 3:
variety Watson et al (17))

There is no denying that cyclic AMP, and now its partner
cyclic GMP, are responsible for a large proportion of what is
interesting in biology. There is no denying also that they
were bound to be considered responsible for activating
lymphocytes. There is every reason to suppose that a second
messenger should, in principle, exist for lymphocytes (vide
supra) but how good is the evidence that it is cyclic AMP or

Table 4

RESPONSE OF NU/NU SPLEEN B LYMPHOCYTES
TO POLYCLONAL MITOGENS

Mitogen[3]	Response c/min[1]	
	Untreated	$\alpha\Theta$ and filtered[2]
Normal CBA control	3,100	1,400
ConA	33,000	2,100
PWM	23,000	n.t.
LPS	18,000	n.t.
LPS + ME	28,700	35,000
Nu/nu [2] control	2,100	1,900
ConA	3,200	2,100
PWM	19,000	25,000
LPS	16,700	12,000
LPS + 2% T cells [4]	n.t.	11,000
LPS + ME [5]	34,000	35,000

1. (^{3}H)-thymidine uptake (48-64 hrs) Duplicate cultures
2. Filtered through cotton wool columns at 37°
3. Optimal concentration only
4. 5% CBA spleen cells (=2% T cells)
5. 5×10^{-4} M, Mercaptoethanol
n.t.-not tested

cyclic GMP. The relevant reported facts are as follows:
1) cAMP itself and drugs/or hormones that increase intra-cellular cAMP levels suppress T cell proliferative and functional responses (see 37 fr refs.).

2) cGMP but not cAMP levels in mixed T-B populations increase impressively within 30 minutes of adding an optimal mitogenic concentration of a T cell mitogen (38).

3) Daily feeding of cultures with cGMP considerably facilitates the response of T cell deprived suspensions to SRBC and rescues normal spleen cells from cAMP induced suppression of the SRBC response (17).

Our relevant information is that
1) cAMP but not cGMP suppresses both T and B proliferative responses to polyclonal mitogens (Fig.2). However in contrast to other systems (39,40) cAMP induced suppression could not be reversed by cGMP (Fig.3). This result contrasts with the competitive effects reported by Watson et al (17).

2) Dibutyryl cAMP, cGMP and carbomylcholine which raises intracellular cGMP levels in lymphocytes (14) are not B or T polyclonal mitogens (Fig.4).

3) cGMP does not facilitate a B lymphocyte response to ConA (Fig.5), anti-Ig or a TI antigen, TNP-KLH (Feldmann and Greaves, unpublished observations). Some weak amplification of SRBC responses were observed but it is possible that both these and the more impressive responses reported by Watson et al (17) reflect an amplification of weak T cell independent response to SRBC. It seems possible therefore that some of the cAMP effects on lymphocytes may be misleading, possibly non-physiological and/or non-specific, and that cGMP is not a true 'second messenger' (note that a second messenger for hormones can replace the hormone itself). We are attracted by the possibility that cAMP and cGMP may regulate proliferation rates and the expression of different functions in lymphocytes, but remain unconvinced that they operate crucially in the early phase of initiation to either directly activate the cell, or provide a second signal to complement that provided by another non-stimulatory ligand.

5. Complement activation as an obligatory second signal generator Model 3, variety Dukor (16))
Since virtually all TI antigens and polyclonal mitogens share the common property of activating C3 by the alternate pathway, it is very reasonable to propose that such activity might contribute to B cell stimulation. We have already presented elsewhere evidence that C3 does not seem to be essential for spleen B lymphocyte responses to polyclonal B lymphocyte mitogens (42). Thus, optimal LPS responses can

Figure 2. INHIBITION OF T AND B PROLIFERATIVE RESPONSES BY
DIBUTYRYL CYCLIC 3' 5' ADENOSINE MONOPHOSPHATE (cAMP)

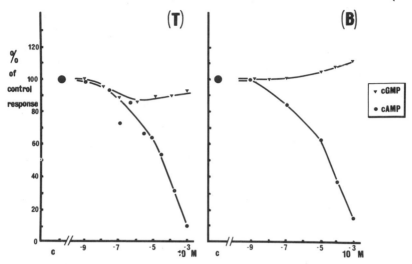

Spleen T cells activated by ConA, B cells by LPS.
Nucleotides added in single dose at 0 hrs simultaneously with
polyclonal mitogen. Responses assayed by (3H) uptake 48 to
69 hrs of culture (under Group B conditions - see Table 3).

Figure 3. ATTEMPT TO REVERSE cAMP INHIBITION OF POLYCLONAL
MITOGEN RESPONSES WITH cGMP

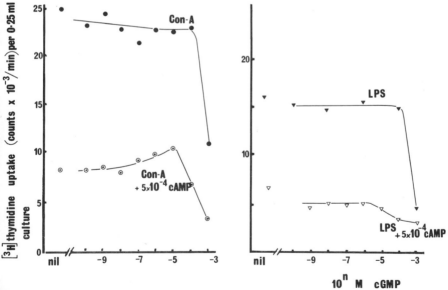

Mitogens and cyclic nucleotides added at 0 hrs. cGMP added
in single dose or in daily pulses gave identical results.

Figure 4. FAILURE OF CYCLIC NUCLEOTIDES AND CARBOMYLCHOLINE
TO ACTIVATE MOUSE SPLEEN LYMPHOCYTES

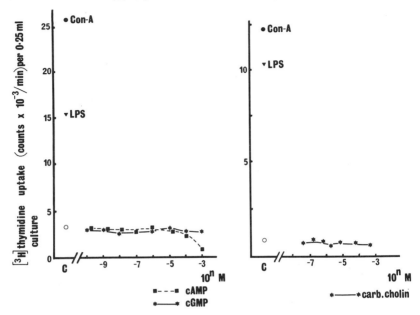

In repeat experiments cultures were pulsed with 10^{-4} to
10^{-6}M cGMP each day. No responses were observed.

Figure 5 A.   B LYMPHOCYTES DO NOT RESPOND TO ConA PLUS cGMP

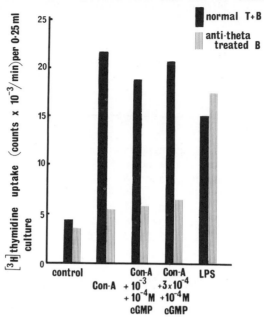

Two pulses of cGMP given as indicated

Figure 5 B.   B LYMPHOCYTES DO NOT RESPOND TO ANTI-Ig PLUS cGMP

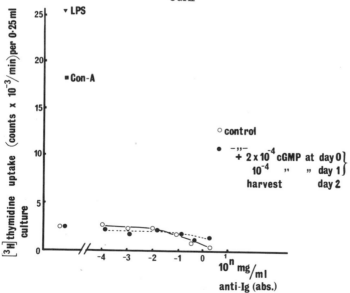

Purified anti–IgM antibodies (react with effectively all
B lymphocytes as assessed by indirect immunofluorescence)
Normal CBA spleen culture.

be induced in macrophage depleted cultures in the absence of any foreign serum source of functional C3 and in the presence of antibodies to neutralise any internally generated mouse C3. Furthemore the LPS used in these experiments was itself devoid of detectable complement inactivating activity (Table 5). These results find a clear parallel with responses to TI antigens in vitro (43) which are also complement independent. It is however possible that activated C3 can play an important role in polyclonal mitogen responses of lymph node (as opposed to spleen) B lymphocytes and for responses to TD antigens (43). However in these situations it is not clear whether complement involvement reflects a necessity for <u>some</u> B cells (IgG programmed?) to receive a second signal from this source or whether some other potentiation or antigen presentation effects are involved.

6. <u>Why is it that anti-Ig does not stimulate mouse B lymphocytes</u>?
Hidden in Fig 5b is a point for discussion which is that anti-Ig itself does not appear to stimulate B cells in the mouse. This has been reported before (1) and is a crucial point in relation to all three models. We have tried over the past four years to stimulate mouse B cells with a large variety of antisera to mouse light and heavy chains and although some weak responses were recorded (44) we have never seen any responses with purified antibodies to whole Ig, k chain or μ chain (Janossy, Greaves and Cooper, unpublished). Furthermore we have not been able so far to convert anti-Ig to a polyclonal stimulator for mouse B lymphocytes by increasing the extent of cross-linkage involved either by adding a second anti-anti-immunoglobulin or by coupling the anti-mouse immunoglobulin antibodies to sepharose particles. We have also been able to detect no shift at all in the LPS dose response curve following anti-Ig treatment, indicating that B cells are quite oblivious to cross-linkage and resultant modulation of their surface associated immuno-globulin. There are several possible interpretations of these observations.
1) That we should try harder since it obviously works well in the rabbit (45,46) and possibly in the chicken as well (47).
2) Cross-linkage of antigen receptors by anti-immuno-globulin in the mouse does not successfully mimic the effects of antigen binding to these same molecules,
3) The rabbit response is not in fact due to direct activation solely via surface immunoglobulin and the reason

Table 5

MITOGENICITY IN C3 DEPLETED MOUSE SPLEEN CULTURES

	10% FCS[1]	5% human serum[1]	serum free[2]
control (unstimulated)	10.000	11.200	1.000
Concanavalin-A	136.000	90.400	
LPS mR 345 [3]	79.000	63.000	153.000
" + anti-mouse c3 [4] (0.04-4 µg/ml)	58.000- -77.000		165.000
" ⌈ cotton wool filtered cells in zymosan treated and heat inactivated serum	70.000		
" ⎮ + anti-mouse C3 (0.4-5 µg/ml)	70.400- -79.000	50.200	
" ⎮ + anti-human C3 (5-40 µg/ml)		49.400- -55.800	

Results are expressed as c.p.m./ml cultures.
1 ^{3}H-thymidine 4 µCi/ml culture, 50 mCi/mmol, 48-64 h.
2   "   2 µCi/ml culture, 5 Ci/mmol, 24-48 h.
3 LPS mR 345 (a preparation from Salmonella mR 345) was unable to destroy
  haemolytic complement when tested with serum from colostrum-free piglets
  (Galonos et al., Eur.J.Biochem. 19, 143 (1971) and Janossy et al., Nature
  New Biology 245, 108 (1973)). Other LPS preparations, with complement inactivating capacity, have also been studied and gave similar results as shown
  above.
4 This preparation of anti-mouse C3 inhibits antihapten response to TNP-KLH and
  DNP-FγG but not to DNP-POL (Feldmann & Pepys, in press).

we failed in the mouse reflects an inability of immunoglobulins to directly initiate an activation or tolergenic
sequence. The latter view accords with the Coutinho-Möller
hypothesis (Model 2) and conflicts with our results (vide
supra) using insolubilized haptens.

Exit

Three currently 'popular' models of B lymphocyte
activation have been discussed principally from the point of
view of using polyclonal mitogens as probes. The evidence
presented, or rather interpretations of data, would appear
to make all three doubtful as completely satisfactory
explanations of the mechanism of activation of all B
lymphocytes by immunogens and polyclonal mitogens. At least
part of the current confusion may relate to insufficient
consideration being given to actually defining what is
meant by 'triggering' or 'activation'. The common usage of
'triggering' to denote activation is an unfortunate choice
since it implies a magic (all or none) switch on or off of
cells. Lymphocytes do not 'switch on' to an antigen or polyclonal mitogen as a muscle or post-synaptic junction responds
to neuropharmacological ligands, neither do they give the
moderately quick regulatory responses of many of the target
cells for polypeptide and peptide hormones. Numerous
sequential steps intervene between the initial binding of
antigen or polyclonal mitogen to whatever cell surface
molecules are the true receptors, and eventual overt responsiveness (cf. growth hormone response?). These include early
changes in membrane permeability and phospholipid turnover,
and enhanced translational activity (-although these changes
have only been well studied in lectin activated T cells,
see refs. 1,48). At what point do we decide that a cell is
activated? At what stages are activated cells subject to
regulatory influences? It already seems clear that products
of activated T cells considered to be mitogens (12) or
second signal generators (14) for B cells could well be
potentiation factors operating post-inductively in the
activation sequence. Thus, such factors (and cGMP also –
ref. 17) can exert their influences during the second and
third days in culture after initial antigen-lymphocyte
interaction (49). When such 'factors' are applied to 'pure'
B cells following challenge with completely T cell dependent
ligands (vide supra and ref. 15) then no response is seen.
It is of course quite legitimate to consider these potentiation mechanisms as second 'signals' essential for full
productive activation of B cells. They should however be
distinguished from initiating events. Unfortunately many of

the experimental systems currently employed are inadequate for this purpose. Other soluble factors may operate closely to the critical initiating events as suggested by Schraders' work with supernatants of activated macrophages (15).

Finally can we really assume, as implied by all three models discussed above, that B lymphocytes responding to DNP on Polymerized flagellin (TI response) and DNP-monomeric flagellin (TD response) are identical? Similarly, are all B cells programmed for IgM, IgG and other Ig classes subject to the same rules for activation? It would be surprising if the membrane associated initiating events were radically different; however B cells subsets (within clones of a given specificity) could well differ considerably in the extent to which their expression of activation is dependent upon secondary potentiation or amplification mechanisms.

We have already discussed above (see under - 'insoluble ligands') evidence which suggests that some IgM and IgG secreting precursor cells may have different requirements for full activation.

Recent comparative studies (Doenhoff and Janossy, in preparation) suggest also that qualitative differences exist between B lymphocytes in spleen versus lymph node. Mouse lymph node B lymphocytes respond less well to LPS and PWM than spleen B cells. A similar anatomical compartmentalis-ation of responder B cells has also been seen with human cells (50). These results suggest that B lymphocytes in different sites may have differing requirements for activ-ation and/or that ancillary potentiating cells are more abundant in spleen than lymph node cultures. These possibilities have been investigated by mixing syngeneic spleen (T6) and lymph node (lac) cells at varying proportions and analysing the responding dividing cells by chromosome analysis. The rationale of the experiment was that when equivalent numbers of spleen and lymph node B cells were present in cultures then they should have the same opportunity to benefit from any accessory amplification mechanisms derived from the 'high responder' spleen population. The results (Fig 6) show that lymph node cells are considerably less responsive than spleen cells in such mixtures. In control studies a 50:50 contribution to responding cells were found as expected when T6 spleen and lac spleen were mixed.

The discrepancy between splenic and lymph node LPS response is only marginally less when corrections are made for differing proportions of B cells in the respective unmixed suspensions and when the experiments were repeated using T cell depleted populations (i.e. anti-θ treated).

Figure 6. RELATIVE RESPONSES OF SPLEEN AND LYMPH NODE
LYMPHOCYTES TO POLYCLONAL MITOGENS

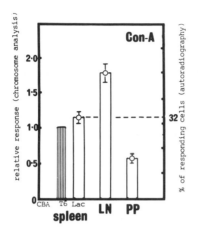 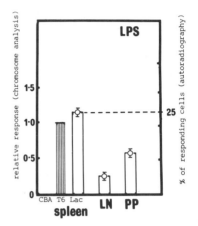

Spleen cells from CBA-T6T6 mice were mixed in varying proportions (75/25, 50/50, 25/75) with cells from either spleens
or lymph nodes orPeyers patches of CBA-LAC mice. After 2
days stimulation with either Con-A or LPS colcemid was
added (0.1 µg/ml final concentration) and the relative percentage of dividing T6T6 and Lac cells was examined in
smears prepared 16 hrs later. The data are expressed as
relative response (r) of Lac cells according to the formula
$(r = \frac{\% \text{ of Lac mitoses}}{\% \text{ of T6 mitoses}})$. Standard error of mean is shown.
Data are collated from 5 different experiments. Data taken
from Doenhoff,MJ. and Janossy, G. (in preparation).

Absolute estimates of Con-A and LPS responsive cells in
CBA-LAC spleen have also been investigated by autoradiography. Cells were incubated for 24 hrs after which [3]H-
thymidine and colcemid were added. The cultures were then
incubated for a further 24 hrs. Smears were prepared from
cell pellets by the stripping film technique. The percentages shown represent ratios of labelled cells to the total
cell number present. The total of surviving plus dead cells
was >90% of the number of the initial culture. The data are
from 5 different experiments.

Although the two different approaches are not strictly
comparable, the data provide approximate estimations of
potentially mitogen responsive cells

These results suggest that the <u>relative</u> response capacity of spleen versus lymph node   lymphocytes is approximately 5:1. An estimate of the <u>proportion</u> of LPS responsive B cells in spleen versus lymph node has also been determined by auto-radiographic analysis of colcemid containing cultures (19). The results (Fig. 6) when corrected for B cell proportions indicated that 50% of spleen B lymphocytes respond to an optimal dose of LPS whereas only 16% of lymph node B cells respond. This would appear to constitute reasonable evidence for B lymphocyte subsets differing in tissue distribution and responsiveness to polyclonal mitogens (and TI antigens?) and parallels earlier observations of T lymphocyte subsets (51). This B cell heterogeneity may also be reflected in programming for synthesis of different Ig classes (vide supra) and in recirculation capacity (52). 'Normal' spleen secretes principally IgM and 'normal' lymph node IgG (Parkhouse, personal communication) and when equivalent numbers of spleen and lymph node B cells are activated by LPS the former population is much more active in Ig synthesis, and this is almost entirely IgM (Parkhouse and Janossy, unpublished observations). Qualitatively distinct B lymphocytes undoubtedly exist and regardless of whether there are distinct separate populations or overlapping members of a single linear developmental pathway, it seems likely that they do not have identical requirements for activation. Fig 7 outlines our current incomplete working hypothesis.

ACKNOWLEDGMENTS

Work reported in this paper was supported by the Imperial Cancer Research Fund, the Medical Research Council Drs Humphrey, Parker and Pepys participated in several of the experiments reported. We are grateful to Miss J. Snajdr and Mr B. de Sousa for technical support.

REFERENCES

1. Greaves, M.F. and Janossy, G., Transpl. Rev. <u>11</u>, 87 (1972).
2. Andersson, J., Sjöberg, O. and Möller, G., Transpl. Rev. <u>11</u>, 132 (1972).
3. Janossy, G., Shohat, M., Greaves, M.F. and Dourmashkin, R.R., Immunology <u>24</u>, 211 (1973).
4. Parkhouse, R.M.E., Janossy, G. and Greaves, M.F., Nature New Biology <u>235</u>, 21 (1972).
5. Andersson, J. and Melchers, F., Proc.Natl.Acad.Sci.USA <u>70</u>, 416 (1973).
6. Andersson, J., Sjöberg, O. and Möller, G., Eur.J.Immunol. <u>2</u>, 349 (1972).

Fig 7. B LYMPHOCYTE HETEROGENEITY AND
ACTIVATION MECHANISMS

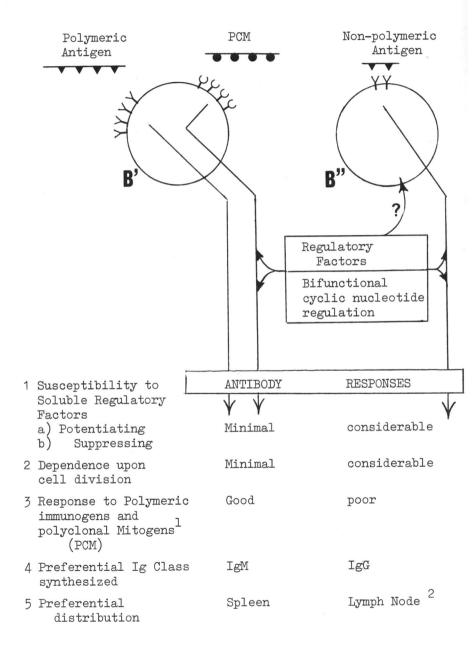

	ANTIBODY	RESPONSES
1 Susceptibility to Soluble Regulatory Factors a) Potentiating b) Suppressing	Minimal	considerable
2 Dependence upon cell division	Minimal	considerable
3 Response to Polymeric immunogens and polyclonal Mitogens[1] (PCM)	Good	poor
4 Preferential Ig Class synthesized	IgM	IgG
5 Preferential distribution	Spleen	Lymph Node [2]

Fig 7 legend.

1. This preferential response might reflect either
   a) Differential capacity of the stimulants to evoke
   production of amplification factor(s), and/or
   b) Different membrane properties of B^1 vesus B^{11} cells
   which determine whether or not the binding of a ligand
   of a particular valency initiates the activation
   sequence.

2. These cells could be immunologically experienced
   'memory' B cells (cf. 52)

7. Remold, H.G., Transpl. Rev. 10, 152 (1972).
8. Andersson, J., Möller, G. and Sjöberg, O., Eur.J.Immunol. 2, 99 (1972).
9. Möller, G., Sjöberg, O., and Andersson, J., Eur.J.Imminol. 2, 586 (1972).
10. Asherson, G.L., Ferluga, J. and Janossy, G., Clin.Exptl. Immunol. 15, 573 (1973).
11. Coutinho, A., Gronowicz, E., Bullock, W., and Möller, G., J.Exp.Med. 139, 74 (1974).
12. Coutinho, A. and Möller, G, Scand, J. Immunol.(in press).
13. Ashman, R.F., Kaplan, A.B. and Metzgar, H., Immunochem. 8, 627 (1971).
14. Watson, J., Trenkner, E. and Cohn, M., J.Exp.Med. 138, 699 (1973).
15. Schrader, J., J.Exp.Med. 138, 1466 (1973).
16. Dukor, P. and Hartmann, K.H., Cell. Immunol. 7, 349 (1973))
17. Watson, J., Epstein, R. and Cohn, M., Nature, 246, 405 (1973).
18. Janossy, G. and Greaves, M.F., Clin.Exptl.Immunol. 10, 525 (1972).
19. Janossy, G., Greaves, M.F., Doenhoff, M.J. and Snajdr, J., Clin.Exptl.Immunol. 14, 581 (1973).
20. Feldmann, M. and Basten, A., J.Exp.Med. 34, 103 (1971).
21. Feldmann, M., Eur.J.Immunol. 2, 130 (1972).
22. Feldmann, M. and Nossal, G.J.V., Transpl. Rev. 12, 3 (1972).
23. Greaves, M.F. and Bauminger, S., Nature New Biology, 235, 57, (1972).
24. Andersson, J., Edelman, G.M., Möller, G. and Sjöberg, O., Eur.J.Immunol 2, 233 (1972).
25. Feldmann, M., Greaves, M.F., Parker, D. and Rittenberg, M.B., Eur.J.Immunol. (in press).
26. Osborne, D.P. and Katz, D., J.Immunol. 111, 1164 (1973).
27. Dukor, P., Schumann, G., Gisler, R.H., Dierich, M., König, W., Hadding, U. and Bitter-Suermann, D., J.Exp. Med. 139, 337 (1974).
28. Coutinho, A. and Möller, G., Nature New Biology 245, 12 (1972).
29 Janossy, G., Greaves, M.F., Doenhoff, M.J. and Snajdr, J. Clin. Exptl. Immunol. 14, 581 (1973).
30. Ling, N.R., In, 'New Concepts in Allergy and Clinical Immunology' (Eds.) U. Serafini and A.W. Frankland, p. 187, Excepta Medica, Amsterdam (1971).
31. Schellekens, P.Tha. and Eijsvoogel, V.P., Clin.Exptl. Immunol. 3, 561 (1968).
32. Coutinho, A., Möller, G., Andersson, J. and Bullock, W.W. Eur.J.Immunol. 3, 299

33. Melchers, F. and Andersson, J., Transpl. Rev. 14, 76 (1973).
34. Feldmann, M., Contemporary Topics in Molecular Immunology Vol 3 (in press).
35. Kagnoff, M.F., Billings, P. and Cohn, M., J.Exp.Med., 139, 407 (1974).
36. Riepschel, E.P., Kim, Y.B., Watson, B.W., Gallanos, C., Lüderitz, O. and Westphal, O., Infect.Immun. 8, 173(1973).
37. Greaves, M.F., FEBS 26, 17 (1972).
38. Hadden, J.W., Hadden, E.M., Haddox, M.K. and Goldberg, N.D., Proc.Natl.Acad.Sci. 69, 3024 (1972).
39. Goldberg, N., Haddox, M.K., Hartle, D.K. and Haddon, J.W., In, 'Proceedings of IV International Congress of Pharmacology' Karger, Basel, p. 146 (1972).
40. Kram, R. and Tomkins, G.M., Proc.Natl.Acad.Sci.USA 70, 1659 (1973).
41. Illiano, G., Tell, G.P.E., Siegel, M.I. and Cuatrecasas, P., Proc.Natl.Acad.Sci.USA 70, 2443 (1973).
42. Janossy, G., Humphrey, J.H., Pepys, M.B. and Greaves, M.F., Nature New Biology 245, 108 (1973).
43. Feldmann, M. and Pepys, M.B., Nature New Biology (In press).
44. Greaves, M.F., Transpl. Rev. 5, 45 (1970).
45. Sell, S., Transpl. Rev. 5, 19 (1970).
46. Fanger, M.W., Hart, D.A., Wells, J.V. and Nisonoff, A., J.Immunol. 105, 1484.
47. Kirchner, H. and Oppenheim, J.J., Cell. Immunol. 3 695 (1972).
48. Cooper, H.L., Transpl. Rev. 11, 3 (1972).
49. Schimpl, A. and Wecker, E., J.Exp.Med. 137, 547 (1973)
50. Greaves, M.F., Janossy, G. and Doenhoff, M., J.Exp.Med. (In press).
51. Stobo, J.D., Transpl. Rev. 11, 60 (1972).
52. Strober, S. and Dilley, J., J.Exp.Med. 137, 1275 (1973).

THE ORGANIZATION OF IMMUNOGLOBULIN GENES

P. Leder, T. Honjo, S. Packman, D. Swan,

M. Nau and B. Norman

Laboratory of Molecular Genetics
National Institute of Child Health and Human Development
National Institutes of Health
Bethesda, Maryland 20014

ABSTRACT. In order to distinguish among various models which have been advanced to account for the diversity of antibody molecules, we must know how the constant and variable regions of immunoglobulins are represented in the somatic genome. For this purpose, we have purified mRNA corresponding to a mouse kappa immunoglobulin light chain from the myeloma tumor, MOPC-41. This mRNA directs the enzymatic synthesis of highly radioactive DNA (cDNA). This cDNA, which should correspond to the constant region of the kappa chain, was assessed for reiteration frequency using hybridization kinetic analysis and was found to be represented approximately three times per haploid genome. This result tends to rule out germ line hypotheses which require many copies of the constant region gene. It also requires the postulation of a recombinational mechanism to join constant and variable region sequences.

Hybridization kinetic analyses designed to assess the entire light chain sequence (C and V regions) made use of ^{125}I-MOPC-41 mRNA. These revealed a major component of relatively unique frequency and a minor (~ 20%) component with a reiteration frequency of approximately 30-50 copies per haploid genome. Careful analysis of the extent of hybridization of this mRNA to DNA prepared from several tumors and tissues, thermal profiles, and relevant competition studies, while sensitive, do not permit us to distinguish unambiguously between a germ line model and the type of somatic mutation model which permits germ line genes corresponding to each kappa subgroup. Our results do, however, clearly rule out the existence of thousands of variable region sequences so closely related to the MOPC-41 V-region as to permit extensive, stable cross hybridization.

INTRODUCTION

Remarkable structural studies carried out over the last decade have defined the constant and variable sequences of antibody molecules and have provided a useful insight into the basis of the specificity of the antigen antibody interaction. These studies, in fact, have also raised a problem that is now central to modern immunology: How can one account genetically for the diversity necessary to encode the variable regions of antibodies?

On the basis of much structural, genetic and serologic evidence, several useful hypotheses have been advanced to explain the origin of this diversity and the organization of immunoglobulin genes (1-17). These hypotheses fall into three general classes, represented diagramatically in Table 1+. The first, which we call the <u>stringent germ line hypothesis</u>, requires approximately 1,000 variable gene sequences alternating with 1,000 constant region sequences (14). Since this is a germ line model, each cell in the organism, immunocytes and non-immunocytes, would have precisely the same genetic complement. The second type of model, the <u>recombinational germ line hypothesis</u> (3, 8, 16), would also require approximately 1,000 light chain variable region sequences, but would require only a few copies, less than 10, of the constant region sequence which would recombine at some level with the appropriate variable region in a specific immunocyte clone. Again, since we are speaking of a germ line hypothesis, each cell in the organism would have an identical number of sequences in the genome.

The <u>somatic mutation hypothesis</u> (1, 2, 4, 5, 7, 9, 10) in its most modern form (13) requires a germ line gene corresponding to each of the variable region subgroups defined by structural studies of immunoglobulin molecules. These basic subgroup germ line genes are held to undergo mutation during the somatic development of immunocyte clones. This hypothesis would require fewer copies of genes corresponding to

---

+ Assume 10^6 different antibody molecules

TABLE 1

PREDICTED FREQUENCIES OF LIGHT CHAIN CONSTANT AND VARIABLE GENE
SEQUENCES IN CLONED IMMUNOCYTE DNA

		Theoretical Gene Frequency		Expected Frequency as Determined by Hybridization with MOPC-41 Light Chain mRNA	
		Variable	Constant	Variable	Constant
Stringent Germ Line Hypothesis					
DNA Source					
MOPC-41	$\underline{V_{41}}\ \underline{C_k}\ \underline{V_2}\ \underline{C_k}\ \underline{V_3}\ \underline{C_k}\ \cdots$	~1000	~1000	<50	~1000
Other	$\underline{V_{41}}\ \underline{C_k}\ \underline{V_2}\ \underline{C_k}\ \underline{V_3}\ \underline{C_k}\ \cdots$	~1000	~1000	<50	~1000
Recombinational Germ Line Hypothesis					
DNA Source					
MOPC-41	$\underline{V_{41}}\ \underline{V_2}\ \underline{V_3}\ \underline{V_4}\ \cdots\ \underline{V_{10^2-10^3}}\ \underline{C_k}$	~1000	<10	<50	<10
Other	$\underline{V_{41}}\ \underline{V_2}\ \underline{V_3}\ \underline{V_4}\ \cdots\ \underline{V_{10^2-10^3}}\ \underline{C_k}$	~1000	<10	<50	<10
Somatic Mutation Hypothesis					
DNA Source					
MOPC-41	$\boxed{\underline{V_{41}}}\ \underline{V_2}\ \underline{V_3}\ \underline{V_4}\ \cdots\ \underline{V_{10-10^2}}\ \underline{C_k}$	<100	<10	<<50	<10
Other	$\boxed{\underline{V_1}}\ \underline{V_2}\ \underline{V_3}\ \underline{V_4}\ \cdots\ \underline{V_{10-10^2}}\ \underline{C_k}$	<100	<10	<<50*	<10

* According to the somatic mutation hypothesis, the gene sequence corresponding to the variable region of the MOPC–41 immunocyte should differ from the comparable sequence in other clones. Therefore, hybrids of the MOPC–41 variable region mRNA and the comparable DNA regions derived from other clones should be mismatched and incomplete were this hypothesis correct.

variable regions, let us say about 100, but these somatically mutated genes would clearly differ from one another amongst immunocyte clones. The somatic mutation hypothesis does not require a smaller number of constant region genes but we have incorporated this feature into the model for convenience.

THE EXPERIMENTAL APPROACH

Obviously these hypotheses have predictive value in terms of the number of genes to be expected to encode constant and variable region sequences and in the relationship between these sequences amongst various immunocyte clones. In order to assess these properties experimentally, we have employed hybridization techniques which depend upon the availability of pure immunoglobulin mRNA. Using the cell-free system as an assay for the purification of the message (18), our intention was to obtain a homogeneous mRNA molecule corresponding to an immunoglobulin light chain which could be used as a hybridization probe for the quantitation of immunoglobulin light chain genes and for assessing the relationship of these genes to one another in a variety of myeloma tumors. Our initial studies depended upon the extraction of a kappa-type light chain mRNA from membrane-bound polysomes derived from MOPC-41 myeloma tumors, kindly supplied by Dr. Michael Potter (18).

PURIFICATION OF MOPC-41 LIGHT CHAIN mRNA

The light chain mRNA was purified using techniques which we had previously developed for the purification of globin mRNA from mammalian reticulocytes (18, 19). In addition to the isolation of membrane-bound polysomes from myeloma tumors referred to above, it also involved chromatography of the crude polysomal RNA on oligo(dT)-cellulose as well as repeated centrifugation on sucrose gradients under relatively denaturing conditions (40). The results of this purification procedure were analyzed at various stages of purification by formamide gel electrophoresis (Figure 1) (20, 21). As shown, the final sucrose gradient centrifugation yields an mRNA fraction which is homogeneous by this criterion.

The purification procedures allow us to characterize certain features of the immunoglobulin mRNA as well. The fact that it can be purified by annealing to oligo(dT)-cellulose suggested that it contains a poly(A) sequence (18). This expectation has been confirmed (21-23). The properties of the

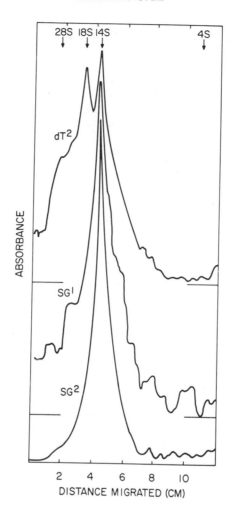

Fig. 1.   Analysis of MOPC-41 RNA on denaturing acrylamide gels.   0.2 A^{260} dT^2, 0.1 A^{260} SG^1 and 0.05 A^{260} SG^2 RNAs were dialyzed overnight against H$_2$O, lyophilized, dissolved in 15 μl deionized, buffered formamide (containing 5 mM barbital, 0.02% bromophenol blue, 20% sucrose, set to apparent pH 9). Samples were applied to 5% acrylamide gels (6 mm x 100 mm) and run 5 hrs at 100 V according to the method of Staynov et al. (20).   Gels were stained overnight with Stains-All, de-stained in H$_2$O and light and scanned at 600 mμ in a Gil-ford spectrophotometer.   dT^2 represents RNA from a second chromatography on oligo(dT)-cellulose.   SG^1 and SG^2 are pool-ed peak RNA fractions from the first and second sucrose grad-ient centrifugations, respectively (40).

mRNA on formamide gel electrophoresis, a technique which provides a reasonably accurate assessment of chain length, indicates that this light chain mRNA consists of approximately
1300 nucleotides, a value somewhat greater than that proposed
for other immunoglobulin mRNAs (21, 23). Assuming that approximately 200 of these bases comprise the poly(A) region
(23), the MOPC-41 mRNA still contains almost twice as many
bases as would be required to encode the secreted form of the
light chain molecule. A portion, at least 150 bases (24), of
this sequence is required to encode the extra amino acids seen
in the putative precursor form of the light chain synthesized
in vitro.

SYNTHESIS OF DNA COMPLIMENTARY TO MOPC-41 mRNA

mRNA isolated from the MOPC-41 tumor can be transcribed
into DNA of very high specific activity using the avian mye-
loblastosis virus RNA-dependent DNA polymerase (22, 25). This
property provides a very valuable hybridization probe, both
for the quantitation of immunoglobulin genes and for the
analysis of the purity of our immunoglobulin mRNA preparation.
Our most recent studies using the MOPC-41 mRNA have resulted
in the synthesis of ^{3}H-cDNA which very precisely co-migrates
with a standard DNA molecule 630 bases in length upon alkaline
sucrose gradient centrifugation.

Because the RNA-dependent DNA polymerase requires a
primer for the synthesis of cDNA, one can phase the enzyme
to ensure synthesis from the 3' end of the mRNA - template
by annealing an oligo(dT) primer to the 3' poly(A) end of the
molecule. The product synthesized in such a reaction can be
represented diagramatically as shown in Table 2. The ^{3}H-cDNA,
630 bases in length, should extend through the region of the
myeloma mRNA which encodes the constant region, possibly including a portion of the variable region as well as an untranslated sequence between the constant region and the
poly(A) sequence. If this were the case, we would expect
that the MOPC-41 ^{3}H-cDNA probe would form an extensive and
stable hybrid with an mRNA derived from another kappa chain
subgroup. That this is indeed the case is shown in Table 3.
The hybrid formed between MOPC-41 ^{3}H-cDNA and its homologous
mRNA has thermal denaturation characteristics (Tm) virtually
identical to that formed between MOPC-41 ^{3}H-cDNA and a heterologous (different subgroup) mRNA. The fact that the extent
of hybridization of the MOPC-41 ^{3}H-cDNA probe with its homologous mRNA is 20% greater than that when hybridized to heterologous kappa mRNA could be due to some extention of the probe

TABLE 2

DIAGRAMATIC REPRESENTATION OF MOPC-41 mRNA

AND ITS COMPLEMENTARY ³H-cDNA

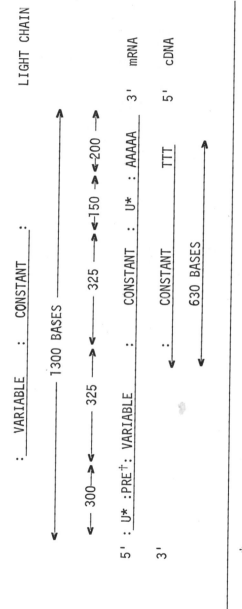

† Precursor sequence

* Putative untranslated sequence

305

TABLE 3

CROSS-HYBRIDIZATION BETWEEN MOPC-41 ^{3}H-cDNA AND LIGHT

CHAIN mRNA DERIVED FROM A DIFFERENT SUBGROUP

SOURCE OF LIGHT CHAIN mRNA	MAXIMUM EXTENT OF HYBRID FORMATION	Tm
MOPC-41	93%	85°
MPC-11 (456)	71%	84.5°

Hybridization reactions and assays were carried out as indicated in the legend to Figure 2. Thermal denaturation was assayed using hydroxyapatite elution as described previously (26).

into the variable region or to sequence differences located in the untranslated region of both mRNA molecules.

The purity of the mRNA with respect to constant region sequence also can be assessed using hybridization kinetic analysis (Figure 2). Since the total complexity (or chain length) of the alpha and beta globin mRNAs is approximately 1200 bases and the complexity of the immunoglobulin molecule is approximately 1300 bases, probes for globin and immunoglobulin, 500 and 600 bases in length, respectively, should hybridize at approximately the same $Crt_{1/2}$ value*. The observed $Crt_{1/2}$ of 5.5 and 6.5 x 10^{-4} for each of these analyses is consistent with the relative homogeneity of the immunoglobulin probe.

GENETIC REPRESENTATION OF THE KAPPA CONSTANT REGION SEQUENCE

Inasmuch as the mRNA template upon which the ^{3}H-cDNA was synthesized is homogeneous by the above mentioned criteria and the ^{3}H-cDNA cross-hybridizes with constant region sequences found in other kappa subgroups, hybridization kinetic analysis of this probe should reveal the frequency with which this sequence occurs in any genome in question. Again, the stringent germ line hypothesis requires many copies of the constant region gene, whereas the recombinational models require only few copies (cf. Table 1).

The relevant experiment is shown in Figure 3. For comparison, the hybridization kinetics of mouse globin cDNA, a relatively unique sequence, is shown. The $Cot_{1/2}$ value of the MOPC-41 immunoglobulin probe is 1100, a value consistent with approximately 3 copies of the sequence per haploid genome. This value can also be calculated by taking advantage of the extent of hybridization at very high Cot values and the results obtained are virtually identical (30). This analysis has been carried out using DNA derived from a number of kappa and lambda myeloma tumors as well as other differentiated mouse tissue and the values obtained are essentially identical (32). Thus, the result rules out a <u>stringent germ line hypothesis</u> which would require many copies of the constant region genome.

---

* This relationship is defined by Britten and Kohne (29) in which the Cot (concentration of the polynucleotide times time of incubation) is directly proportional to the complexity (C = number of bases) of the polynucleotide under analysis (Cot (or Crt) = KC).

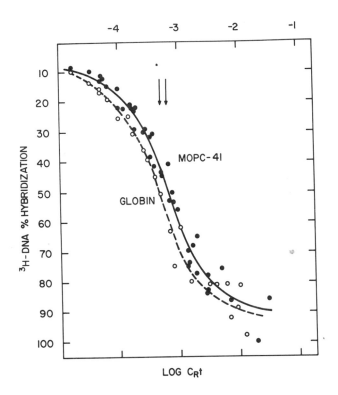

Fig. 2. Hybridization of purified mouse globin and MOPC-41 light chain mRNAs and their respective ^{3}H-cDNAs. The hybridization reaction was carried out in 0.6 M NaCl - 0.2 mM EDTA - 1.5 mM Tris·HCl, pH 7.2 at 75°. mRNA is present at 10 to 100-fold excess over cDNA. Aliquots were taken at time intervals for the assay of the hybrid formed by S_1 nuclease digestion (27, 28).

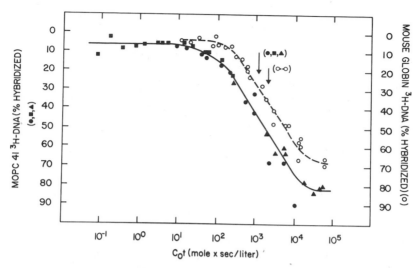

Fig. 3. Kinetics of annealing of MOPC-41 ^{3}H-cDNA to a vast excess of total cellular MOPC-41 DNA. Hybridization kinetics of MOPC-41 ^{3}H-cDNA were carried out in the presence of up to a 1.2 x 10^7-fold excess of unlabeled, sheared MOPC-41 cellular DNA. [For comparison, the kinetics of hybridization, under similar conditions, of mouse globin ^{3}H-cDNA with MOPC-41 cellular DNA are shown.] The cDNA and cellular DNA were prepared as described (25, 30), with the former having a specific activity of 4.6 x 10^7 dpm/μg, and a base length of 630 by alkaline sucrose gradient centrifugation. The hybridization procedure and S$_1$ nuclease assays were as described (30), and were performed at DNA concentrations and salt concentrations appropriate for each portion of the kinetic curve (see below). The Cot values on the abscissa are those that would obtain at 0.18 M Na$^+$ (31). Cot$_{1/2}$ for MOPC-41 DNA x MOPC-41 DNA equals 1130. Cot$_{1/2}$ for globin cDNA x MOPC-41 DNA equals 2100. The filled symbols represent MOPC-41 cDNA x MOPC-41 DNA: (■) 0.99 mg/ml DNA, 0.18 M Na$^+$; (●) 9.9 mg/ml DNA, 0.54 M Na ; (▲) 9.9 mg/ml DNA, 1.06 M Na$^+$; (O) results for globin cDNA x MOPC-41 DNA.

GENETIC REPRESENTATION OF THE VARIABLE SEQUENCE

The remaining hypotheses, recombinational germ line and somatic mutation, differ from one another in the number of variable region sequences which they require and the divergent requirements for genetic identity in different somatic cells. Referring again to Table 1, we may now ask what results we might expect from hybridization analysis were either of the models correct. The differences between variable regions amongst the subgroups are so great (generally greater than 30%) that from our own observations using interspecies globin mRNA hybridization, we would not expect that there would be stable hybrid formation between sequences of different subgroups (26). Inasmuch as sequences which are homologous in over 80% of their amino acids form less stable hybrids which further require higher Cots for their formation, we might expect some cross-hybridization to occur between sequences that represent immunoglobulin molecules of the same subgroup. Were each subgroup to include approximately 50 variable sequences, a not unreasonable expectation, the germ line hypothesis would require an observed reiteration frequency of 50 or fewer copies for the variable region. Were the somatic mutation hypothesis correct and the subgroup represented by a single germ line gene, we would see expected $Cot_{1/2}$ values consistent with the unique representation of this gene, assuming its sequence were close enough to provide a stable hybrid. A further expectation would be that this sequence would differ among different cloned immunocytes and among different organs. We might, thus, expect that hybrid formed between mRNA from one clone and DNA from another would be less stable and hybridization less extensive, were the somatic mutation hypothesis correct.

The extent of hybridization is easily measured by the amount of [125]I mRNA which eventually forms hybrid in the presence of unlabeled cellular DNA. The congruity (absence of mismatching) of this hybrid can be assessed using thermal denaturation analysis. The difficulty, as we shall see, in ruling out the somatic mutation hypothesis results from our inability to determine the extent of hybridization and thermal denaturation at an accuracy which would reflect a 10-15% or smaller difference between somatic genes.

The hybridization kinetic analysis of ^{125}I MOPC-41 mRNA in the presence of vast excesses of homologous MOPC-41 DNA is shown in Figure 4. For comparison, an analogous analysis using ^{125}I mouse globin mRNA is shown in the same figure. The major portion of the ^{125}I-mRNA hybridizes with a rela-

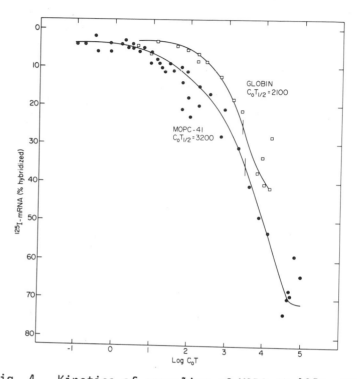

Fig. 4. Kinetics of annealing of MOPC-41 ^{125}I-mRNA to a vast excess of total, cellular MOPC-41 DNA. Hybridization kinetics of MOPC-41 [125]I mRNA in the presence of up to a 2.94 x 10^6-fold excess of unlabeled, sheared MOPC-41 cellular DNA. [For comparison are shown the results of the hybridization of mouse globin [125]I mRNA with mouse spleen DNA.] Cellular DNA was prepared as described (30). MOPC-41 mRNA was prepared as described (40). Iodination was performed according to the procedure of Prensky et al. (41); specific activity of the MOPC-41 [125]I mRNA is $\overline{3.2 \times 10^6}$ cpm/µg. Hybridzation was performed at 65°-67°C in 1.04 M Na^+ - 0.02 M Tris-Cl, pH 7.0, with 0.18 M Na^+ used at the lower Cot values. DNA concentration was 10 mg/ml, with 0.94 mg/ml used at the lower Cot values. Cot values on the abscissa are those that would be obtained at 0.18 M Na^+ (31) in a DNA-DNA reannealing reaction. At each time point, aliquots were diluted 100-fold into 2 x SSC (0.3 M NaCl - 30 mM Na-citrate), and assayed (37° x 40 min.) for resistance to 60 µg/ml RNase A, according to the procedure of Melli et al. (42). Reaction mixtures were acid-precipitated and collected onto GFC glass fiber filters. Filters were eluted with NCS, and counted in solution in a standard toluene-fluor mixture in a Beckman LS-250 β-scintillation spectrometer. The symbols represent: (●) MOPC-41 [125]I mRNA x MOPC-41 DNA, $Cot_{1/2}$ equals 3200, (○) mouse globin [125]I mRNA x mouse spleen DNA, $Cot_{1/2}$ equals 2100.

tively unique $Cot_{1/2}$ (3200). There is <u>no</u> very highly reiterated material. In contrast to previous studies, the Cot curve
is not obviously biphasic (33-39). Nevertheless, approximately 20% of the [125]I mRNA does hybridize over the range of Cot
between 2 and 600-800. One would assign a reiteration frequency to this material of 30 to 50 copies per haploid genome,
though it is difficult to feel secure about this number. It
<u>is</u> important to note that [125]I <u>globin</u> mRNA does <u>not</u> contain
these moderately reiterated sequences. The extent of hybridization, the amount of hybrid formed when the reaction is complete, is approximately 70%.

A similar analysis has been done using the MOPC-41 [125]I
mRNA and DNA derived from a myeloma of a different subgroup,
MOPC-265 (Fig. 5). The results are quite similar: a portion
of the material is moderately reiterated, the major component
is relatively unique and the extent of hybridization is approximately 66%.

An uncritical interpretation of this data would view them
as being entirely consistent with the recombinational germ
line hypothesis. There is a portion of the mRNA which is
moderately reiterated, consistent with the number of genes one
might expect in a single subgroup. The extent of hybridization does not differ significantly when one views the hybridization of a specific kappa mRNA to homologous and heterologous subgroup DNA. Still, it is clear that the extent of
hybridization can only be estimated within a wide margin of
error (10-15%). Thus, we might easily overlook a significant
difference in extent of hybridization. And further, what
evidence is there to suggest that the moderately reiterated
RNA in fact corresponds to the variable region? Unfortunately, there is none, save hopeful inference. We have carried
out preliminary competition experiments using RNAs of various
subgroups. These studies have been complicated by an unexpected effect of the added competing RNA in slowing the
rate of hybrid formation and thus altering the apparent reiteration frequency. It is clear that additional experiments
are necessary.

Additional information is available, however, from the
thermal denaturation analysis of mRNA-DNA hybrids formed
with subgroup-homologous and heterologous DNAs. Thermal
denaturation studies shown in Figure 6 indicate that there
is not a significant difference between the thermal denaturation profiles formed between homologous RNA-DNA hybrids

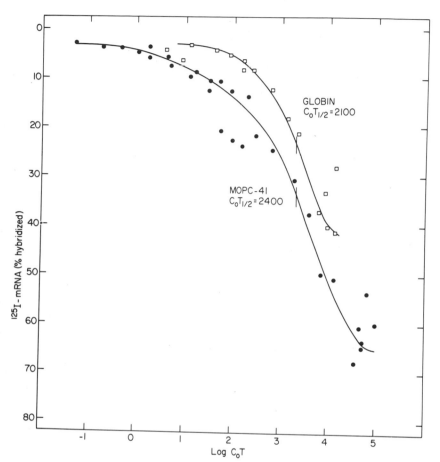

Fig. 5.   Kinetics of annealing of MOPC-41 ^{125}I-mRNA to a vast excess of total, cellular MOPC-265 DNA.   Hybridization kinetics of MOPC-41 [125]I mRNA in the presence of up to a 2.9 x 10[6]-fold excess of unlabeled, sheared MOPC-265 cellular DNA. Procedures are as described in the legend to Figure 4.   The symbols represent: (●) MOPC-41 ^{125}I-mRNA x MOPC-265 DNA, Cot$_{1/2}$ equals 2400, (O) globin (mouse) [125]I mRNA x mouse spleen DNA, Cot$_{1/2}$ equals 2100.

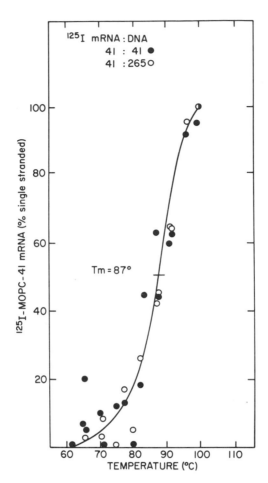

Fig. 6. Thermal denaturation of hybrids formed between MOPC-41 ^{125}I-mRNA and DNA from MOPC-41 and MOPC-265 tumors. Kinetics of melting of MOPC-41 [125]I mRNA:DNA hybrids. Hybrids were formed in 1.04 M Na[+] as described in the legend to Figure 4 and diluted 4 fold at the initial temperature of the melt curve. The reaction mixture was kept in a glass test tube in a Haake circulating water bath, and kept at each temperature for 8-10 min. prior to sampling. At each temperature, aliquots were withdrawn, diluted 50 fold into 2 x SSC and assayed for resistance to 60 µg/ml RNase A, as described in the legend to Figure 4. The ordinate represents the % of the total cpm made single-stranded during the melting.

(MOPC-41:MOPC-41) and heterologous RNA-DNA hybrids
(MOPC-41:265, different subgroups). While 20% of the hybrid
dissociates at temperatures below 80°, this is consistent with
the cross-hybridization which might occur between variable
regions of the same subgroup as expected by the recombinational germ line hypothesis. The congruity of these melt
profiles suggests that the hybrids formed are essentially
equivalent, a further expectation of the germ line hypothesis.
But we must keep in mind the limits of this analysis and recognize that a small sequence difference ($\sim$ 10% in only a portion of the mRNA) might provide melt differences beyond the
limits of detection of the technique. Therefore, until we can
view directly the properties of the variable sequence, we must
reserve final judgement.

CONCLUSIONS

These studies differ from those which have preceded it in
that they are based upon the utilization of a specific immunoglobulin messenger RNA which is homogeneous by several criteria. Possibly reflecting this difference, the hybridization
kinetic analyses which are obtained also differ from a number of earlier studies. In particular, our analyses indicate
that the kappa constant region is represented approximately
3 times per haploid mouse genome and that this gene frequency
does not change in a variety of mouse tumors and organs.
*Such a result rules out a stringent germ line hypothesis which
would require extensive reiteration of a constant region sequence.* This conclusion, of course, is consistent with much
genetic and serologic evidence.

Distinguishing between recombinational germ line and
somatic mutation hypotheses is more difficult. Our results
certainly indicate that there are no very highly reiterated
(thousands of copies per haploid genome) sequences present
in our purified kappa light chain mRNA. The mRNA preparation
contains a moderately reiterated sequence (50 to 30 copies)
and a major component which is clearly unique. This result
coupled with the observed extents of hybridization and the
thermal denaturation characteristics of hybrids formed between MOPC-41 mRNA and DNA from subgroup homologous and
heterologous tumor are possibly more supportive of the germ
line hypothesis, but a rather restricted somatic mutation
hypothesis involving many germ line subgroup genes cannot be
ruled out. The extension of these studies, particularly
competition experiments carried out between mRNAs in different subgroups, should shed more light on these possibilities.

315

ACKNOWLEDGMENTS

We are most grateful to Ms. Catherine Kunkle for her expert assistance in the preparation of this manuscript. We are very grateful to Dr. Michael Potter for supplying the tumors used in these studies.

REFERENCES

1. J. Lederberg, Science 129, 1649 (1959).
2. F.M. Burnet, The Clonal Selection Theory of Acquired Immunity (Cambridge University Press, 1959).
3. W.J. Dreyer and J.C. Bennett, Proc. Nat. Acad. Sci. USA 54, 864 (1965).
4. S. Brenner and C. Milstein, Nature 211, 242 (1966).
5. E.S. Lennox and M.A. Cohn, Rev. Biochem. 365 (1967).
6. O. Smithies, Science 157, 267 (1967).
7. M. Cohn, in Nucleic Acids in Immunology, (edit. by D.J. Plescia and W. Braun), 671 (Springer Berlin, 1968).
8. L. Hood and D. Talmage, Science N.Y. 168, 325 (1970).
9. N. Jerne, in Immune Surveillance (edit. by R.T. Smith and M. Landy) pp. 345-363 (Academic Press, New York, 1970).
10. J.A. Gally and G.M. Edelman, Nature 227, 341 (1970).
11. M. Cohn, Cell. Immun. 1, 461 (1971).
12. N.K. Jerne, Eur. J. Immul. 1, 1 (1971).
13. M. Cohn, Ann. N.Y. Acad. Sci. 190, 529 (1971).
14. D.D. Brown, in Molecular Genetics and Developmental Biology (edit. by M. Sussman), pp. 101-125 (Prentice-Hall, Inc., Englewood Cliffs, New Jersey, 1972).
15. J.A. Gally and G.M. Edelman, Ann. Rev. of Genetics 6, 1 (1972).
16. L.E. Hood, Fed. Proc. 31, 177 (1972).
17. H. Wigzell, Scan. J. Imm. 4, 199 (1973).
18. D. Swan, H. Aviv and P. Leder, Proc. Nat. Acad. Sci. USA 69, 1967 (1972).
19. H. Aviv and P. Leder, Proc. Nat. Acad. Sci. USA 69, 1408 (1972).
20. D.Z. Staynov, J.C. Pinder and W.B. Gratzer, Nature New Biol. 235, 108 (1972).
21. I. Schechter, Proc. Nat. Acad. Sci. USA 70, 2256 (1973).
22. C.H. Faust, Jr., H. Diggelman and B. Mach, Biochemistry 12, 925 (1973).
23. G.G. Brownlee, E.M. Cartwright, N.J. Cowan, J.M. Jarvis and C. Milstein, Nature New Biol. 244, 236 (1973).

24. D. McKean, T. Honjo, D. Swan, M. Nau and P. Leder, unpublished results.
25. H. Aviv, S. Packman, D. Swan, J. Ross and P. Leder, Nature New Biol 241, 174 (1973).
26. P. Leder, J. Ross, J. Gielen, S. Packman, Y. Ikawa, H. Aviv and D. Swan, Cold Spring Harb. Symp. on Quant. Biol. 38 (1973) in press.
27. J. Ross, H. Aviv, E. Scolnick and P. Leder, Proc. Nat. Acad. Sci. USA 69, 264 (1972).
28. J. Ross, H. Aviv and P. Leder, Arch. Biochem and Biophys. 158, 494 (1973).
29. R.J. Britten and D.E. Kohne, Science 161, 529 (1968).
30. S. Packman, H. Aviv, J. Ross and P. Leder, Biochem. Biophys. Res. Commun. 49, 813 (1972).
31. R.J. Britten and J. Smith, Carnegie Institution of Washington Yearbook 68, 378 (1970).
32. S. Packman, T. Honjo, D. Swan and P. Leder, unpublished observations.
33. U. Storb, J. of Immunol. 108, 755 (1972).
34. T.L. Delovitch and C. Baglioni, Proc. Nat. Acad. Sci. USA 70, 173 (1973).
35. E. Premkumar, M. Shoyab and A.R. Williamson, Proc. Nat. Acad. Sci. USA 71, 99 (1974).
36. A. Bernardini and S. Tonegawa, FEBS Lett. (1974) in press.
37. T.H. Rabbits and J.O. Bishop, FEBS Lett. (1974) in press.
38. U. Storb, Biochem. Biophys. Res. Commun. (1974) in press.
39. S. Tonegawa, A. Bernardini, B.J. Weimann and C. Steinberg, FEBS Lett. (1974) in press.
40. T. Honjo, S. Packman, D. Swan, M. Nau and P. Leder, submitted to Proc. Nat. Acad. Sci. USA.
41. W. Prensky, D.M. Steffensen and W.L. Hughes, Proc. Nat. Acad. Sci. USA 70, 1860 (1973).
42. M. Melli, C. Whitfield, K.V. Rao, M. Richardson and J.O. Bishop, Nature New Biol. 231, 8 (1971).

QUANTITATIVE ESTIMATION OF THE mRNA
FOR H-CHAIN IMMUNOGLOBULIN

Ronald H. Stevens*

National Institute for Medical Research
Mill Hill, London, England

ABSTRACT. The interaction between immunoglobulin and the
mRNA for H-chain immunoglobulin has been used to develop a
quantitative assay for H-chain mRNA. Soluable complexes of
immunoglobulin and H-chain mRNA can be effectively retained
by nitrocellulose filters while the uncomplexed mRNA passes
through the filter. Concentrations of H mRNA were determined by titering increasing concentrations of total mRNA
against a fixed concentration of antibody or, increasing
concentrations of immunoglobulin against a fixed concentration of mRNA, and assaying the samples for the protein-RNA
complex. A value of 6500-7500 H-chain mRNA molecules/cell
was determined for exponentially growing 5563 mouse myeloma cells.

INTRODUCTION

During differentiation of activated lymphocytes alterations in gene expression occur which result in the formation of mature immunoglobulin secreting plasma cells. The
synthesis, assembly and secretion of immunoglobulin have
been areas of extensive research during recent years owing
largely to the ability to isolate and minutely characterize
the individual heavy (H) and (L) chain immunoglobulin proteins (1). In direct contrast, however, little information
has been obtained on the intracellular mechanisms regulating synthesis and secretion of immunoglobulin.

It is clear that production of immunoglobulin can be
regulated at multiple levels within eukaryotic cells including a) transcription of the proper genes into RNA
copies, b) processing of these copies within the nucleus

---

* Present address: Department of Microbiology and
Immunology, University of California, Los Angeles,
California 90024

to allow subsequent c) transport of the mRNA into the cytoplasm where d) translation into protein can occur. Although
differentiation in lymphocytes would be expected to utilize
all available forms of controls, few regulatory mechanisms
have been characterized in lymphoid tissue and these have
represented controls on mRNA translation (2,3). The study
of the mechanisms regulating the transcription, nuclear
processing and transport of heavy and light chain mRNA molecules has been more difficult, and in many respects this has
resulted from the inability to easily and quantitatively obtain specific heavy and light chain mRNA molecules free from
other mRNA contamination.

Recent advances in the isolation and characterization
of mRNA have allowed partial purification and cell-free
translation of the mRNA for heavy (4,5) and light (6,7,8,9)
chain immunoglobulin proteins. In particular, the discovery
of a strong, specific binding between immunoglobulin and H-
chain mRNA has provided a powerful, sensitive assay for investigating the intracellular sequence of events leading
from the genes for H-chain to the production and active
translation of H-chain mRNA (10,11).

RESULTS AND DISCUSSION

The interaction between immunoglobulin and H-chain mRNA
was initially detected as a translational control of H-chain
protein synthesis in mouse plasmacytoma cells (5563) (2).
When 5563 myeloma cells were incubated at 27°, secretion of
immunoglobulin ceased although synthesis and assembly of H
and L chains into 7S immunoglobulin occurred normally but at
a reduced rate. This led to an increase in the intracellular level of immunoglobulin and resulted in a visible dis-
tortion of the rough and smooth endoplasmic reticulum. Con-
commitant with the increased intracellular build-up of immunoglobulin was the selective repression of H-chain synthesis (figure 1). After 2-3 hours at 27°, H-chain synthesis
was reduced approximately 80%, whereas L-chain synthesis
showed little reduction. Subsequent cell-free experiments
demonstrated that the H-chain repression resulted from the
direct interaction between immunoglobulin and H-chain mRNA
(10). These observations in turn led to the development of
a procedure for isolating highly purified heavy chain mRNA.

Most mRNA molecules in eukaryotic cells have been shown
to contain an adenylate-rich segment of 150-200 nucleotides
on the 3' and of the molecules (12,13,14). The ability of
this polyA region to hybridize with polyU or oligo dT immobilized on cellulose, enables mRNA to be conveniently

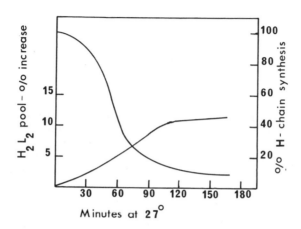

Fig. 1. Repression of H-chain synthesis by increased intracellular levels of immunoglobulin 5563 myeloma cells were incubated at 37° and at various time intervals, samples were removed, incubated with ^{35}S-methionine and the synthesis of H and L chain immunoglobulins were measured by specific immune precipitation. The increase in the intracellular immunoglobulin pool was calculated from the pool size at 37° and the relative rates of immunoglobulin synthesis at 27 and 37 degrees. From reference 2.

Fig. 2.   Flow scheme for immune isolation of H-chain
mRNA. A culture of 5563 myeloma cells was labeled overnight with ^{3}H-uridine (100 μCi/ml), collected by centrifugation and washed with PBS (140 mM NaCl, 3 mM KCl, 1 mM MgCl$_2$,
5 mM phosphate buffer, pH 7.4). The cells were lysed with
extraction buffer (100 mM Na acetate, 200 mM NaCl, 2 mM
MeDTA, 0.1% sodium dodecyl sulfate, pH 5.0 with acetic acid)
and the RNA isolated by two extractions with phenol (redis-
tilled) chloroform-isoamyl alcohol 3:1:0.05, and precipitated overnight (-20°) with two volumes of ethanol. The
RNA was resuspended in binding buffer (500 mM KCl, 10 mM
Tris, pH 7.4) and passed through a 1 ml column of oligo-dT
cellulose. The ribosomal RNA was eluted with 15 ml. of
binding buffer and the mRNA was subsequently eluted with
10 mM Tris-HCl buffer, pH 7.4. The ribosomal RNA and the
messenger RNA fractions were ethanol precipitated, and resuspended in PBS (0°). 50 micrograms purified 5563 immunoglobulin was added to both RNA fractions and the mixture
incubated on ice for 4 minutes. An equivalent amount of
purified rabbit anti-5563 immunoglobulin was then added and
the mixtures incubated a further four minutes at 0°. The
immune precipitates containing the bound H-chain mRNA were
collected by centrifugation and washed twice with PBS. The
immune precipitates were dissolved in extraction buffer
containing 70% dimethyl sulphoxide and the released RNA
analyzed by acrylamide gel electrophoresis.

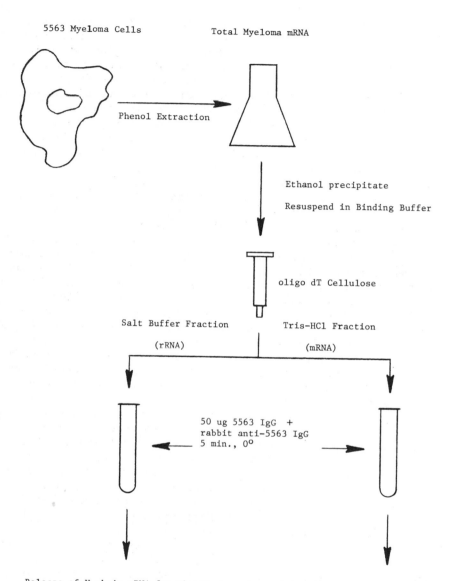

5563 Myeloma Cells

Total Myeloma mRNA

Phenol Extraction

Ethanol precipitate

Resuspend in Binding Buffer

oligo dT Cellulose

Salt Buffer Fraction

(rRNA)

Tris-HCl Fraction

(mRNA)

50 ug 5563 IgG +
rabbit anti-5563 IgG
5 min., 0°

Release of H chain mRNA for electrophoresis or injection into oocytes

Figure 2. See legend on page 322.

separated from cellular ribosomal RNA or mRNA lacking the polyA region. Utilizing the interaction between immunoglobulin and H-chain mRNA, it is possible to isolate H-chain mRNA from both the polyA (+) and polyA (-) RNA fractions. A scheme for this isolation procedure is shown in figure 2. Myeloma cells were initially separated into nuclei and cytoplasm with NP-40 detergent and total RNA isolated by conventional techniques. Separation into RNA which contained polyA and RNA which was devoid of polyA was accomplished by fractionation on either cellulose (15) or oligo dT cellulose (7) columns. Both RNA fractions [polyA (+) and (-)] were adjusted to the proper ionic conditions and 50 μg of 5563 immunoglobulin was added (all solutions were maintained at 0° throughout the procedure). Binding of H-chain mRNA to the 5563 immunoglobulin is rapid and nearly quantitative. The RNA-Ig complex was then precipitated by an excess rabbit anti-5563 antiserum. The resulting immune precipitates containing bound H-chain mRNA were collected by centrifugation, washed and the H-chain mRNA released by resuspending the precipitates in a disassociating buffer. Electrophoretic analysis of the released mRNA demonstrated a single peak of molecular weight 6×10^5 from the polyA (-) mRNA, and a single peak of 3×10^5 molecular weight from polyA (+) RNA (figure 3). The significant enrichment of a single species of mRNA was demonstrated by a comparison of the electrophoretic profiles of the antibody precipitated RNA with that of total 5563 polyA (+) RNA (figure 4).

A mRNA molecule coding for a protein containing 450 amino acid residues can be calculated to have a minimum molecular weight of approximately 4×10^5 and therefore the polyA (+) RNA would appear to be of insufficient size to code for heavy chain protein. Nevertheless, both the polyA (+) and polyA (-) immune fractionated mRNA peaks contained total information for heavy chain protein as demonstrated by the translation in oocytes from Xenopus laevis of both RNA species into complete H-chain protein (figure 5). The apparent discrepancy in mobility on acrylamide gels between the two H-chain mRNA molecules appeared to arise from the presence or absence of polyA sequences on the H-chain mRNA, the presence confirming a more rapid mobility of the RNA in acrylamide gels. This was demonstrated by sucrose density gradient centrifugation in which both mRNA species were shown to sediment with a molecular weight of 6×10^5.

Total myeloma RNA analyzed by the above procedure revealed an additional peak of 2.5×10^6 molecular weight which was confined to the nucleus and eventually confirmed as a nuclear precursor to cytoplasmic H-chain mRNA (16).

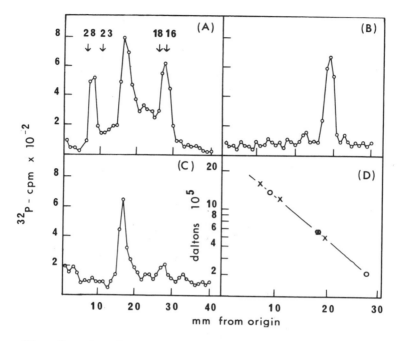

Fig. 3. Acrylamide gel analysis of antibody-bound RNA. Myeloma cells (10^7/ml) were labeled for 6 hr with [^{32}P] orthophosphate (100 μCi/ml), and total and cytoplasmic RNA were isolated. Total cellular RNA (A), cytoplasmic RNA enriched in mRNA (B), and cytoplasmic RNA enriched in rRNA (C) were treated 5 min at 0° with 5563 myeloma protein and anti-5563 antiserum, and the precipitates were washed twice with solution A. ^{3}H-labeled 28S and 18S ribosomal RNA from myeloma cells and 23S and 16S ribosomal RNA from *E. coli* were added to the precipitates, which were then made 2% with respect to SDS. The mixtures were layered upon 4% acrylamide gels containing SDS, and electrophoresis was conducted at 10 mA per gel for 90 min at room temperature. The gels were sliced into 1-mm sections and hydrolyzed with concentrated NH_4OH; the radioactivity was determined by scintillation counting. ^{32}P, O———O. The relationship between mobility and molecular weight for myeloma 28S and 18S and E. coli 23S and 16S ribosomal RNA (X) is shown in Fig. 3D. The mobilities of the three RNA bands (I, II, and III) are plotted on this line (0) to estimate apparent molecular weights.

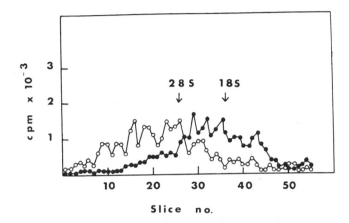

Fig. 4. Electrophoretic analysis of mRNA fractions
from nuclei and cytoplasm. The nuclear (O) and cytoplasmic
(●) mRNA were resuspended in electrophoresis buffer
(0.04 M Tris, 0.02 M sodium acetate, 2 mM EDTA, 0.5%
SDS, pH 7.4) and mixed with $^{32}PO_4$-labelled ribosomal marker
RNA. Electrophoresis on 2.6% acrylamide gels and radioactivity determinations determinations were performed as
described.

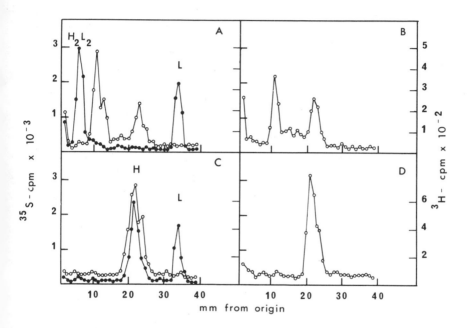

Fig. 5. Translation products of specifically purified
RNA. Oocytes from *Xenopus laevis* were injected with purified
RNA from bands II or III. The oocytes were homogenized after
24 hr of incubation at room temperature, and synthesized
5563 protein was precipitated by direct antibody precipitation with anti-5563 antiserum. The precipitates were washed
four times with phosphate-buffered saline (pH, 7.4), [3]H-
labeled 5563 marker protein was added, and the precipitates
were dissolved in 2% SDS. The samples were divided into two
portions: one portion was alkylated with iodoactamide
(0.15 M) and the other portion was reduced with mercaptoethanol (0.1 M) before alkylation. Unreduced and reduced
samples from oocytes injected with RNA from band II (A and
C, respectively) or from oocytes injected with RNA from
band III (B and D, respectively) were analyzed by electrophoresis on 7.5% acrylamide gels containing SDS. After
electrophoresis the gels were sliced into 1-mm sections and
hydrolyzed, and their radioactivity was determined. [35]S,
O——O; [3]H ●——●.

QUANTITATION OF H-CHAIN mRNA

The potential and usefulness of the immunoglobulin precipitation technique for isolating H-chain mRNA could be
considerably expanded where quantitative measurements of H-
chain mRNA possible.

All immunoglobulins tested to date appear capable of
binding to heavy chain messenger RNA (17). This has included highly purified preparations of rabbit anti-dinitro-
phenol (DNP) immunoglobulin (18) prepared by affinity chro-
motography (19).

It has been known for several years that purified RNA
or native DNA will pass unhindered through nitrocellulose
filters. When proteins are specifically bound to the nucleic acids the protein-nucleic acid complex becomes retained by the nitrocellulose filter (20,21). This procedure
has been elegantly used for studying the lac (22,23) and
bacteriophage lambda repressor-operator systems (24,25), and
forms the basis for the quantitative assay for H-chain mRNA
(26).

A flow diagram of the nitrocellulose filter binding
assay is shown in figure 6. Solutions of total mRNA and
immunoglobulin were mixed in the required proportions in PBS
and allowed to reach equilibrium. DNP-ovalbumin was added
and the solutions immediately passed through nitrocellulose
filters and washed. Control samples consisted of total mRNA
which was interacted with DNP-ovalbumin and passed through
the nitrocellulose filters. The DNP-ovalbumin does not
directly participate in the reaction, but the formation of
a larger protein-nucleic acid complex allows more reproducible binding. When preparations of radioactive myeloma mRNA
were mixed with increasing amounts of purified rabbit anti-
DNP-IgG, and allowed to attain equilibrium, increasing
amounts of mRNA became bound to the nitrocellulose filter
presumably due to the formation of an antibody-H-chain mRNA
complex. The amount of RNA bound to the filter eventually
reached a plateau saturating at approximately 3-4% of the
input mRNA (figure 7). In theory, assuming stochiometric
binding, the concentration of H-chain mRNA in the total mRNA
sample, can be determined from the concentration of the
immunoglobulin at saturation. This emphasizes the need for
highly purified immunoglobulin preparations. One-half
saturation of 20 µl mRNA preparation occurred at 6×10^{-13} M
anti-DNP immunoglobulin and therefore the concentration of
H-chain mRNA in the 20 µl sample was 1.2×10^{-12} M.

The above statements are conditional subject to the
method being specific for H-chain mRNA, that the filter

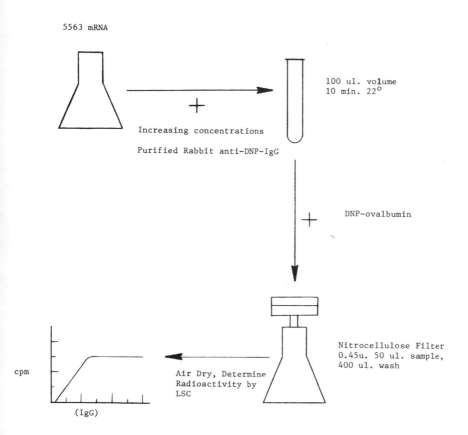

Fig. 6. Flow scheme for nitrocellulose filter binding assay. Total radioactive mRNA from 5563 myeloma cells was extracted and separated into mRNA and rRNA fractions as in figure 2. The mRNA fraction was adjusted to the ionic conditions of PBS, and, in a total volume of 100 µl., a constant amount of mRNA was interacted with increasing concentrations of rabbit anti-DNP-IgG. The mixtures were incubated 7 min. at 22° to attain equilibrium. An excess DNP ovalbumin was added and duplicate 50 µl aliquots were filtered through nitrocellulose filters (Millipore, 0.45 µ, type HA), washed with 400 µl PBS, dried and the bound radioactivity determined by liquid scintillation counting.

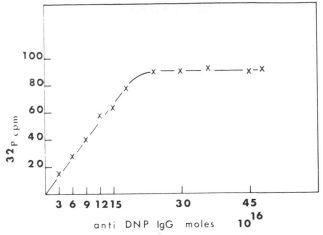

Fig. 7. Quantitation of H chain mRNA using nitrocellulose filters 5563 mRNA (1.2 x 10^5 cpm/µg), 0.15 µg
added per sample) samples were mixed with increasing amounts
of rabbit anti-DNP antibody in total sample volumes of
100 1. Following 5 min incubation at 22°, 5 µl DNP-ovalbumin was added to each sample which were then divided into
two 50 µl aliquots, filtered and the radioactivity determined. Each point is the average of two determinations.

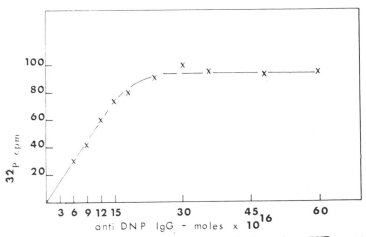

Fig. 8. Quantitation of H chain mRNA using DNP cysta-
mine columns. DNP-acrylamide beads were prepared and equilibrated with PBS and 2 ml columns prepared as in Materials
and Methods. 5563 mRNA (0.15 µg/sample, 1.2 x 10^5 cpm per
µg) was mixed with increasing amounts of rabbit anti-DNP
antiserum in a total sample volume of 200 µl. The mixtures were incubated at 22° for 5 min and 100 µl aliquots
were applied to DNP-cystamine columns. The columns were
washed and the radioactivity determined as in Materials
and Methods.

doesn't disturb the equilibrium, that the RNA-IgG is sufficiently strong and that there are single independent binding
sites on H-chain mRNA and the immunoglobulin. Many of the
above objections could be removed by performing an identical
saturation experiment but using a column of DNP-acrylamide
to trap the RNA-immunoglobulin complex. In this way, any
artifactual binding of RNA to the nitrocellulose filter
could be eliminated (figure 8). A comparison of figures of
7 and 8 reveals similar saturation curves using either DNP-
acrylamide or nitrocellulose filters to trap the immunoglobulin-H-chain mRNA complex; each giving the same concentration of bound mRNA in the 20 µl sample. These results
suggested that the saturation curve obtained with nitrocellulose filters was not generated by artifactual binding.

The presence of H-chain mRNA in the mRNA bound to the
DNP-acrylamide column was demonstrated by eluting the antibody-bound RNA from the DNP-acrylamide column and assaying
for mRNA activity in the oocyte translation assay (27).
Figure 9 shows that total mRNA stimulates both heavy and
light chain protein synthesis within the oocyte (3% of total
protein synthesis) whereas the mRNA eluted from the DNP
acrylamide column stimulated the synthesis of only H-chain
protein (55% of total protein synthesis). It appears,
therefore, that like the antibody precipitation technique
for isolating H-chain mRNA, the DNP-acrylamide column and
nitrocellulose filters when used in conjunction with rabbit
antiserum are specific for isolating H-chain mRNA.

The nitrocellulose filter binding assay has been initially used to quantitate H-chain mRNA in 5563 myeloma
cells. In table I, separate determinations of the amount
of H-chain mRNA per 5563 myeloma cell has been determined
using several techniques, which have included performing
the assay with constant amount of mRNA and increasing
amounts of immunoglobulin or constant amount of immunoglobulin with increasing amounts of mRNA. Furthermore, the
assays have been performed by trapping the H-chain mRNA-
immunoglobulin complex on either nitrocellulose filters or
DNP-acrylamide columns. All methods provide reproducible
values of H-chain mRNA ranging from 6900-8500 molecules
per cell with an average of 7400. This value correlates
well with the actual quantity of H-chain protein produced
by 5563 cells.

KINETICS OF IMMUNOGLOBULIN-H-CHAIN mRNA BINDING

The ability to quantitatively and reproducibly trap
the immunoglobulin-H-chain mRNA complex can be used to in-

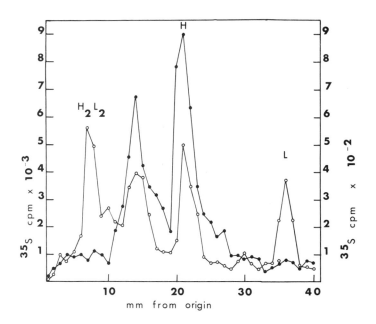

Fig. 9.   5563 products from oocytes injected with RNA
prepared by DNP-affinity chromatography.   Total mRNA from
myeloma cells was resuspended in PBS and mixed with 10^{-11}
moles rabbit anti DNP-IgG.   The mixture was incubated on
ice for 10 min and passed through a column of DNP-cystamine
immobilized on polyacrylamide beads.   The bound mRNA was
eluted from the column with acetate buffer containing
0.1% SDS and phenol extracted.   Total 5563 mRNA or the mRNA
which remained bound to the DNP affinity column (both from
5×10^{6} cells) was injected into oocytes from *Xenopus
laevis* and the 5563 protein precipitated with specific antiserum.   The washed antibody precipitates were dissolved by
heating to 100° in 2% SDS and analyzed by electrophoresis
on 7% acrylamide gels containing SDS.   -0-0- products from
oocytes injected with total mRNA -•-•- products from
oocytes injected with mRNA bound to DNP-cystamine column.

Table 1. Quantitation of H-chain mRNA in 5563 cells.
Cultured 5563 myeloma cells were labelled overnight with
^{32}P-orthophosphate and messenger RNA enriched RNA fractions
prepared. Samples of RNA were mixed with increasing
amounts of anti-DNP antibody and analyzed on columns of
acrylamide beads containing bound DNP-cystamine (Expt. 1)
or nitrocellulose filters (Expt. 4). Alternatively,
increasing amounts of radioactive RNA were added to constant
amounts of anti-DNP antibody and the resulting protein-
RNA complexes analyzed on columns of acrylamide beads
containing DNP-cystalyzed on columns of acrylamide beads
containing DNP-cystamine (Expt. 2) or nitrocellulose
filters (Expts. 3,5).

Determination of H-chain mRNA in 5563 cells

Expt.	Assay	No. cells	Moles H-chain mRNA	Molecules H-chain mRNA per cell
1	DNP column	6.1×10^6	7.0×10^{-14}	7000
	Increasing IgG			
2	DNP column	3.7×10^7	4.5×10^{-13}	7300
	Increasing RNA			
3	Filter	8.0×10^6	9.2×10^{-14}	6900
	Increasing RNA			
4	Filter	6.1×10^6	7.5×10^{-14}	7450
	Increasing IgG			
5	Filter	5.3×10^7	7.5×10^{-13}	8500
	Increasing RNA			
Average				7400

333

vestigate the nature of the interaction between H–chain mRNA
and immunoglobulin. Preliminary results will be briefly
summarized.

The interaction appears to follow the kinetics of a
second order reaction as expressed in equation 1 where HR
is the concentration of heavy chain mRNA, Ig is the concentration of immunoglobulin and HRIg is the concentration of
the RNA–immunoglobulin complex.

$$HR + IgG \underset{k_b}{\overset{k_a}{\rightleftharpoons}} HRIg \quad (1)$$

The association (k_a) disassociation (k_d) and equilibrium ($K_{equ} = k_d/k_a$) were 8.4×10^8 M^{-1} sec^{-1},
2.4×10^{-4} sec^{-1} and 2.65×10^{-13} M respectively. The
association kinetics of the reaction were determined by
mixing accurately known quantities of immunoglobulin and H–
chain mRNA and sampling the reaction mixture at various time
intervals for the formation of the HIg complex (figure 10)
by filtering through nitrocellulose filters. The kinetic
data can be replotted in a linear form and the association
constant determined from the slope of the resulting line
(26). Similarly the disassociation constant of the reaction
was determined by allowing total formation of the HIg complex, adding a 20–fold excess nonradioactive H–chain mRNA
and measuring the loss of radioactivity from the HIg complex. The excess unlabelled mRNA prevents the reformation
of the released radioactive H–chain mRNA with IgG. The loss
of complex radioactivity thus represents the disassociation
of the HIg' complex. The $T_{1/2}$ of the complex at room temperature is approximately 40 minutes which corresponds to a
k_d of 2.4×10^{-4} sec^{-1}.

Comparison of the interaction between H–chain mRNA with
immunoglobulin with other well documented nucleic acid–protein interactions reveals several similarities (table II).
All the interacting proteins are multi–subunited and appear
to bind to double stranded regions of the nucleic acids;
preliminary results suggest that this is also true for the
immunoglobulin–H–chain mRNA interaction.

From the limited information available on nucleic acid–
protein interaction, it is interesting to note that the
interaction between immunoglobulin and H–chain mRNA falls
within the range of the more stable regulatory interactions.
The main in vivo function of this strong and specific interaction is unknown. As discussed earlier, the interaction
can apparently function as a feedback control mechanism
regulating the translation of H–chain mRNA. Whether the

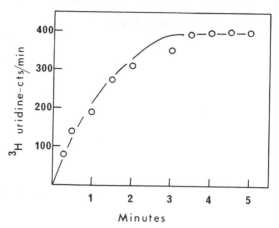

Fig. 10. Kinetics of IgG-H chain mRNA association. Rabbit anti-DNP IgG (8 x 10^{-15} moles) and radioactive 5563 mRNA containing 4 x 10^{-15} moles H chain mRNA were combined in a total volume of 1.0 ml. At selected time intervals, 100 μl aliquots were removed and mixed with 50 μg DNP ovalbumin. Duplicate 50 μl samples were immediately filtered, washed and the radioactivity determined. Non-specific binding of radioactive RNA to DNP-ovalbumin and nitrocellulose filters (0.2% of input radioactivity) were subtracted from each sample.

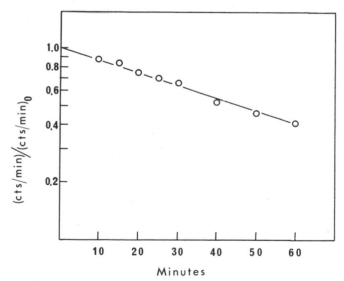

Fig. 11. Determination of the Disassociation Constant (k_d) Radioactive 5563 H chain mRNA (5 x 10^{-12}M) and rabbit anti DNP-IgG (6 x 10^{-12}M) were incubated at room temperature for 10 min to reach equilibrium. A 20-fold excess non-radioactive H chain mRNA was added and at selective time intervals 50 μl samples were removed, mixed with DNP-OA (10μg) and filtered through nitrocellulose filters.

Table 2. Comparison of regulatory protein-nucleic acid associations.

Interaction	Repressor	Binding site	K_{equ}	Ref
lac-operon-repressor	Tetramer 40,000 m.w. subunits	DNA ds	$1\text{-}2 \times 10^{-13}$ M	22,23
lambda, 434 phage operator-repressors	Dimer, 29,000 m.w. subunits	DNA ds	$3\text{-}4 \times 10^{-14}$ M	24,25
MS2, R17 phage synthetase repression	Coat protein 14,000 m.w. subunits	RNA, ds?	-	29
7S immunoglobulin-H chain mRNA	7S immunoglobulin 75,000 dimer of H-L	RNA ds?	$2\text{-}3 \times 10^{-13}$ M	2,10,11
tRNA–tRNA syntethase (Methionine)	Tetramer, 45,000 m.w. subunits	RNA ds?	$0.2\text{-}1 \times 10^{-6}$ M	28

feedback repression is the sole function of the interaction appears unlikely from the strength, specificity and yet generality of the reaction between many immunoglobulin and heavy chain mRNA molecules. The immunoglobulin and heavy chain mRNA in plasma cells are normally separated by membrane. Conditions where immunoglobulin would be allowed to freely interact with H-chain mRNA would appear restricted to the early stages of lymphocyte differentiation into plasma cells. At these times there is little well developed endoplasmic reticulum and interaction of the synthesized immunoglobulin with H-chain mRNA may occur more easily. Whether resting lymphocytes are indeed the site of action and whether the immunoglobulin-H-chain mRNA interaction functions to activate or modulate the humoral immune response must await further investigation.

REFERENCES

1. M. J. Bevan, R. M. E. Parkhouse, A. R. Williamson, Prog. Biophys. and Mol. Biol. 25, 133 (1972).
2. R. H. Stevens and A. R. Williamson, J. Mol. Biol. 78, 505 (1973).
3. R. H. Stevens, Eur. J. Biochem. in press (1974).
4. R. H. Stevens and A. R. Williamson, Nature 239, 143 (1972).
5. N. J. Cowan and L. Milstein, Eur. J. Biochem. (1973).
6. J. Staunezer and R. C. Huang, Nature New Biol. 230, 172 (1971).
7. D. Swan, H. Aviv and P. Leder, Proc. Nat. Acad. Sci. 69, 1967.
8. B. Mach, C. H. Faust, and P. Vassalli, Proc. Nat. Acad. Sci. 70, 451 (1973).
9. S. Tonegawa and I. Baldi, Biochem. Biophys. Res. Comm. 51, 81 (1973).
10. R. H. Stevens and A. R. Williamson, J. Mol. Biol. 78, 517 (1973).
11. R. H. Stevens and A. R. Williamson, Proc. Nat. Acad. Sci. 70, 1127 (1973).
12. J. Darnell, R. Wall and R. Tushinski, Proc. Nat. Acad. Sci. 68, 1321 (1971).
13. M. Edmonds, M. Vaughan and H. Nakuzato, Proc. Nat. Acad. Sci. 68, 1336 (1971).
14. W. Jelinek, M. Adesnik, M. Salditt, P. Sheiness, R. Wall, G. Molloy, L. Philipson and J. E. Parnell, J. Mol. Biol. 73, 515 (1973).

15. P. A. Kitos, L. Saxon, and H. Amos, *Biochem. Biophys. Res. Comm. 47*, 1426–37 (1972).

16. R. H. Stevens and A. R. Williamson, *Nature New Biology 245*, 101 (1973).

17. R. Premkumar, R. H. Stevens and A. R. Williamson, *in preparation.*

18. R. L. Valentine and N. M. Green, *J. Mol. Biol. 27*, 615.

19. H. Eisen, W. Gray, J. R. Little and E. Summers *in Methods in Immunology and Immunochemistry, vol. 1*, 351, Academic Press, New York & London (1967).

20. O. W. Jones and P. Berg, *J. Mol. Biol. 22*, 199 (1966).

21. H. Kuno and H. Kihara, *Nature 215*, 974 (1967).

22. A. D. Riggs, H. Suzuki and S. Bourgeois, *J. Mol. Biol. 48*, 67 (1970).

23. A. D. Riggs, S. Bourgeois and M. Cohn, *J. Mol. Biol. 53*, 401 (1970).

24. P. Chadwick, V. Pirrotta, R. Steinberg, N. Hopkins and M. Ptashne, *Cold Springs Harbor Symp. Quant. Biol. 35*, 283 (1970).

25. T. Maniatis and M. Ptashne, *Nature 46*, 133 (1973).

26. R. H. Stevens, *J. Mol. Biol.* manuscript submitted.

27. C. Lane, G. Marbaix, and J. Gurdon, *J. Mol. Biol. 61*, 73 (1971).

28. Bruton and Hartley, *J. Mol. Biol. 52*, 165 (1970).

29. T. Sugiyama, *Cold Spring Harbor Symp. Quant. Biol. 34* 687 (1969).

30. R. Pulbecco and M. Vogt, *J. Exp. Med. 99*, 167–182 (1954).

MUTATIONS IN MOUSE MYELOMA CELLS

Barbara K. Birshtein, Jean-Louis Preud'homme,*
and Matthew D. Scharff

Department of Cell Biology
Albert Einstein College of Medicine
Bronx, New York 10461

ABSTRACT. Cultured mouse myeloma cells of the MPC-11 tumor, which synthesizes an IgG2b molecule, have been cloned in vitro. An antiserum directed against the Fc portion of the molecule was used to detect variants which 1) no longer synthesized H chains; 2) no longer secreted H chains; 3) synthesized an altered H chain. All variants spontaneously arising in the parent population had lost the ability to synthesize H chains. Mutagenesis with the acridine mustard, ICR-191, and with the phenyalanine mustard, Melphalan, increased the incidence of variants 10-20 fold till they comprised 3-6% of the population. Two-thirds of the variants arising after mutagenesis were like spontaneously arising variants, but the remainder synthesized an altered H chain. Some variant H chains were smaller then the parent; other variant H chains were of the same size or larger, but now had the γ 2a serotype. Peptide maps confirmed structural differences. Variants of one type gave rise to variants of another type after exposure to culture and cloning. Preliminary chemical characterization has confirmed that one short H chain variant does not contain a normal Fc.

INTRODUCTION

Experimentally induced mutations have been elegantly used in bacteria to explore the sequence of metabolic pathways and their controls. We would like to use a similar approach to deal with the interactions that take place in cells having more than one chromosome and which have many cell organelles engaged in the synthesis and export of certain products. A good system is that of immunoglobulin synthesis since a great deal is known about the biology of

---

* Present address: Laboratoire d'Immunochimie, University De Paris, Faculte De Medecine, Institut De Recherches Sur Les Maladies Du Sang, Hospital Saine-Louis, 2, Place du Docteur-Fournier, Paris-Xe, FRANCE

339

the lymphocyte, that cell which is committed to the synthesis of a single immunoglobulin, and about the chemistry of antibodies.

In particular, we have used a myeloma tumor -- the result of a malignancy of a plasma cell -- to yield a cultured cell line which continues to synthesize and secrete large quantities of a single homogeneous immunoglobulin molecule. This cell line has been mutagenized with agents such as the acridine mustard, ICR-191, and the phenyalanine mustard, Melphalan, to yield variants which synthesize an immunoglobulin different from the parent. Both biological and chemical studies are underway to characterize these variants.

ISOLATION OF VARIANTS

The tumor MPC-11, which synthesizes an IgG_{2b} molecule, was adapted to grow in vitro (1,2). Cultured cells were cloned at different times to yield a less heterogeneous cell source for experiments. Cells were grown in Dulbecco's modified Eagle's medium containing 20% horse serum and supplemented with non-essential amino acids, glutamine, and antibiotics. Mutagens were added to the medium at a dose of $1\mu g/ml$, for 24 hours, after which cells were transferred to medium without the mutagen. After an additional 24 hrs., cells were cloned in soft agar (3,4).

Screening of the cloned cells was done with a rabbit antiserum directed against the Fc or C-terminal half of the MPC-11 molecule. Those clones which normally synthesized and secreted the MPC-11 molecules were obscured by the resulting antigen-antibody precipitate. "Unstained" clones were selected as presumptive variants. These variants might: 1) no longer synthesize H chains; 2) no longer secret H chains; 3) make an altered H chain.

Unstained variants arose spontaneously in a clone of the MPC-11 cell line at a rate of 1.1×10^{-3}/cell/generation (3). Stained and unstained clones were retrieved from the agar, grown to mass culture, and analyzed by electrophoresis of radiolabeled cell proteins on acrylamide gels containing sodium dodecylsulfate (SDS) (5). Cells were incubated with ^{14}C or ^{3}H-valine, threonine, and leucine for 10 minutes to label intracellular proteins and for 3 hours to label secreted proteins (1). Immunoglobulin components were isolated by immunological precipitation using an indirect technique. These precipitates were solubilized by treating with SDS and analyzed by electrophoresis on acrylamide gels containing SDS either

directly or after complete reduction of the disulfide bridges
to effect separation of light and heavy chains (1). When
spontaneously arising variants were analyzed in this way,
they were found to be synthesizing only L chains, having
discontinued H chain synthesis (3).

Parental cells were then treated with a variety of
mutagens. X-irradiation and ethyl methanesulfonate were
ineffective mutagens, while nitrosoguanidine only doubled
the incidence of variants. On the other hand, the acridine
mustard ICR-191 and the phenylalanine mustard, Melphalan,
increased the incidence of variants 10-20 fold till they
constituted up to 3-6% of the mutagenized clones (6,7).

Serological classification of the variant clones by
Ouchterlony analysis has enormously facilitated our screening of hundreds of variants. Ouchterlony analysis was done
on both cytoplasmic and secreted proteins by a simple procedure. About 3 mls of a logarithmically growing cell
culture (5-15 x 10^5 cells/ml) were spun to pellet the cells.
The supernatant (secretions) was removed for analysis. The
cell pellet was lysed with the addition of 0.05 ml of an iso-
tonic buffer containing 0.5% NP-40. Nuclei were pelleted by
centrifugation and the resulting cytoplasmic lysate and the
secretions, which had been originally set aside, were tested
in agar diffusion analysis with a variety of antisera. An
antiserum against the completely reduced and alkylated heavy
chain (anti-H (CRA)) showed reactivity with the cytoplasmic
lysates of ~1/3 of the variant clones derived after mutagenesis.

SDS acrylamide gel electrophoresis of those variant
clones which contained H chain detectable by Ouchterlony
analysis showed that the H chains differed from the parent
in size and in their ability to polymerize with light chain.
Those clones (the remaining two-thirds) whose cytoplasmic
lysates were negative with anti-H (CRA) were found to resemble spontaneously occurring variants in that they synthesized
only light chains.

We have focused our attention on those variants synthesizing altered heavy chains and have grouped these variants on
the basis of their assembly patterns, the size of the chain
and serology. The classification is shown in Table 1.

SHORT-CHAIN VARIANTS

Six variants have been found which synthesize heavy
chains smaller than the parent. These can be divided into
two groups: Type 1, which synthesizes a chain of 50,000 MW
(as compared to the parent of 55,000 MW) and Type 2, which

Table 1

VARIANT H CHAINS, THEIR SIZE, SEROLOGICAL CHARACTERISTICS, AND PEPTIDE MAP PROFILES

	H Chain Size	Cytoplasm				Secretions		Tryptic-chymotryptic peaks in common with parent
		Anti-Fc	Anti-H(CRA)*	Anti-γ2b	Anti-Fab	Anti-Fc	Anti-H(CRA)	
Parent	55,000	+	+	+	+	+	+	
Small Chain								
Type 1 (3)	50,000	-	+	-	+	-	-	26/30
Type 2 (3)	44,000	-	+	-	+	-	+	27/35
γ2a Serotype								
a) (1)	75,000	+	+	-	+	-	-	18/34
b) (3)	55,000	+	+	-	+	-	N.D.	18/34

*CRA means completely reduced and alkylated

synthesizes a H chain of 44,000 MW. A representative of each type was radiolabeled and the Ig components analyzed on SDS-acrylamide gels. As shown in Figure 1, the assembly patterns (lefthand panels) are distinctive and show that the H chain of Type 1 variants do not polymerize as well as the H chain of Type 2. The right hand panels show that after reduction and alkylation, the II chains of Type 2 are smaller than those of Type 1 and both are smaller than the parent.

To ascertain whether these differences in the size of the chains and in the assembly patterns reflected structural differences, we analyzed variant H chains by comparative peptide mapping. ^{14}C-labeled variant and ^{3}H-labeled parent H chains were isolated from SDS-acrylamide gels electrophoresis of completely reduced and alkylated molecules and then mixed. SDS was removed from the molecules after which the H chain mixture was digested with trypsin and chymotrypsin. Peptides were resolved by ion exchange chromatography on a cation exchange column with a linear pyridine-acetate gradient.

An experiment comparing a Type 1 variant H chain with the parent H chain is shown in Figure 2. The maps are very similar: arrows mark those 6 peaks which differ in the maps. The variant lacks 4 peaks contained in the parent, and the parent contains 2 small peaks not seen in the variant. Maps comparing a Type 2 variant H chain with the parent H chain show more differences, but the overall patterns remain quite similar. When the variant H chain types are compared with each other, it is found that all peaks of the 44,000 MW chain map are contained in the map of the 50,000 MW chain. Maps of two Type 2 variants, one derived directly from Melphalan treatment, and one derived from a Type 1 - ICR variant after culture, were identical with the exception of one or two small peaks.

VARIANTS OF THE γ 2a SEROTYPE

Five variants have been derived after Melphalan or ICR mutagenesis which continue to make H chains of the same size or larger than the parent. These variants were screened by Ouchterlony analysis with a variety of antisera and, in particular, were found to have lost the γ 2b serotype of the parent and to have gained a γ2a serotype. A summary of the serological data is found in Table 1.

When variants were radiolabeled and the Ig components examined by SDS-acrylamide gel electrophoresis, the resulting assembly patterns differed from the parent and from the short-chain variants as shown in Figure 3. The major

343

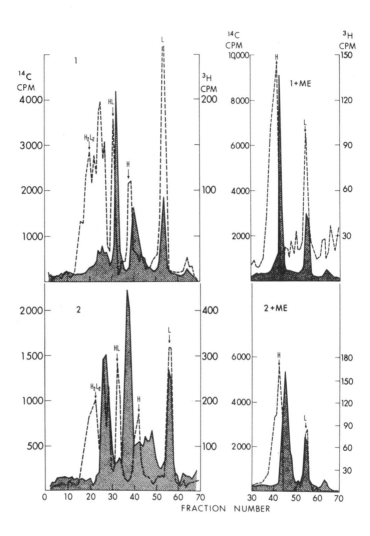

Figure 1. SDS-acrylamide gel electropherograms of a Type 1 (top) and Type 2 (bottom) variant, each compared to the parent. Radiolabel of immunoglobulin components in cytoplasm: left without, right with, complete reduction of the disulfide bridges. The shaded areas mark the variants. The dotted lines mark the parent.

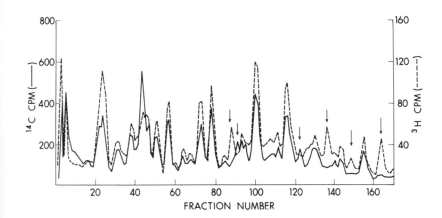

Figure 2. Comparative peptide maps of the H chains of a Type 1 variant (14C-solid line) and parent (3H-dashed line). The peptides were derived from successive enzyatic cleavages with trypsin and chymotrypsin and resolved as described in the text.

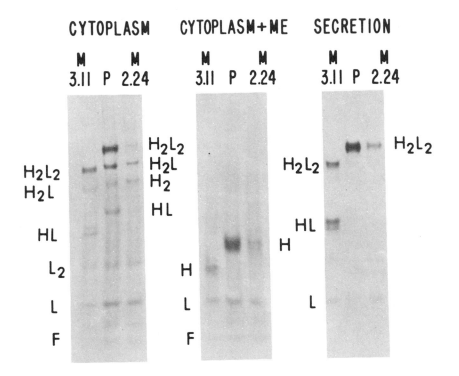

Figure 3. Autoradiogram of the SDS-acrylamide gel electropherogram of two variants derived after Melphalan mutagenesis. M3.11 is a Type 2 variant. M2.24 is a γ 2a-normal sized variant. P is parent. Left panel - Cytoplasmic Ig components after 10 min. label. Middle panel. Cytoplasmic Ig after reduction and aklylation. Right panel. Secreted Ig after 3 hr. labeling time.

346

difference is the lack of HL in the cytoplasms of these γ 2a variants as compared to the parent, a characteristic feature of the assembly patterns of known IgG_{2a} tumors and cell lines (8).

A comparative peptide map of one normal-sized γ 2a variant H chain with the parent H chain showed some similarities but the overall maps were quite different from each other. The numbers of peaks shared in the two maps are tabulated in Table 1 for both these and the maps of short chain variants to help give an estimate of structural similarities and differences.

RELATIONSHIPS BETWEEN VARIANTS

At various times, especially with our first experience with short chain variants of the Type 1 class, variants have been found to be unstable in that they lost the ability to synthesize heavy chains. In an effort to retrieve those few cells which might be continuing variant H chain synthesis from a population of cells, most of which continued to synthesize only L chains, variants were recloned. In most instances, analysis of the resulting subclones showed them either to be resembling the original variant or producing only L chains.

However, in three instances, we have seen a change in the phenotype of the variant other than loss of chain synthesis. When a Type 1 variant, which synthesizes a 50,000 MW H chain (Figure 1) was recloned and clones were overlayed with an antiserum directed against completely reduced and alkylated H chains, most clones were "unstained" and were found to be like the original variant or like spontaneous L chain producers. One-third of the clones were "stained" with these antisera; these were found to synthesize a 44,000 MW H chain and were of the Type 2 phenotype. We have recently begun to repeat the observation with another Type 1 variant and have retrieved 16 stained clones from a Petri dish containing 478 unstained clones.

Another change in phenotype has been documented by Dr. Saija Koskimies in an experiment in which the variant synthesizing a H chain of 75,000 MW with the γ 2a serotype was recloned. The overlay antisera used in this instance was rabbit anti-Fc since the original variant was unstained with this antiserum. One stained clone was found among 660 unstained clones. When grown to mass culture and analyzed, it was found to synthesize and secrete a variant H chain of the γ 2a serotype but of normal size (55,000).

347

STRUCTURAL STUDIES

We are trying to define the various structural defects in an attempt to understand the genetic basis of individual variants and to cope with these interesting inter-relationships.

All variants retain tumorogenicity but only those of normal size and having the γ 2a serotype secrete paraprotein of any quantity into the serum. Consequently, sequence studies have focused on the parent MPC-11 protein, which can be isolated easily and rapidly from the serum of mice bearing tumors. The rationale is the following: we hope to work out preparative methods of dealing with fragments of the parent molecule, both to determine the general structure and to pave the way for amino acid sequence determinations on relevant portions. At the same time, we are looking for analytical methods of dealing with these same portions of the molecule to facilitate screening variant chains which may be available only in radiolabel quantities.

The parent MPC-11 molecule (H_2L_2) was cleaved at methionine residues with CNBr. The digest was fractionated on Sephadex G-100 equilibrated with 8 M urea, 0.1M in formic acid: two major pools were found. When pool II was subjected to complete reduction and alkylation to break any disulfide bridges, and filtered through a column of Sephadex G-50, equilibrated in 0.05 M. NH_4HCO_3 three fragments were found. Together, these constituted approximately 200 residues and were held together by two disulfide bridges. One fragment contained no homoserine or alanine which identified it as the C-terminal fragment of the H chain. (The C-terminal CNBr fragment of K chains contains alanine).[9] These 3 fragments then accounted for practically all the Fc region.

SDS-acrylamide gel electrophoresis of the initial CNBr digest showed good separation of the "Fc" from larger fragments. Consequently, we used this method as an analytical tool for comparing a Type 2 variant which synthesizes a 44,000 MW H chain and the parent. Both parent and variant cells were labeled with ^{14}C-valine, threonine, and leucine, and H_2L_2 was isolated. The H_2L_2 of each was digested with CNBr and the digest subjected to electrophoresis on SDS-acrylamide gels. The radioautograph showed that the Type 2 variant protein completely lacked a fragment of the size of the parent Fc. Small fragments from this region were probably lost during electrophoresis, but hopefully they can be found by gel filtration of the CNBr digest.

DISCUSSION

We should like to call the variants described here "mutants". They arise after mutagenesis, their phenotypes are generally stable and they produce heavy chains which differ functionally, serologically, and chemically from the parent chain and from each other.

The inability of rabbit anti-Fc to detect these variants suggests that the lesion lies somewhere in the C-terminal half of the chain. In addition, the preliminary structural evidence presented here confirms this finding for one short chain variant. The methods we have described would seem to be generally applicable in screening other variants. However, our findings raise, perhaps, more questions than they answer:

1) Why should variants in Ig production arise at such a high incidence - 3 - 6% when the mutation rate in bacteria is orders of magnitudes lower, say 10^{-6}? Does this indicate something special about mammalian cells? Other investigators have noted difficulties in finding mutants of cultured mammalian cells, (10,11) but recently workers have been successful in isolating variants of the enzyme hypoxanthine-guanosine phosphoribosyl transferase, (HGPRT) (12,13) α -amanitin resistant variants, (14) and variants expressing a change in a tRNA synthetase, (15) all of which seem to meet the criteria of real mutants.

The high incidence of variants we see is specific for immunoglobulin synthesis; variants resistant to drugs arise at an incidence of less than 1 in 10^6 cells (6). One might have originally thought that the variability we detect was caused by mechanisms of somatic mutation, but these mechanisms have been postulated to account for the hypervariability associated with antigen binding, not for differences in the C-terminal half of H chain. Variants spontaneously arising in another cultured mouse myeloma cell line were also found to affect the constant regions (16). What, then, are we observing? Are there nuances connected with the use of a heteroploid cell line which account for these results? Are we observing variability in the genetic control of this multigene system?

2) That the short chain variant H chains seem so similar to the parent suggests that they are related to it by a deletion, either internal or C-terminal. Deletions of part of the gene coding for the present protein can account for both types of alterations. In addition, a C-terminal dele-

tion can be the result of a single base change which yields
a nonsense codon thus terminating the protein, or the result
of a frameshift mutation caused by the intercalation of an
acridine into the DNA. Sequence studies of the short chain
variants whould distinguish these possibilities. We can
likewise speculate on the derivation of variants which now
express the γ2a serotype. Since the peptide maps of two
γ 2a variant H chains are not identical, the possibility
that a strict translocation mechanism is responsible can be
ruled out. However, a recombinational event may well account
for these variants, or alternatively, the turning off of one
gene and turning on of a new gene in this multigene system.

3) What the relationship is between the variants in which
one gives rise to another after exposure to our culture
conditions and cloning is also curious. We are carefully
examining these newly arising variants in hopes that they
will provide us more information about the initial genetic
event.

Here, we provide evidence for structural gene mutations
in a mouse myeloma cell line. However, we puzzle over the
high incidence of variants, their effect on the Fc as contrasted to the antigen-binding-site, and the switch in
serotypes and in phenotypes. Hopefully, further observations
which can be grounded in structural correlates, will help us
to try to understand the genetic controls operating in immunoglobulin synthesis.

ACKNOWLEDGMENTS

This work was supported by funds from the National
Institutes of Health (AI 5231, AI 10702, and CA 12152), and
the National Science Foundation (GB 29560). B.K.B. was a
fellow of the New York Heart Association. J-L.P. was
supported by the French National Institutes of Health and
Medical Research (INSERM) and a National Institutes of
Health John E. Fogarty International Fellowship #1F05TW-1862.
We thank Ms. Lucille Frank and Ms. Theresa Jasek for
their expert technical assistance.

REFERENCES

1. Laskov, R., and Scharff, M.D., *J*. *Exp*. *Med*. 131, 515
   (1970).
2. Laskov, R., Lanzerotti, R., and Scharff, M.D., *J*. *Mol*.
   Biol. 56, 327 (1971).

3. Coffino, P., and Scharff, M.D., Proc. Nat. Acad. Sci. U.S.A., 68, 219 (1971).
4. Coffino, P., Baumal, R., Laskov, R., and Scharff, M.D., J. Cell Physiol. 79, 429 (1972).
5. Maizel, J.V., Jr., Methods in Virology, (K. Maramorosh and H. Koprowski, eds.) 5, 179 (1971).
6. Baumal, R., Birshtein, B.K., Coffino, P., and Scharff, M.D., Science 182, 164 (1973).
7. Preud'homme, J.-L., Buxbaum, J., and Scharff, M.D., Nature 245, 320 (1973).
8. Baumal, R., Potter, M., and Scharff, M.D., J. Exp. Med. 134, 1316 (1971).
9. Svasti, J., and Milstein, C., Biochem. J. 128, 427 (1972).
10. Harris, M., J. Cell. Physiol. 78, 177 (1971).
11. Metzger-Freed, L., Nature New Biol. 235, 245 (1972).
12. Beaudet, A.L., Roufa, D.J., and Caskey, C.T., Proc. Nat. Acad. Sci. U.S.A., 70, 320 (1973).
13. Sharp, J.D., Capecchi, N.E., and Capecchi, M.R., Proc. Nat. Acad. Sci. U.S.A., 70, 3145 (1973).
14. Chan, V.L., Whitmore, G.F., and Siminovitch, L., Proc. Nat. Acad. Sci. U.S.A., 69, 3119 (1972).
15. Thompson, L.H., Harkins, J.L., and Stanners, C.P., Proc. Nat. Acad. Sci. 70, 3094 (1972).
16. Secher, D.S., Cotton, R.G.H., and Milstein, C., FEBS Letters 37, 311 (1973).

SPONTANEOUS MUTATION IN IMMUNOGLOBULIN GENES

David S. Secher, Richard G. H. Cotton, Nicholas J. Cowan
and Cesar Milstein

MRC Laboratory of Molecular Biology
Hills Road, Cambridge, CB2 2QH, U. K.

ABSTRACT. Using a new method for screening animal cells in
tissue culture, 7,000 clones of a mouse myeloma cell line
(P3K) have been examined for the spontaneous occurrence of
variants with defects in Ig synthesis. Variants which
failed to secrete Ig were found at a high frequency. At a
lower frequency variants which secreted an Ig of altered
isoelectric point were detected. Analysis of these proteins
and of mRNA suggested that such variants arise as a result
of mutations in the structural genes coding for Ig H-chains.
This constitutes the first case in which a somatic mutation
in a structural gene has been correlated with an alteration
in amino acid sequence.

INTRODUCTION

The contribution of somatic mutation to the generation
of antibody diversity has been the basis of a number of
theories devised to explain the enormous diversity observed
(1,2,3). A knowledge of the rate and mechanisms of somatic
mutation in Ig genes is thus crucial to the evaluation of
its biological role. Yet the available data is surprisingly limited. Much higher spontaneous rates have been reported for mammalian cells in culture than for single gene
loci in prokaryotic organsism (4,5). However the loss of a
function in a mammalian somatic cell has yet to be correlated with an altered protein sequence.

METHODS

We therefore initiated a search for spontaneous
mutations in Ig structural genes. The system chosen was
the mouse myeloma cell line, P3K, which secretes a homogenous (γ_1,κ) protein (6). In order to screen large
numbers of cells for rare variants it was necessary to
develop a simple and sensitive technique for examining the
products of clones. The technique, which has been described
in detail elsewhere (7,8), involves the cloning in soft agar
of cells from an aged spinner culture and the subsequent
analysis of the secreted protein by incorporation of [14]C-

lysine and isoelectric focusing on polyacrylamide starch gels. Radioautography of the dried gels revealed a series of bands, in the pH range 6–8, characteristic of P3K Ig.

7,000 clones have now been screened and a number of variant clones detected. The most common form of spontaneous variant were those which failed to secrete Ig, or Ig-chains. This type of variation occurred at a frequency of about 10^{-4}/cell/generation. This is of the same order as the frequency of occurrence of L-chain producers in the myeloma line MPC-11 (9).

A less common variation involved an alteration in the isoelectric point of the secreted Ig. Such variants were detected at a frequency of about 10^{-5}/cell/generation and two of these (IF-1 and IF-2) have been studied in detail (10). SDS-gel electrophoresis and peptide mapping of tryptic and peptic digests of internally labelled variant proteins suggested that the alteration in isoelectric point was caused by a deletion of part of the H-chain, the C-terminal domain (C_H3) in the case of IF-1. Analysis of the carbohydrate moiety of IF-1 H-chain showed that this was also altered (11). To show that the modified carbohydrate and the apparent C-terminal deletion were the result of a defect in the Ig H-chain structural gene and not to differences in post-translational modifications of otherwise identical polypeptides, the newly synthesized, intracellular myeloma protein was examined in IF-1 and P3K cells and shown to be different (10).

As final evidence that the primary translation product in IF-1 cells differs from that in P3K, Ig mRNA was partially purified and examined using techniques in use in our laboratory for purification (12) and translation in a cell-free system (13,14) of Ig mRNAs. This showed a difference between IF-1 and P3K mRNAs coding for H-chain (10) and thus the mutation in IF-1 is expressed at the level of mRNA.

In the case of IF-2, fingerprinting evidence showed on internal deletion of about 100 residues encompassing approximately the C_H1 domain. A striking resemblence to certain H-chain disease proteins was noted and the involvement of residue 216 (Eu numbering) was also suggested (10).

DISCUSSION

The observation of large deletions in this study and also, after mutagenesis, in that of Birshtein et al. (this symposium) remains a puzzle. Our screening system is capable of detecting single charge changes and yet no such

simple substitutions have been detected. We hope that
further characterization of these and other spontaneous
mutants will provide an insight into the nature of somatic
mutation in Ig genes.

ACKNOWLEDGMENT

D.S.S. is a Fellow of the Salters' Company, London.

REFERENCES

1. Milstein, C. and Pink, J. R. L., Progr. Biophys. Molec.
   Biol. 21, 209 (1970).
2. Cohn, M., Ann. N. Y. Acad. Sci. 190, 529 (1971).
3. Jerne, N. K., Europ. J. Immunol. 1, 1 (1971).
4. Breslow, R. E. and Goldsby, R. A., Exp. Cell. Res. 55,
   339 (1969).
5. Lieberman, I. and Ove, P., Proc. Nat. Acad. Sci. U. S.
   45, 872 (1959).
6. Horibata, K. and Harris, A. W., Exp. Cell Res. 60, 61
   (1970).
7. Cotton, R. G. H., Secher, D. S. and Milstein, C., Europ.
   J. Immunol. 3, 135 (1973).
8. Milstein, C., Cotton, R. G. H. and Secher, D. S., Ann.
   Immunol. (Inst. Pasteur) 125C, 287 (1974).
9. Coffino, P. and Scharff, M. D., Proc. Nat. Acad. Sci.
   U. S. 68, 219 (1971).
10. Secher, D. S., Cotton, R. G. H. and Milstein, C. FEBS
    Lett. 37, 311 (1973).
11. Cowan, N. J., Secher, D. S., Cotton, R. G. H. and
    Milstein, C., FEBS Lett. 30, 343 (1973).
12. Brownlee, G. G., Cartwright, E. M., Cowan, N. J.,
    Jarvis, J. M. and Milstein, C. Nature New Biol. 244,
    236 (1973).
13. Brownlee, G. G., Harrison, T. M., Matthews, M. B. and
    C. Milstein. FEBS Lett. 23, 244 (1972).
14. Cowan, N. J. and Milstein, C., Eur. J. Biochem. 36, 1
    (1973).

BIOGRAPHY OF THE B CELL

Norman R. Klinman, Joan L. Press, Allan R. Pickard,
Robert T. Woodland and A. Faye Dewey

Department of Pathology,
Medical School
University of Pennsylvania
Philadelphia, Pennsylvania 19174

ABSTRACT. The in vitro stimulation of isolated B cells in fragment
cultures has permitted the analysis of splenic B cells obtained from
neonates and immune or non-immune adults with respect to several
characteristics including a) specificity and hapten inhibitability of
stimulation, b) dependence of stimulation on antigen concentration
and carrier recognition, c) burst size and longevity of clones derived
from stimulated cells, and d) immunoglobulin class and affinity of the
antibody produced by such clones. The results indicate that there exist
at least three types of B cells one of which predominates in spleens of
neonates (neonatal B cells), a second which predominates in spleens of
non-immune adults (primary B cells) and a third predominating in
spleens of immune mice (secondary B cells).

INTRODUCTION

Methodology is currently available which should enable a comprehensive analysis of antibody forming precursor cell populations
(B cells). Perhaps the most fruitful approach to this analysis has been
the study of the clonal progeny of isolated B cells antigenically stimulated in vivo or in vitro (1-8). Utilizing the latter technique it has recently been possible to characterize and enumerate B cells specific for
several defined antigenic determinants (5,9). In the course of these
studies, it has been noted that B cells have markedly different characteristics depending on the stage of development or antigenic history of
the donor animal (5,9,10,11). The majority of B cells derived from
neonatal and non-immune adult mice differ from one another and from
those derived from immune adult mice in properties which include the
specificity and hapten inhibitability of antigenic stimulation (5,12),
the dependence of stimulation on carrier recognition (5,10), the burst
size and longevity of clones derived from stimulated cells (5,11,13),
and the immunoglobulin class and affinity of antibody derived from
such clones (5,14). These differences indicate that the life history of

the B cell population of an individual includes at least three distinguishable cell types. This finding may have important implications for the function of the immune response and should therefore be considered in any analysis of the stimulation or specificity of humoral responses.

METHODS

1.) Animals and Immunization.

Balb/c mice were used at 8 weeks of age. Mice were immunized by injection of 0.1 mg of antigen emulsified in complete Freund's adjuvant intraperitoneally. Recipient mice were immunized with hemocyanin 4 to 8 weeks prior to use.

2.) In Vitro cloning and radioimmunoassay.

The methods used for obtaining splenic foci in vitro and the radioimmunoassay used to detect antibody produced by positive foci were carried out as previously described (4,5).

3.) Detection of antibody producing cells.

Antibody forming cells within fragment cultures were enumerated as plaque forming cells using a modification of the techniques described by Mishell and Dutton (15). TNP coupled sheep erythrocytes prepared by the method of Rittenberg and Pratt (16) served as the target cells. The methodology utilized to analyze fragment cultures for plaque forming cells is described in detail elsewhere (17).

4.) Antigen Binding Cells.

Antigen binding cells were enumerated by methods described previously by Davie, et al (18,19).

5.) Characterization of Antibody.

The affinity of antibody produced by fragment cultures was measured by equilibrium dialysis utilizing a method previously described (1,3). The immunoglobulin class of antibody produced by fragment cultures was analyzed utilizing mono-specific anti-heavy chain antibody (14,20).

RESULTS AND DISCUSSION

Table I summarizes the results obtained when B cell populations derived from neonatal, non-immune adult, and immune adult Balb/c mice are compared. The comparative parameters of clonal precursor cells have been categorized as either characteristics of and requisites for B cell stimulation; or as the qualitative and quantitative properties of the clones derived from such stimulated B cells.

It has been shown previously that the antigen dose dependence of stimulation is similar for B cells derived from the three donor sources (5,9,11). For several other parameters, however, there are striking differences in precursor cells derived from immune mice as compared to precursor cells from neonatal and non-immune adult mice. In the absence of a mechanism for carrier recognition, which is presumably mediated by T cells, only B cells which have been derived from immune mice have the capacity to be stimulated by soluble hapten protein complexes (5,10,21). Although the efficiency of stimulation of these cells is low, this nonetheless constitutes an absolute difference in the stimulation of clonal precursor cells derived from immune mice, compared to neonatal and non-immune adult precursor cell stimulation.

In addition to being stimulated in the absence of carrier recognition, B cells obtained from the spleens of immune mice differ from those of neonatal or non-immune adult donors in the sensitivity of stimulation to hapten inhibition. While the stimulation of B cells from immune mice is poorly inhibited by free hapten (5), the majority of B cells from non-immune adult and neonatal donors are readily inhibited by free hapten concentrations only slightly higher than the hapten concentration presented on the immunogen (5).

In terms of antigen dose dependence and hapten inhibition of stimulation, there is no significant difference between B cells obtained from neonatal or non-immune adult mice (9,11). It is noteworthy, however, that 20 to 40% of neonatal and non-immune adult splenic B cells are not readily inhibited by free hapten. This finding may imply that this is an intrinsic property of a subpopulation of non-immune B cells in general, which is perhaps the result of specificity directed against determinants other than the hapten alone. The finding that stimulation of cells derived from immune mice was inhibited

TABLE I

Comparative Properties of B Cells in Spleens of Immune, Non-Immune and Neonatal Balb/c Mice

Source of donor spleen cells	Frequency of DNP Specific B Cell		Parameters of Stimulation[1]				Clonal Properties						
							cells			antibody			
	Per total lymphoid cells	Per immunoglobulin bearing cells (B cells)	Cloning effic.	Overlap stim. by TNP	Inhib. of stim. by 5×10^6 M DNP lysine	Stim. without T cells or carrier rec.	Burst size (cell divisions)	Max.av. ab.Prod. day (ηg)	in vitro half life (days)	Mean Ko 7°C	μ only	γ_1 only	$\mu + \gamma_1$
non-immune 8-12 wk old Balb/c male	$1/10-12 \times 10^3$	$1/5-6 \times 10^3$	3-4%	<5%	60-80%	<1%	-	3	12-14	2.8×10^6	16%	42%	16%
Balb/c male immunized with DNP-Hy	$1/3-4 \times 10^3$	$1/1.5-2 \times 10^3$	3-4%	30-40%	20-30%	10-15%	8-10	8	20-30	14.3×10^6	<5%	68%	14%
Neonatal Balb/c 0-5 days after birth	$1/12-14 \times 10^3$	$1/3-4 \times 10^3$	-	<10%	60-80%	<2%	-	1.5	7-9	-	50-70%	-	-

1) All stimulation at 5×10^{-7} M DNP-Hy or TNP-Hy.

360

poorly by hapten has been interpreted as indicating that receptors of secondary cells may be functionally multivalent while those of primary cells may be functionally monovalent (5). This difference may also be reflected in the fact that the affinity of antibody produced by clones derived from non-immune B cells shows a much stricter antigen dose dependence than the affinity of antibody produced by clones derived from immune B cells (5). It was therefore reasoned that the multivalence of the receptors of cells derived from immune donors should make such receptors more avid, thus stimulation should be less affinity dependent. This diminished affinity dependence was verified by an analysis of the specificity of stimulation of B cells derived from immune and non-immune donors. It was found that the B cells derived from non-immune mice that responded to TNP were essentially distinct from those which responded to DNP in that the stimulation with both antigens together yielded a number of clones equivalent to the sum of clones produced by stimulation with either antigen alone (12). Thus, in this regard, there was little overlap stimulation of non-immune B cells by determinants highly cross-reactive at the level of humoral antibody. In contrast, TNP-Hy apparently stimulated 30-40 percent of the DNP specific precursor cells derived from clones previously immunized with DNP since the stimulation with both antigens together was not additive. This diminution of immune B cell stimulation specificity is consistent with recent findings of Cramer and Braun (22), who showed that B cells from non-immune mice specific for streptococcal group A antigen could not be stimulated by group A variant antigen. However, B cells of the same clone could be stimulated by group A variant antigen if the cells were derived from mice previously immunized to the group A antigen. The specificity of stimulation of B cells derived from neonatal mice is analogous to that of B cells derived from non-immune adult donors in the lack of overlap stimulation of the same B cells by DNP and TNP. These results are consistent with the notion that the stimulation of B cells derived from non-immune mice is exquisitely specific. This is verified by the finding that within the B cell population of neonatal mice the cells stimulated by DNP and TNP consist of small definable sets which can be identified by iso-electric focusing and appear to be distinct from one another (23).

While B cells derived from neonates and non-immune adults appear similar to one another in the characteristics of their stimulation, and while both differ markedly from B cells derived from immune mice, analysis of the characteristics of the clones derived from these cells clearly distinguished them. An analysis of the maximum average amount of antibody produced per day indicates that clones derived from spleen cells of immune mice release a maximum average of 8 nanograms of antibody per day, while those derived from B cells of non-immune donors release a maximum average of 3 nanograms a day and those from neonates 1.5 nanograms per day (5,11). Analysis of the plaque forming cells within fragments containing a stimulated clone indicate that stimulated B cells from immune mice undergo at least 8 to 10 divisions (13). If the rate of antibody production is similar for cells derived from non-immune and neonatal animals, then these differences in daily antibody production reflect a variation in the average proliferative ability of stimulated non-immune, neonatal and immune B cells. Estimates of proliferative ability suggest non-immune B cells undergo 6 to 8 divisions after stimulation while those derived from neonatal mice undergo only 4 to 6 divisions. Conversely an equivalence in average proliferative ability would suggest discrepancies in the rate of production of antibody by the progeny of these precursor cells. So that, while the progeny of immune B cells produce an average maximum of 20×10^3 antibody molecules per second per cell, the progeny of B cells derived from non-immune or neonatal mice may have a lower rate of production (13). In addition, the clones derived from cells of immune donors continue to produce antibody in culture up to two months after stimulation, while those derived from non-immune mice usually cease antibody production within one month and those derived from neonatal mice rarely produce detectable antibody for more than 21 days after stimulation (4,5,11).

These differences noted in the character of cell clones derived from B cells of non-immune, immune and neonatal donors are also reflected in differences in the quality of the antibody they produce. Clones derived from spleen cells of immune donors produce antibody with an average association constant approximately 5 fold higher than that of cells derived from non-immune donors, although it should be noted that the range of affinities of antibodies derived from the latter span much of the affinity range of the precursor cells derived from immune mice (5). 82% of the clones derived from immune donor B cells yield antibody of the γ_1 heavy chain class, while 16% of these clones also produce antibody of the μ heavy chain class (14). Few, if any, clones derived from spleens of immune mice produce only IgM antibody. 58% of the clones derived from non-immune donor B cells produce antibody of the γ_1 heavy chain class and again 16% of the clones make both IgG 1 and IgM antibodies. Significantly, 16% of the clones derived from non-immune B cell populations produce anti-body solely of the IgM class (14). It is striking that a majority of the clones derived from neonatal spleen cells give rise to clones produc-ing only IgM antibody.

These findings clearly delineate the majority of B cells derived from immune donors from those of non-immune donors, and to a lesser extent differentiate the majority of B cells in neonatal spleens from the majority of B cells in spleens of non-immune adults. Thus three general categories of B cells can now be described. In neonates, a cell predominates (neonatal B cell) which has stimulatory character-istics much like the B cells predominating in non-immune adults (primary B cells). However, the neonatal precursor cell gives rise to progeny which produce antibody for a short duration and which is mainly of the μ heavy chain class. Progeny of primary B cells produce antibody for a longer duration than that of neonatal clones, and the antibody is predominantly of the γ_1 but also of the μ heavy chain class. The third category of B cells is the cell which predominates in immune mice (secondary B cell). The secondary B cell differs from the neo-natal and primary B cell in that its stimulation can occur in the ab-sence of carrier recognition; its stimulation is resistant to inhibition by free hapten; and its stimulation manifests less specificity than the stimulation of primary B cells. Clones derived from secondary B cells produced the greatest amount of antibody for the longest time, and the antibody is of high affinity and almost never solely IgM.

Cells of the neonatal type appear to predominate well into the third week of life and are gradually replaced by primary type B cells. Primary B cells appear to predominate thereafter, unless contact is made with antigen. Subsequent to antigen stimulation primary type B cells appear to be diminished with kinetics reflecting the appearance of plaque forming cells (24). Precursor cells (presumably of the secondary type), are generated much more slowly and reach a maxi-mum level at 2 to 3 weeks, persisting at or near this level for several months (24).

By comparing the increment in antigen binding cells with the increment in precursor cell frequency several months after immuni-zation, it has been possible to measure the cloning efficiency and hence the absolute precursor frequency. These data are presented in the first three columns of Table I (25). Assuming that the increment in antigen binding cells long after immunization is due to an increase in specific B cells, then the efficiency of the cloning procedure is three to four percent for secondary cells. Thus, the absolute frequency of DNP specific B cells in spleens of Balb/c mice 3 to 4 months post immunization is $1/3 - 4 \times 10^3$ or $1/1.5 - 2 \times 10^3$ immunoglobulin bearing cells (B cells) (25). If this efficiency also holds for primary and neonatal B cells [whose homing to the spleen are quite similar (11)], then the frequency of DNP specific B cells in the spleens of non-immune adult Balb/c mice is $1/10 - 12 \times 10^3$ cells or $1/5 - 6 \times 10^3$ B cells and $1/3 - 4 \times 10^3$ B cells in a neonate at day two of life. These frequencies are quite similar to those obtained for TNP specific precursors. It is of interest to note that using standard procedures for detecting antigen binding cells, less than 10% of cells with the capacity to bind DNP in a non-immune spleen are actually DNP specific clonal precursor cells (25), verifying the notion that antigen binding may be a necessary but not a sufficient condition for antigenic stimulation (5,9,26).

The fact that the predominant cell populations change so markedly in the course of postnatal development and following immunization must be taken into consideration when analyzing phenomenology involved with antigenic stimulation and tolerance. For example, it is conceivable that neonatal type B cells are particularly susceptible to tolerance induction which would explain the often noted ease of tolerance induction in neonates (27). In addition, the relative ease of stimulation of secondary precursor cells may clearly be responsible for phenomena such as "original antigenic sin" and tolerance breakdown with related antigenic determinants. Thus, primary contact with an antigenic determinant, even in an animal tolerant to a closely related determinant, would yield a population of secondary precursor cells which could then be stimulated by a closely related determinant (even in the absence of carrier recognition) and thus yield antibody with greater affinity for the original immunogen (12).

The finding that these three types of clonal precursor cells differ so markedly in their characteristics and develop, at least in the case of secondary B cells, with kinetics completely distinct from those of the generation of plaque forming cells after stimulation, may indicate that the neonatal and primary cell types are not true progenitors of secondary B cells. Indeed it is conceivable that each cell type is derived independently from a common progenitor and share with each other only the same set of antibody specificities.

REFERENCES

1. N.R. Klinman, Immunochemistry 6:757, (1969).
2. M. Bosma and E. Weiler, J. Immunol. 104:203, (1970).
3. N.R. Klinman, J. Expt. Med. 133:963 (1971).
4. N.R. Klinman and G. Aschinazi, J. Immunol. 106:1338, (1971).
5. N.R. Klinman, J. Expt. Med. 135:241, (1972).
6. B.A. Askonas, A.R. Williamson and B.E.G. Wright, Proc. Nat. Acad. Sci. (U.S.A.), 67:1398, (1970).
7. H.W. Kreth and A.R. Williamson, Eur. J. Immunol. 3:141 (1973).
8. I. Lefkovits, Eur. J. Immunol. 2:360, (1972).
9. J.L. Press and N.R. Klinman, Eur. J. Immunol.(in Press)(1974).
10. R.A. Doughty and N.R. Klinman, J. Immunol. 111:1140 (1973).
11. J.L. Press and N.R. Klinman, J. Immunol. 111:829 (1973).
12. N.R. Klinman, J.L. Press and G.P. Segal, J. Expt. Med. 138:1276, (1973).
13. R.T. Woodland, Fed. Proc. 33:807 (Abst.), (1974).
14. J.L. Press and N.R. Klinman, J. Expt. Med. 138:300 (1973).
15. R.I. Mishell and R.W. Dutton, J. Expt. Med. 126:423, (1967).
16. M.B. Rittenberg and K.L. Pratt, Proc. Soc. Expt. Biol. Med. 132:575, (1969).
17. R.T. Woodland, Doctoral Dissertation Univ. of Pennsylvania (1974).
18. J.M. Davie and W.E. Paul, J. Expt. Med. 134:495, (1971).
19. J.M. Davie, A.S. Rosenthal and W.E. Paul, J. Expt. Med. 134:495, (1971).
20. J.L. Press and N.R. Klinman, Immunochemistry 10:621 (1973).
21. N.R. Klinman and R.A. Doughty, J. Expt. Med. 138:473 (1973).
22. M. Cramer and D.G. Braun, J. Expt. Med. 138:1533 (1973).
23. N.R. Klinman and J.L. Press, Federation Proceedings (in Press) (1974).
24. A.R. Pickard, A. F. Dewey, R.T. Woodland and N.R. Klinman, Manuscript in preparation (1974).
25. A.R. Pickard and N.R. Klinman, Manuscript in preparation (1974).
26. C.J. Elson, J. Singh and R.B. Taylor, Scand. J. Immunol. 2:143 (1973).
27. W.O. Weigle, Adv. in Immunol. 16:61 (1973).

THE GENERATION OF DIVERSITY WITHIN SINGLE CLONES

OF ANTIBODY-FORMING CELLS

A.J. Cunningham and Linda M. Pilarski

Department of Microbiology
The John Curtin School of Medical Research
Canberra, Australia.

ABSTRACT. This paper proposes that most antibody diversity arises by rapid production of variants within clones of antibody-forming cells after antigenic or mitogenic stimulation. Evidence for this comes from cloning experiments in vivo and in vitro, including micromanipulative work where single antibody-forming cells were cultured for 2 days and their progeny shown to be heterogeneous for antibody specificity in some cases.

INTRODUCTION

The most remarkable thing about antibody is its diversity : an animal seems to have the ability to produce antibodies against an almost infinite range of antigens. This leads to a familiar paradox. How can the limited DNA of the antibody loci provide such unlimited adaptability? Somatic mutation theories (1) deal with this problem by assuming that as the lymphoid system develops, there is a vast amount of spontaneous mutation in antibody V-genes. All current theories assume that by the time an animal reaches adulthood, it has its full complement of antibody specificities, present as receptors on competent cells.

There is another possibility which seems to make more sense teleologically. It is one which has often been mentioned, but rarely taken seriously. The animal may produce relatively few receptor specificities spontaneously, and then, when one of these is stimulated by antigen, rapidly generate within the clone a family of related but random variant specificities, from which antigen "selects" those which fit best. Fig. 1 shows the essentials. This idea cuts across several of today's cherished beliefs :

367

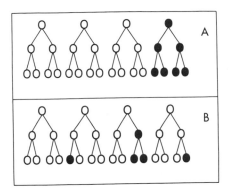

Fig.1. Clonal development of antibody-forming cells of different specificities. The blank circles represent a relatively rare variant. According to conventional views (A), all different types of B cell are present before antigen stimulation, and no significant variation occurs during expansion of a clone. By contrast the "antigen-generated diversity" theory (B) proposes that new variants arise with high frequency within clones most of whose members are releasing a different antibody specificity.

absolute clonal stability (based mainly on the homogeneity of myeloma proteins); the feeling that variation in the relevant DNA could not happen fast enough (because other genes in bacteria and higher animals are relatively stable); and the concept that self-tolerance is established by a purging of self-reactive clones early in ontogeny, after which the repertoire of immunocompetent cells is set for life (2). This last argument is the most important, since if variants are being randomly produced, some of them must have anti-self activity. It is weakened however by newer ideas on possible mechanisms of tolerance (which may also apply to self-tolerance) such as enhancing antibody, suppressor T cells, and the 'one-hit tolerance' model of Bretscher and Cohn (3). Self-reactive variants would certainly appear as variants within immunocyte clones, but it no longer seems impossible that these might be inactivated as they arise.

The concept that "antigen generates diversity" has been fully discussed elsewhere (4) along with the extensive but indirect evidence in the literature which supports it. Several points must be made here. First, it is a theory at the level of phenotype rather than genotype : it predicts high-rate clonal variation but does not say whether this occurs by mutation or switching from one gene to another (we prefer the former). Second, as our experiments will show, variation is stimulated by mitogen as well as by antigen, although in this case there is presumably less selection of higher affinity variants. Third, the receptors on immunocytes present before antigen may have low individual affinity for a random antigen, but multipoint binding may raise the avidity of the bond between cell and antigen to a level sufficient to stimulate the cell. Finally it is important to point out that some considerable diversity must exist before deliberate antigenic stimulation, since the emerging immune system is faced with a great variety of self antigens which will tolerise some cells but must leave others. "Priming" of the immune system by self antigens along the lines suggested by Jerne (5) seems feasible to us.

There are two main predictions of the theory that antigen generates diversity. The first is that during an immune response, entirely new antibody specificities should appear. We have presented some evidence for this elsewhere (6). The second prediction, that variants are generated within single clones, is the subject of this paper. We will outline four experimental tests of this proposition.

METHODS

These will be described briefly, since details have been given elsewhere (6, 7).

CBA mice were used throughout this work, lethally irradiated (850r) animals acting as "recipients" for in vivo experiments, and the spleen cells from animals over 8 weeks old being cultured for the in vitro experiments. The antigens used were heterologous erythrocytes. Sheep red cells were obtained from six merinos. Red cells (rbc) from goat, cow, pig and horse were needed in some experiments (see below).

Limit dilution cultures.

The polyacrylamide "rafts" of Marbrook and Haskill (8) were used. These allowed separate microcultures of 36 pellets of cells in one dish. Numbers of spleen cells could be adjusted so that only a proportion of wells was positive. This level was reached with around 10^4 spleen cells per well. The medium outside the raft was 8 ml of Eagles minimal essential, with 10% foetal calf serum added and $10^{-5}M$ 2-mercaptoethanol, plus sufficient bicarbonate to ensure a pH of 7.3 in an atmosphere containing 10% CO_2. The 2 ml of medium inside the raft was the same except that it also contained HEPES buffer at 2 x $10^{-3}M$ and lipopolysaccharide from E. coli (0128:B12) at a final concentration of 7 - 10 μgm/ml.

Cultures were incubated for 1 - 4 days at 37°C. Wells were harvested by sucking out the cells with a fine pipette, dispensing this medium as a drop on a piece of "Parafilm", and mixing complement and rbc in suitable amounts before directly transferring the mixture to a slide chamber for a haemolytic plaque assay (9).

Single-cell cultures

Mass cultures of CBA spleen cells (10^7/raft) were cultured for 1 day, after which they contained about 100 plaque-forming cells (PFC) when assayed against sheep rbc. These PFC were identified by incubating the spleen cells with complement in a lawn of rbc in small drops under oil, and individual active cells were micromanipulated out, as described elsewhere (10). This manipulation was done under sterile conditions in medium 199 containing HEPES buffer and foetal calf serum. Such PFC were then pipetted (observed at X40) into empty wells in new rafts, or into wells containing about 1000 sheep rbc and 100 heavily irradiated (5000r) syngeneic spleen cells from normal animals. Cultures were incubated for 2 days after which the progeny of the initial PFC were removed (often they formed a small ball of from 2 - 12 cells), separated by sucking up and down in a micropipette or by mild trypsin treatment, and reassayed for their plaque-forming abilities (7).

Detecting small differences in specificity of antibody released by different individual cells in a clone

The specificity of antibody from single cells was characterised by its cross-reactivity, using a modified version of the haemolytic plaque technique (9). Briefly, it involves testing antibody plaque-forming cells (PFC) not against a single type of rbc, but on a mixture of two types. These may be from different species, (11, 12), or alternatively, one may use erythrocytes from two different individual sheep. Plaques can be classified as clear (both red cells lysed), partial (only one lysed) or "sombreros" (13) with different degrees of lysis of both indicators (fig. 2). Plaque morphology depends on specificity of antibody and not simply on the amount, since the morphology is faithfully maintained as the plaque grows in size with incubation. There are also

371

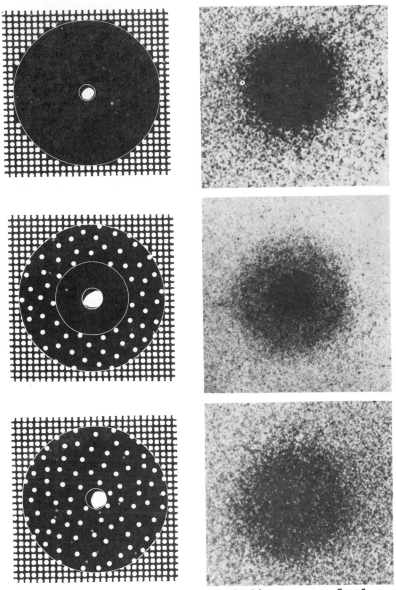

Fig.2. Photographs and diagrams of clear, "sombrero" and partial plaques each produced by a single cell in a mixed monolayer containing erythrocytes from two different sheep. In the diagrams, squares and circles represent the different erythrocyte types. Magnification is dark-field, so areas of complete lysis appear black, and of partial lysis, grey. The actual diameter of the plaques was about 0.6 mm.

good reasons for believing that differences in cross-reactivity reflect differences in V-region structure of the antibody released, and not variation in other properties of the molecule, such as class. In our experiments plaques were always direct, produced early in a response (1 - 3 days) and obtained from cultures stimulated with bacterial lipopolysaccharide (7), all conditions which favour IgM over other classes. Differences in C region which might, for example, affect complement-fixing ability, would be expected to influence all specificities equally. We have also shown by direct experiment that the proportion of clear and partial plaques on mixed monolayers is independent of the complement concentration over a wide range (unpublished).

There is another apparently possible interpretation of the difference between clear and partial plaques : the partials might be caused by a single type of antibody, and the clears by 2 antibodies, each able to lyse only one of the erythrocyte types. A sombrero would form around a cell which produced 2 antibodies in different amounts. We have not disproved this, although it would not affect our **main** argument which is simply that different antibody specificities may be made by different members of the same clone. However it can be shown to be very unlikely by the following line of reasoning. If a sombrero plaque is a "double-producer", so also is a clear, the difference being that a clear plaque is made by 2 different antibodies in similar amounts. Clear plaques can also be seen on mixtures of erythrocytes from 6 different sheep (unpublished), a kind of indicator layer on which different antibody-forming cells score as anywhere from very faint partials to completely clear (i.e. it appears that individual cells may lyse from 1 or 2 of the erythrocytes to all 6). If lysis of 2 rbc necessarily implies 2 antibodies, then lysis of 6 implies 6. This could be extended to any number of indicators, which points up the logical absurdity of claims that lysis of more than one erythrocyte type means more than one antibody.

RESULTS

This section describes 4 different experimental tests of the prediction that single clones may contain cells producing different antibodies.

Test 1. When spleen cell suspensions are cultured in vitro at limiting dilutions, antibody-forming cells of different specificities should often occur together.

The polyacrylamide raft method of Marbrook and Haskill (8) is a simple way of doing limit dilution cultures. When about 10^4 mouse spleen cells are cultured in each well of these rafts, most of the wells contain no PFC at all against sheep rbc, while a proportion have from 1 to about 30 plaques (most commonly 1 - 10). There are several reasons for believing that all the PFC in each positive well belong to the same clone i.e. come from one initial B cell (with the proviso that a certain chance association of two or more precursor cells is expected, and can be calculated from the Poisson distribution):

(1) There is a linear one-hit dose/response relationship between the frequency of positive wells (corrected for overlap) and the number of cells cultured. This implies that only one cell type is limiting.

(2) Cells are grown in the presence of E. coli lipopolysaccharide, which is thought to stimulate B cells directly (14). So it is probably the presence or absence of a B cell of anti-sheep specificity which determines whether or not plaques develop in a well.

(3) Spleen cells of nude mice respond as well as spleen cells from normal CBA mice. This fact, and point (2) above, make it very unlikely that it is T cells which are limiting in the wells, with B cells present in excess.

If the PFC in a raft are assayed not on rbc from a single sheep but on a mixture of rbc from two different sheep (see Methods), then it is

easy to distinguish two specificity "types" :
those PFC which lyse both rbc, giving clear
plaques, and those which lyse only one, producing
partial plaques (fig. 2). According to conventional ideas, all members of a clone should
release the same antibody, so all should make
either clear or partial plaques. Single wells
containing both types are expected only at low
frequency, due to chance association of two precursors. We tested this on several different rbc
mixtures, and consistently found a higher association than chance would dictate. Examples are
given in fig. 3 and table 1. Table 1 also shows
experiments to control for non-random distribution of precursors. Here, half the contents of
each well were assayed separately on each of two
very dissimilar rbc, sheep and horse, demonstrating that there was no significant tendency for
quite different antibody specificities to occur
together. That is, anti-horse and anti-sheep
plaques did not appear together with significant
frequency, while clear and partial plaques on a
micture of 2 sheep rbc did.

The simplest explanation for the association
of PFC with different (although related) specificities is that both kinds of PFC come from the
same initial precursor. The control experiments
also seem to show that variations within a clone,
while presumably random, produce small rather
than large changes in antibody specificity. This
suggests mutation rather than a switch from one
pre-existing gene to another as the mechanism of
variation.

Test 2. Cells producing antibodies of rare specificities will make smaller sub-clones than cells
producing common specificities.

According to conventional ideas, all types
of precursor cell exist before stimulation. That
is, cells whose progeny will make antibody with,
for example, very high affinity, or unusual cross-
reactivity, are present in the animal before it
is stimulated with antigen or mitogen, although
in relatively small numbers. Stimulation with
mitogen in vitro should induce these cells to
form clones of the same average size as clones
releasing common specificities (see fig. 1). By

375

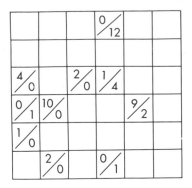

Fig.3. Plaque assays on the 36 wells of a raft containing 4 x 10⁵ mouse spleen cells which was cultured for three days. The contents of each well was assayed on a mixture of erythrocytes from two different sheep : numbers of plaques showing partial lysis are recorded above the diagonal line, and numbers of clear plaques below the line.

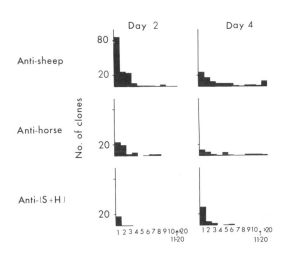

Fig.4. The frequency of clones of different sizes. Several experiments have been pooled to compare the size ranges of similar numbers of clones with anti-sheep, anti-horse, and anti-(sheep + horse) specificities. PFC with the highly cross-reactive specificity occur in relatively small aggregates.

TABLE 1

REPRESENTATIVE EXPERIMENTS SHOWING A SIGNIFICANT
TENDENCY FOR RELATED ANTIBODY SPECIFICITIES TO
OCCUR TOGETHER IN THE SAME CULTURE WELL, WHILE
UNRELATED SPECIFICITIES DID NOT ASSOCIATE (see
text).

Test A: Association of clear and partial plaques
when each well was tested on a mixed monolayer of
sheep "1" plus sheep "2" (a total of 31 experiments of this kind were done).

	Expt 1	Expt 2
Total number of wells assayed	180	216
Total number of wells containing partial plaques	44	45
Total number of wells containing clear plaques	10	24
Total number of wells containing both kinds of plaques	9	13
χ^2	25	18.2
p	<0.001	<0.001

Test B: Lack of association of anti-sheep and
anti-horse plaques when each well was tested separately on each type of erythrocyte.

	Expt 1	Expt 2
Total number of wells assayed	143	284
Total number of wells containing anti-sheep PFC	92	68
Total number of wells containing anti-horse PFC	63	23
Total number of wells containing both	44	5
χ^2	1.49	0.59
p	<0.3	<0.5

contrast, our theory predicts that there are relatively few types of B cell present before stimulation and that the cells producing less common antibody types arise within clones producing other
specificities. The average number of PFC releas-
sing "rare" antibodies within single wells should
therefore be relatively small.

An example may make this clearer. Antibodies which can lyse sheep rbc must include a
great variety of different V-region structures.
Antibodies which can lyse both sheep and horse
rbc are a subgroup of the former, and must
obviously be much less heterogeneous. PFC producing clear plaques on mixed monolayers of sheep
and horse rbc are much less frequently found than
cells which lyse sheep rbc alone. However, conventional theory predicts that ("sheep + horse")
B cells exist before stimulation, and that clones
of this specificity should reach the same average
size as clones active against sheep alone. Our
model, on the other hand, says that cells making
anti-(sheep + horse) come from progenitors making
different antibodies, although once generated,
they should have an equal chance of being stimulated to proliferate by LPS. Because these unusually cross-reactive PFC arise only during the
course of the culture period, they have less time
to proliferate, and should occur in smaller groups
than the "anti-sheep" or "anti-horse" PFC.

Figure 4 confirms our prediction. A similar result was obtained for another unusually
cross-reactive specificity, (sheep + pig). These
results fit with earlier studies (6) where it was
found that cells producing anti-(sheep + horse) or
anti-(sheep + pig) were often entirely absent from
the spleens of mice injected two days earlier with
Srbc, but were always present at the peak of the
response.

Test 3. A single antibody-forming cell may divide
to give daughter cells producing antibody of different specificities.

Single PFC were isolated, by micromanipula-
tion, from among populations of spleen cells which
had been cultured for one day. These were transferred to different wells in a new polyacrylamide
raft, and cultured for two more days, when they

378

grew into small clones of 1 - 12 cells (most commonly 2 or 4). The progeny were now tested for plaque-forming ability on a mixture of rbc from two different sheep.

93 of 911 transferred cells produced two or more plaque-forming daughter cells (table 2). In most cases, all such progeny made plaques of identical morphology (apart from small differences in size) on the mixed indicator layer, all being partial, or all clear, or all sombreros with apparently identical relative areas of partial and total lysis (figs. 2 and 5). This would appear to act as a good control for the validity of plaque morphology as a marker of antibody specificity : the nature of the plaques seems not to be affected by possible damage during handling, for example. By contrast with the majority of clones, which were homogeneous, in 10 of the 93 there were striking differences in plaque morphology. The diagram (fig. 5) has been drawn from measurements made on members of two clones which were classified as showing variation, and on one representative homogeneous clone.

Test 4. Single clones cultured in vivo may also contain variants.

This work, which is still in progress, will be described only briefly, mainly to show that clonal variation is not an in vitro artefact. The cloning procedure has been described elsewhere (11) : the spleens of lethally irradiated mice which have received limiting numbers (about 10^6) of syngeneic spleen cells and sheep rbc 5 - 8 days earlier are cut transversely into 8 pieces, and each piece is separately assayed for PFC. Large numbers of plaques appear localised in particular areas (fig. 6), against a background of smaller numbers of PFC in other segments. It was shown earlier (11), that these "colonies" of PFC tend to be more homogeneous in their specificity than PFC taken from a pool of spleens containing many colonies. For example, when a colony is tested against sheep and goat rbc mixtures, in most (not all) cases, all of the plaques are clear or all are partial apart from a small proportion of "background" plaques. This is presumptive evidence that all PFC in such a colony belong to one

TABLE 2

CULTURES OF SINGLE PFC

Protocol	No. of transferred cells	Variation within clone	No. of cases where x daughter PFC developed from the transferred cell										
			x = 0	1	2	3	4	5	6	8	10	11	>11
A^+	340	No variation	248	51	18	5	5	1	1	1	0	0	5*
		Variation	–	–	2	2	1	–	–	–	–	–	–
B^+	571	No variation	437	82	30	9	2	2	3	0	1	0	0
		Variation	–	–	4	–	–	–	–	–	–	1**	–

* In all of these cases there were 1 or 2 large plaques and a large number (up to 60) tiny plaque-like areas with no central white cell, which were possibly caused by fragments of cytoplasm shed from antibody-containing cells.

** This clone came from 2 tightly joined cells which were cultured together.

\+ In series B, the PFC was isolated completely before transfer. In A, a small number (approx 50) random non PFC were transferred with the PFC.

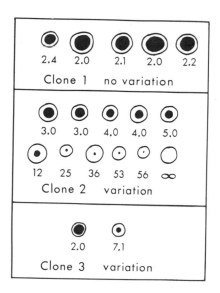

Fig.5. Scale drawing from measurements made on plaques produced by cells in two clones which developed from a single cell (top and bottom), and one which grew from a pair of tightly adherent cells (middle). The plaques were demonstrated on a mixture of erythrocytes from two different sheep. In each case the central black area represents complete lysis of both erythrocytes, while the outer circle is the boundary of partial lysis (see also fig.2). The number under each plaque is the ratio

$$\frac{\text{Area bounded by outside circle}}{\text{Area of total lysis (inner circle)}}$$

The top clone shows the usual picture, all plaques looking almost identical. The lower two are examples where variation occurred within a clone. In the middle case, the two adherent cells initially cultured were probably daughter cells, but even if they were not, there appear to be more than two specificity types among their progeny.

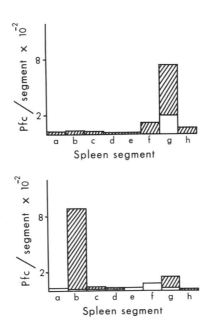

Fig.6. Numbers of PFC in the eight segments of a spleen of 2 irradiated mice into each of which 10⁶ syngeneic spleen cells and sheep erythrocyte antigen had been injected 7 days earlier. The plaque assay was done on a mixture of erythrocytes from two sheep, and the hatched and clear areas represent numbers of PFC producing clear and partial lysis respectively. The lower histogram shows a "pure" colony in segment b, and the upper one, a mixed colony in segment g.

clone. More detailed investigation has shown
that when replicate assays from colonies are
carried out on several different rbc mixtures e.g.
(sheep + goat), (sheep + cow) and particularly
(sheep "1" + sheep "2"), one or more indicator
mixtures can often be found which will demonstrate
at least two specificity types among the members
of the colony (fig. 6). It is particularly intriguing that changing the conditions under which
these clones develop alters the incidence of
variation : for example, daily injection of sheep
rbc antigen into the mouse increases the proportion of "pure" clones (Pilarski and Cunningham,
in preparation).

It is obviously crucial to be sure that
these colonies are true clones. Our main control
has been to inject into irradiated (CBA x C57BL)
Fl mice, a relatively small number (2-6 x 10^6) of
anti-theta-treated CBA spleen cells together with
a larger number (20 x 10^6) of Fl spleen cells.
This produces large number of plaques in each
spleen segment, ensuring that cell types other
than antibody-forming precursors (e.g. T cells)
are not limiting in any one area. When the Fl
plaques are removed by treating with anti-C57BL
alloantisera and complement, a clonal distribution
of CBA plaques is found, with mixtures of specificities in many of these colonies. Since other
cell types were not limiting, it is likely that
such mixed colonies of CBA PFC arose from a single
B cell.

DISCUSSION

Four different pieces of evidence are outlined to support the idea that clones may vary at
a high rate : (1) different specificities occur
together in limit-dilution cultures in vitro;
(2) cells producing relatively rare antibody
specificities occur in small groups, implying
that they may arise from cells originally making
other specificities; (3) single PFC, cultured in
vitro, grow into small clones which sometimes
contain variants; (4) clones of antibody-forming
cells "cultured" in vivo may also be mixed. A
minimum estimate of the rate at which variation
occurs can be made from (1), (3) and (4), by

considering the proportion of clones which are mixed, and the average number of cell divisions per clone. It is roughly one variation event per 30 divisions for the single cell cultures, and one per 60 for the other in vitro work. The rate is difficult to calculate for the in vivo clones because of the high background in these spleens. This is of course a revolutionary (not to say heretical) conclusion in immunology. It is important to emphasise that our results were all obtained with early IgM antibody-forming cells, whereas in nearly all experiments which uphold the concept of clonal stability (e.g. 15, 16, 17) IgG-producing clones or myelomas were studied. It seems quite possible that clones may vary rapidly in their early development and stabilise later. A second factor which probably helped in detecting variants was the method we used. Cross-reactivity of antibody produced by PFC has two main advantages as a specificity marker : first, it can demonstrate a single variant cell within a clone; second, it is possible to adjust the indicator mixture (for example, by using two sheep of the same breed) so that a very small change in antibody specificity will register as a detectable change in plaque morphology, i.e. in the relative extent to which the two indicator cells are lysed. Similar work might be done with closely related haptens, although these seemed to offer no advantages over the more convenient erythrocyte antigens for this kind of work. It is however important that in any attempt to detect variation within a clone, tests of different cells should be cone on closely related antigens : assays on widely different antigens must obviously have a very low probability of success.

There are some hints from the literature that clonal variation may occur under other conditions. Macario et al. (18) cultured fragments of rabbit lymph node at limit dilution (some fragments were unresponsive), and showed that the affinity of the antibody produced by positive pieces increased considerably over the culture period (several weeks). Independent evidence that such fragments contained single clones of specific antibody-forming cells would prove rapid clonal variation. Luzzati et al. (19) found several examples where, in a culture system similar to ours, a single well gave rise to antibody which formed two bands on electrophoresis. A more extensive study would show whether or not such cases were due to chance association of two initial B cells.

Our work deals with antibody phenotype, and permits no definite conclusion about genetic events. However, the finding that closely related specificities occur together in clones more often than distant specificities fits best with the concept of rapid sequential point mutations within a single V-region, producing at each step relatively small changes in activity. There is some support for the idea that point mutations could produce only small changes in activity from the work of Carson and Weigert (20). They showed that when the λ chains of known sequence from a number of different myelomas were combined with the same H chains, those with the most common sequence, and those differing by 1 or by 2 point mutations in the combining site all had similar anti-dextran binding power. Light chains differing by 3 point mutations from the initial sequence had less, but still measurable dextran-binding activity. Overall, the results reported here, when combined with other evidence discussed elsewhere (4, 6) support the theory that many new antibody specificities are created after antigenic (or mitogenic) stimulation. The very rapid rate at which clones of antibody-forming cells generate variants could well provide the major means by which individuals acquire a repertoire of immunocompetent cells against antigens in their environment.

REFERENCES

1. M. Cohn, *Cell. Immunol. 5,* 1 (1972).
2. F.M. Burnet, "*The Clonal Selection Theory of Acquired Immunity*", Camb. Univ. Press, Lond. and N.Y., (1959).
3. P.A. Bretscher and M. Cohn, *Science, 169,* 1042 (1970).
4. A.J. Cunningham, *Contemp. Topics Molec. Immunol. 3,* (1974) in press.

5. N.K. Jerne, *Eur. J. Immunol. 1*, 1 (1971).

6. A.J. Cunningham and L.M. Pilarski, *Eur. J. Immunol.* (1974) in press.

7. A.J. Cunningham and S.A. Fordham, *Nature* (submitted).

8. J. Marbrook and J.S. Haskill, in *"Cellular Interactions in the Immune Response"*, Karger, Basel, p.66 (1971).

9. A.J. Cunningham and A. Szenberg, *Immunol. 14*, 599 (1968).

10. A.J. Cunningham, *Prog. Allergy, 17*, 5 (1973).

11. A.J. Cunningham, *Aust. J. exp. Biol. med. Sci. 47*, 493 (1969).

12. G.J.V. Nossal and H. Lewis, *Immunol. 20*, 739 (1971).

13. A.J. Cunningham and E.E. Sercarz, *Eur. J. Immunol. 1*, 413 (1971).

14. J. Andersson, O. Sjoberg and G. Moller, *Transplant. Rev. 11*, 131 (1972).

15. B.A. Askonas, A.R. Williamson and B.E.G. Wright, *Proc. Natl. Acad. Sci. 67*, 1398 (1970).

16. N.R. Klinman, *J. Immunol. 106*, 1345 (1971).

17. R.G.H. Cotton, D.S. Secher and C. Milstein, *Eur. J. Immunol. 3*, 135 (1973).

18. A.J.L. Macario, E.C. de Macario, C.Franchesi and F. Celada, *J. exp. Med. 136*, 353 (1972).

19. A.L. Luzzati, I. Lefkovits and B. Pernis, *Eur. J. Immunol. 3*, 636 (1973).

20. D. Carson and M. Weigert, *Proc. Natl. Acad. Sci. 70*, 235 (1973).

B MEMORY CELLS IN THE PROPOGATION OF STABLE CLONES OF ANTI-BODY FORMING CELLS

A.R. Williamson[1], A.J. McMichael and I.M. Zitron[2]

N.I.M.R. Mill Hill, London NW7 1AA U.K.

ABSTRACT. Clonal expansion of B cells has been explored during a primary response and during propogation of a single selected clone (S13). In both cases the development of B memory was studied in relation to the generation of antibody forming cells (AFC).

After priming with NIP-BGG it was found that small numbers of clones expanded to give both AFC and memory cells. Memory was detectable, by cell transfer, prior to the peak of AFC. Later in the response recruitment of new clones of memory cells occurs.

In the propogation of a single anti DNP clone, memory was generated as early as 7 days after exposure to antigen. Thus in both systems B memory cells proliferate prior to, or concommitantly with, direct precursors of AFC. A model is proposed where both cell types arise during clonal expansion by virtue of the changing nature of the stimuli reaching the dividing cells.

INTRODUCTION

Memory is a feature of most immune responses. The greater and more rapid response evoked by a second contact with an antigen reveals the existence of a memory of the initial contact. Immune memory has been shown to be mediated by recirculating small lymphocytes (1,2). The recognition of two populations of lymphocyte, one thymus-derived (T cells) and the other (B cells) processed by the bursa or its equivalent, led to the realization that memory could be a property of both cell types.

The secretion of antibody is limited to cells of the B lineage. Antigenic stimulation of B cells gives rise to anti-body-forming cells (AFC) (2,3) and also B memory cells (4,5). In most cases a humoral response requires not only antigenic stimulation of the B cells but also co-operation by 'helper' T-cells. In the T lineage the helper cell is one type of

---

[1] Present address: A.R.W. Department of Biochemistry, The University, Glasgow G12 8QQ.

[2] Present address: I.M.Z. Building 30 Room 327, National Institute of Health, Bethesda, MD. 20014, U.S.A.

effector cell and these can be generated by short-term exposure to antigen (2,6). Long-term exposure to antigen generates a population of T cells which upon re-exposure to antigen can give rise to helper T cells (7). Thus for both T and
B cells effector function and memory appear to be carried by
separate cells. This paper deals with experiments on B memory cells, but a comparison with T memory cells will be drawn
in discussion of possible models.

Specific B memory cells are generated for each clone of
AFC. Propagation of a single clone of AFC by serial transfer
of spleen cells in syngeneic mice requires the antigen-depen-
dant proliferation of specific B memory cells in each generation for transfer to the next generation (8-11). The clonal
nature of memory poses a fascinating problem: how do AFC and
memory cells arise from the same progenitor cell? The present studies were aimed at defining the relative rates of
appearance of AFC and memory cells during clonal expansion
and determining the nature of the control which channels cells
to one population or the other.

Two previous studies (12,13) on the time-course of generation of B memory after primary immunization with foreign
erythrocytes lead to the conclusion that the major increase
in B memory occurs after the peak of AFC has been passed. In
the development of a response to hapten presented on a carrier
protein it was also found that B memory increased over a period of several weeks (4,5). A re-examination of the time-
course of priming with hapten-protein used the number of
primed spleen cells required for a monoclonal response in
irradiated syngeneic recipient mice as a measure of the number of memory cells generated in a given time (14). It was
found that, with $NIP_{4.5}BGG$[1] as the antigen, memory for an
IgG anti-NIP response was first detected at cell transfer on
day 9 after priming. Memory rapidly increased to a plateau
value reached at 4 weeks. The increase in B memory was
accompanied by an increase in the number of different clones
of anti-NIP AFC contributing to the response. This result

---

[1]Abbreviations used in this paper:

NIP: 4-hydroxy-5-iodo-3-nitro-phenacetyl. BGG: Bovine
gamma globulin. CG: Chicken gamma globulin. Cap: amino
caproic acid. DNP: 2:4 dinitrophenyl. OA: ovalbumen.
IEF: Isoelectric focusing. SIII: Pneumococcal polysaccharide type III. iv: intravenous. is: intra splenic.

implies that interpretation of previously determined time-courses of B memory cell generation in relation to the appearance of AFC during clonal expansion could be misleading. To make a valid comparison generation of memory cells and AFC for a single clone must be followed. In this paper we describe the rates of generation of memory cells and AFC from individual virgin (previously unstimulated) progenitor cells. The time course of regeneration of memory cells during the propagation of a single clone is also described. Both sets of data can be described by the same model.

DEVELOPMENT OF CLONAL MEMORY IN A PRIMARY RESPONSE

1. Rate of generation of B-memory cells and AFC.   CBA/H mice (used throughout these experiments) were immunized with alum-precipitated NIP_{56}-BGG (100µg) together with 2×10^9 B.pertussis. These primed mice were used as spleen cell donors for adoptive secondary responses at various times thereafter as shown in Fig. 1. At each time four donor spleens were processed individually: $25^o/o$ of each spleen was assayed for anti-NIP AFC using a hemolytic plaque technique (15); $70^o/o$ of each spleen was transferred by direct intra-splenic injection together with NIP_{56}-BGG (20µg) into irradiated, syngeneic recipients ($10^o/o$ donor spleen-equivalent/recipient). Recipients were bled 14 days after transfer, rechallenged with NIP_{56}-BGG (20µg) on day 21 and bled again on day 28 (Fig. 1). Sera were analysed for IgG antibody by isoelectric focussing using ^{131}I-NIP-Cap as the developing hapten (16).

The results are shown in Fig. 2. The number of AFC are scored separately for IgM and IgG, (no significant numbers of IgG_2 AFC were observed) for each donor at each time point. The number of recipient mice showing IgG anti-NIP isoelectric spectra is scored, with the shading indicative of first or second bleeds, for the group of recipients corresponding to each donor. The two assays show that B memory cells and AFC initially arise at a similar rate during the primary response. Memory cells for IgG producing clones are first detectable on day 4 at which time the first significant number of IgM AFC are detectable. It is not possible to accurately count the number of memory cells. An estimate of the order of magnitude can be made by taking each clonal spectrum appearing in a recipient mouse as representing one B-memory cell and the efficiency of transfer as $1^o/o$ (10,11). By this calculation the number of IgG memory cells generated by day 4 is comparable to the number of IgM AFC. There is a gradual increase in B-memory cells between days 4 and 9 considering data from several experiments. During this time IgM AFC increase to a

389

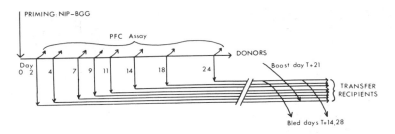

Fig. 1. Experimental design 1: Horizontal lines represent groups of mice; other lines represent procedures. A series of donor mice were primed on day 0 with 100µg alum precipitated NIP$_{56}$BGG with 2 x 10^9 B.pertussis organism, ip. Four donors were killed at each of days 2, 4, 7, 9, 11, 14, 18 and 24. A spleen cell suspension was made from each donor and 25°/o used for a PFC assay; 70°/o was transferred i.s. into 7 sublethally irradiated syngeneic recipients with 20µg NIP$_{56}$BGG per recipient. These were bled and boosted as indicated.

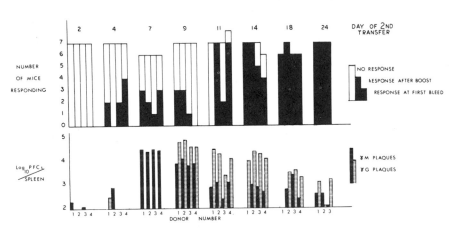

Fig. 2. Rate of Generation of B-memory cells and AFC. The upper histogram shows the number of transfer recipients from each donor that showed a γG anti-NIP response, as judged by IEF. Donors were transferred at various times after priming with NIP$_{56}$BGG. The lower histogram shows the γGl and γM plaque response in the individual donors at the time of transfer. Each donor is directly below its group of recipients in the upper histogram.

390

maximum on day 7 and IgG AFC first appear and rapidly attain a maximum level by day 9. There is a marked increase in memory cells between days 9 and 11 and memory cells continue to increase thereafter as shown in previous studies with hapten-protein conjugates (4,5,14). The previous experiments determining the monoclonal threshold for cell transfer (14) showed that the number of different clones giving rise to memory cells increases rapidly after day 9. The present data was consistant with this increasing recruitment of new clones as judged by the complexity of antibody isoelectric spectra in recipients of cells from donors primed for longer periods.

The present data do not have any bearing on the relationship between IgM AFC and IgG, AFC. We have no means of knowing, in these experiments, whether both class are produced by AFC arising clonally from a single progenitor cell. This becomes important in view of the fact that transferable memory for IgG production preceeds by 3-5 days the appearance of IgG AFC. The isoelectric spectrum of the donor and recipient antibodies does reveal the clonal origins of AFC and memory cells respectively as illustrated in the next experiment.

2. Early B memory is not due to transfer of AFC or their immediate precursors. The experimental design shown in Fig.3 was aimed at looking for the transfer of AFC or pre-AFC. The latter cells, representing an expanded population preceding AFC by one or two divisions, might be capable of giving rise to AFC without requiring further presence of antigen. This possibility is consistant with the finding that DNP-SIII polysaccharide blocks the formation of AFC only when injected prior to day 4 during a secondary response (17). AFC are not known to be transferable but we had to consider the possibility that pre-AFC were responsible for the transfer of responses prior to and during the peak of AFC. The result, shown in Fig. 4, clearly shows that the adoptive secondary responses are consistantly dependent on giving antigen to the recipient mice. In one host receiving cells without additional antigen a faint monoclonal antibody spectrum was observed 15 days, but not 6 days, after transfer. This could be attributed to a trace of antigen carried over with the cells from the donor since very low levels of antigen have been found to elicit detectable antibody in an adoptive secondary response (unpublished observation I.M.Z.).

3. Clonal origin of B memory cells. The data shown in Fig. 4 also includes the number of clones contributing to each secondary response; this number is a subjective estimate based on the antibody isoelectric spectra. Spectra for selected donor

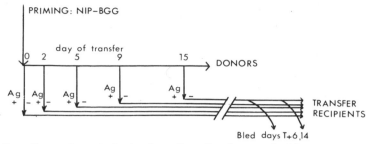

Fig. 3. Experimental design 2. Horizontal lines represent groups of mice and other lines procedures. Donors were primed with $NIP_{56}BGG$ on day 0 and cell transfers performed on days 0, 2, 5, 9, and 15. At each day of transfer a donor spleen was transferred at 20×10^6 cells/recipient i.v., half the recipients receiving antigen ($20\mu g$ $NIP_{56}BGG$) and half receiving no antigen. Recipients were bled 6 and 14 days after transfer.

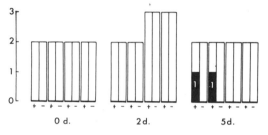

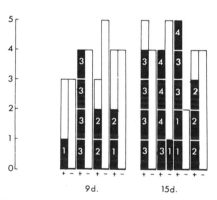

Fig. 4. Early regeneration of memory is not due to transfer of AFCs or their immediate precursors. The height of each column represents the number of mice in each group. Groups from single donors are paired, + indicating transfer with antigen and - transfer without antigen. Solid areas indicate a positive response as judged by IEF and the numbers within each box the number of clone spectra in that recipient. Transfers were carried out at days 0, 2, 5, 9 and 15 after priming.

and recipient sera are shown in Fig. 5. They have been chosen because they illustrate clearly the point made previously with regard to shared clonal origin of memory cells and AFC. Fig. 5A shows the antibody spectra for a single donor and the 8 recipients of cells 9 days after primary antigen, and Fig. 5B for a single donor and 8 recipients 15 days after primary antigen. In each case half of the recipients received antigen with the transferred cells (+) and the other half did not (-). In Fig. 5A it can be seen that all recipients share the same acidic clonal spectrum A and that this clone contributes a major portion of the donor antibody spectrum. In this case clone A antibody was detectable by day 6 after transfer in 3/4 recipients; this early expression is due to memory cells and not pre-AFC since it is not seen in the group not given antigen. Another major clonal pattern (B) is present in the sera of 3/4 recipients bled at day 14 but this antibody is not readily detectable in the donor serum. A third clonal pattern (C) is common to 2 (or 3) recipient spectra (day 14) and is possibly present in the donor spectrum. Fig. 5B clearly shows that the monoclonal antibody made in the donor 15 days after priming is the major antibody species present in all 4 recipients which gave an adoptive secondary response.

Two points should be stressed, on the above evidence: 1) individual clones developing from single virgin precursor cells give rise to both AFC and memory cells 2) the initial rate of production of AFC and memory cells is similar for the major clones observed.

4. Carrier primed helper cells are not limiting in the generation or expression or B-memory cells. The present data indicate the importance of early B memory and consequently raise a doubt as to the adequacy of T-cell helper function early in the primary response. Even though helper cells are rapidly generated (2,6), it might be that such cells are still rate limiting for either the generation of B-memory cells during the early primary response or for expression of B-memory cells in the adoptive secondary response. Both of these possibilities were tested in the experiment outlined in Fig. 6. All donor mice were initially primed with BGG and subsequently given an injection of NIP-BGG or NIP-CG similar to the usual priming schedule. In the mice receiving NIP-BGG excess helper cells are present to cooperate in the generation of B-memory cells and will be transferred to aid expression in recipient mice. The donors receiving NIP-CG must generate CG-specific helper cells at the same time as (or probably before) NIP-specific B-memory cells arise; transfer from these mice is

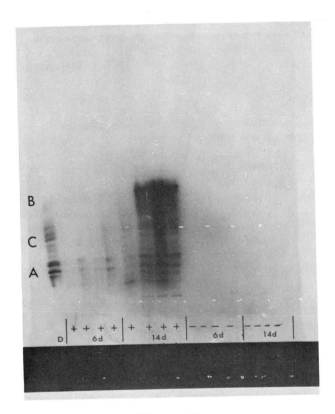

Figure 5a

Fig. 5. Clonal origin of B memory cells. 5A: Anti NIP IEF
spectra of whole sera, developed with NI^{131}P-CAP, from recipients of a 9 day donor. D = Donor serum; 6d = 6 day bleed
of recipients. 14 d = 14 day bleed of recipients; + =
transferred with antigen; - = transfer without antigen.
Three clonal spectrum A, B and C are seen and are shared
between recipients. A and B are also shared with the donor.
The response in recipients in antigen dependent.

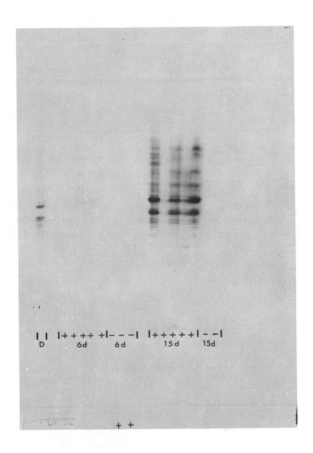

Figure 5b

5B: Anti NIP IEF spectra of whole serum from recipients of
a 15 day donor. Clone spectra are shared between recipients
and one is shared with the donor D. There are 3-4 spectra
per recipient.

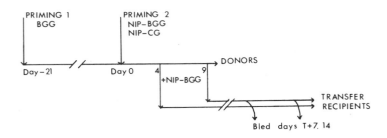

Fig. 6. Experimental design 3. Horizontal lines represent groups of mice and vertical lines procedures. All donors were primed with BGG (100μg alum ppted. + 2 x 10^9 B.pertussis ip) on day-21; on day 0 half were primed with NIP$_{56}$BGG and half with NIP$_4$CG. Transfers were carried out on days 4 and 9 with NIP$_{56}$BGG 20μg in Saline as antigen. Each spleen was transferred to 5 recipients i.v.

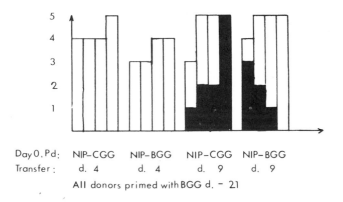

Day 0, Pd:	NIP-CGG	NIP-BGG	NIP-CGG	NIP-BGG
Transfer:	d. 4	d. 4	d. 9	d. 9

All donors primed with BGG d. - 21

Fig. 7. Carrier primed cells are not limiting in early expression of clonal memory. The height of each box represents the number of mice per group and the solid area the number responding, as judged by IEF, 14 days after transfer.

made with NIP-BGG so that expression of B-memory cells will be in the presence of excess specific helper cells.

The result shown in Fig. 7 clearly shows that the presence of carrier-specific helper cells does not enhance either the generation or the expression of B-memory cells. This implies that in the primary response helper cells are not the limiting factor for B-memory cell production. It should be noted that under the present experimental conditions we do not see the expression of virgin anti-NIP clonal progenitor cells in recipient mice even in the presence of excess helper cells.

REGENERATION OF B-MEMORY CELLS IN CLONAL PROPAGATION

A transferable clone of anti-DNP memory cells S13 was used, in passage, to investigate regeneration of memory. This clone had been selected in the course of a partial radioactive suicide experiment (18) and was maintained by serial cell transfer to irradiated recipients (8). It was recognized in each transfer generation by the characteristic, and constant, IEF spectrum of its product, Figure 9. Triggering of the clone had been shown previously to be carrier cell dependent (18) and it is shown here to be antigen dependent (19).

The experimental design is shown in Figure 8. A double transfer system was used with variation of conditions at the first transfer and then a standard second transfer to assay for regeneration of B memory cells. A sufficiency of cells from carrier primed donors was added at both transfers so that B memory alone was being studied. At the first transfer on day 0 memory cells were transferred from a single third transfer generation S13 donor into recipients, either without antigen, or with antigen. DNP SIII was given on day 3 to an additional group that had received antigen on day 0. Antibody production in the recipients was assayed by IEF at day 10, or at the time of retransfer if earlier. The positive control group given antigen on day 0 and bled on day 10 showed an S13 antibody response in all recipients ("26d" in Figure 9). Mice sacrificed at day 7 showed a weak response only, and those killed at day 4 showed no antibody, but a successful transfer is assumed by virtue of the 100°/o take in the positive control group. Mice given DNP SIII on day 3 after antigen on day 0 showed no antibody, as expected (17). Mice given no

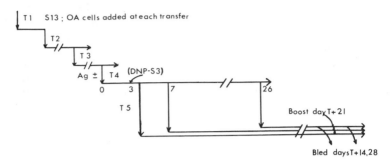

Fig. 8. Experimental design 4. Horizontal lines represent groups of mice, and vertical lines cell transfer. A third transfer (T3) generation S13 mouse was used as a spleen donor for 25 recipients on day 0. 20 of these received cells with antigen (DNP-OA) and 5 of these were also given DNP SIII (DNP-S3) on day 3. Second transfers were carried out on days 4, 7, and 26 for donors that received antigen;on day 26 for those that also received DNP SIII; and on day 26 for those that received no antigen. Second transfer (T$_5$) recipients were bled 14 and 28 days after transfer, and were boosted on day 21 with DNP-OA.

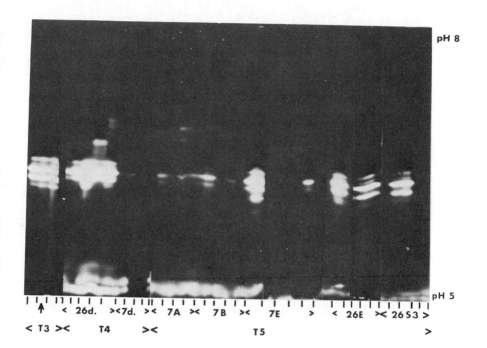

Fig. 9. Regeneration of memory for a selected clone S13. IEF spectra of whole serum, developed with DI^{131}P-DNP-Lys, at transfer generations 3, 4 and 5 (T_3, T_4 and T_5). The original donor for the first transfer is arrowed. Recipients of this transfer that received antigen are shown. Those marked "26d" were bled at 10 days prior to transfer at 26 days and those marked "7d" were bled at the time of sacrifice for retransfer on day 7.

   Recipients (T_5) of cells from these donors are shown. 7A, 7B and 7E received cells from donors 7 days after antigen and 26E from donors 26 days after antigen. (A, B and E indicate the numbers of cells transferred, see Fig. 10). Also shown are recipients 26S3 from donors given antigen on day 0 and DNP S$\overline{\text{III}}$ (DNPS3) on day 3. These donors had failed to make an S13 anti DNP antibody response.

   All clonal spectra are characteristic of the clone S13 apart from faint additional bands in two "26d" mice and one "7A" mouse.

399

antigen on day 0 showed no antibody at day 10.

The second transfers were carried out as described in Fig. 10 with each pool of five donor spleens being distributed in a standard way. These transfers were carried out at various time intervals after the first transfer (Fig. 8). These recipients were bled and assayed by IEF 14 days later. A positive response was the appearance of the S13 IEF spectrum in the serum (Fig. 9), and the number of positive mice in each group is shown in Fig. 10. Thus the assay for clonal memory after the first transfer (fourth clone generation) was the production of antibody after the second transfer (fifth clone generation).

Retransfer at day 4 after antigen and on day 26 after no antigen resulted in no detectable memory. At day 7 however there was clearly specific S13 memory and this was only marginally inferior to the memory at day 26. Thus the number of memory cells generated during 7 days is sufficient to give transfer of the clone S13 using 40°/o or 20°/o of a spleen equivalent i.v. or 20°/o i.s.

When DNP SIII was given on day 3 after the first transfer with antigen, no antibody was produced. However retransfer at day 26 showed a successful take of the clone. As the number of memory cells generated by day 4 had been insufficient to allow retransfer, this suggests that DNP SIII given on day 3 allows some regeneration of memory cells to continue, while blocking AFC production. Retransfer of these memory cells with a single wash procedure removed them from this block and allowed antigen driven proliferation to AFCs in the recipients.

DISCUSSION

Comparing the present data with previous experiments mentioned in the introduction, the major difference lies in the interpretation. Other workers (12,13) observed early B-memory but, in the light of the prolonged increase in B-memory continuing after the peak of AFC and the plateau level of T-memory cells, the initial rise in B-memory cells was not seen as a significant event. We have been able to follow B-memory development as a clonal event by using the isoelectric spectrum of serum antibody as a clonal marker. This has shown us that early memory is due to the generation of many memory cells within each of a small number of clones. The later large increase in B-memory is due to the continued recruitment and expansion of new clones.

A model consistent with the available evidence and providing a hypothetical basis for the control of clonal expansion towards either AFC or memory cells is presented in Fig. 11.

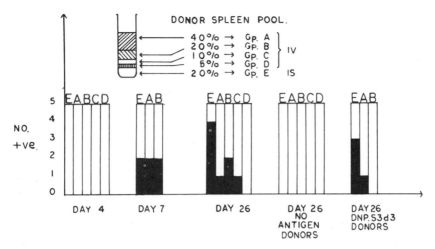

Fig. 10. Regeneration of memory for a selected clone S13;
2nd transfer (T_5). The response in 2nd transfer recipients
from each group of donors is shown. The height of the column
indicates the number of mice in each recipient group and the
solid area the number of mice showing S13 antibody, judged by
IEF. Donors on days 4, 7 and 26 had all been given antigen
when they received S13 cells on day 0 unless otherwise indicated. The group on the extreme right was given antigen on
day 0 and DNP SIII (DNPS3) on day 3.

The distribution of the donor pool of 5 spleens is
indicated in the upper part of this diagram. Cell suspensions
A-D were injected i.v. and E by direct intra splenic injection. The same method of distribution was performed at each
of the times shown. 50µg of DNP-OA per recipient was added
to the suspension prior to cell transfer. 4×10^6 cells from
OA primed donors were also mixed prior to injection.

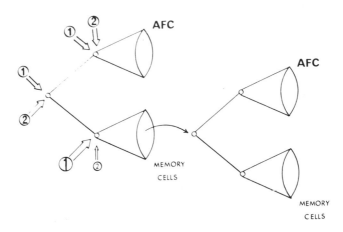

Fig. 11. A model for the clonal development of AFC and memory cells. The initial cell shown is not necessarily the original progenitor cell; it may represent one of a set of cells derived by clonal expansion, driven by signals (1) and (2). Cells up to this point in clonal expansion are capable of giving rise to either AFC or memory cells according to the nature of the continuing stimulus. It is proposed that a change of stimulus guides cells along one or other pathway. In this case a diminution of signal 2 relative to signal 1 is shown favouring memory. This model is reminiscent of the symmetrical division model of Byers and Sercarz (28).

Our data show that, in the expansion of a stable IgG producing clone either from an original virgin progenitor cell or
from a memory cell (a product of a previous clonal expansion),
generation of memory cells occurs simultaneously with, or
preceeds AFC generation. Thus, in the primary response a
large clone of AFC appears to be accompanied by a large number of specific clonal memory cells. The reverse is not necessarily true. Memory cell generation does not have to be
accompanied by production of AFC in appreciable numbers.
During priming, the prolonged build up of B-memory for a
large number of different clones probably entails the expansion of clones of memory cells with little flow of cells into
the AFC category for each clone. In agreement with this, it
has been pointed out recently that, using an assay of memory
in vitro and antibody affinity as a clonal marker, the memory
was expressed for clones not making a detectable contribution
to the primary antibody (20). The idea that priming (i.e.
memory) can be achieved without antibody production is not
new in immunology but could be often explained as T-cell
helper memory. The present finding that memory cells capable
of giving rise to IgG AFC are detectable 3-5 days prior to
the appearance of IgG AFC shows that there is an inherent
potential for generating B-memory cells without antibody production.

The experiment in which DNP SIII was given during the
expansion of clone S13 shows that memory cell production can
be deliberately dissociated from AFC production. The mode of
action of DNP SIII is not yet well defined. DNP SIII was
shown to provide an efficient specific inhibition of anti-DNP
antibody production (17) and it apparently acts by masking
B-cell receptors thus interfering with the delivery of the
T-cell stimulus (signal (2)) via carrier protein epitopes.
DNP SIII can be viewed as a paralytic agent in that it should
only be able to give signal (1) of the two signals postulated
to make up the inductive stimulus (21). It has been shown
that DNP SIII provides signal (1), by giving signal (2) with
allogeneic cells when an anti-DNP response is elicited (22).
Our finding that DNP SIII does not block the memory response
suggests that excess signal (1) may be the factor favouring
clonal expansion toward memory cells. Other circumstantial
evidence is in line with the idea that a high signal (1):
signal (2) ratio favours memory cell production. In T-cell
depleted mice a priming dose of antigen leads to the generation of B-memory cells but no AFC (23). Presenting B-memory
cells with hapten on a heterologous carrier protein at doses
which just give low levels of antibody production (i.e. signal (2) will be very weak) results in good regeneration of

B-memory cells (24). The effect of different doses of antigen on the generation of clonal AFC and memory cells (discussed in following article, 25) is also consistant with the
hypothesis shown in Fig. 11.

The hypothesis explains the prolonged build up of B-
memory as new progenitor cells are recruited. The presence
of antibody will tend to mask antigen, permitting interaction
with one cell, say a B-cell, but making cell-cell cooperation
more difficult. The effect would be to reduce the probability of signal (2) being given but, at the high antigen doses
which favour B-memory, signal (1) would be readily available.
Watson et al (26) have presented evidence for the proposal
that a balance of signals (1) and (2) is necessary for generating AFC; this encourages us to investigate further the
idea that a different balance of signals leads to memory cell
production.

Finally the generation of T-memory cells will be compared with the model for B-memory. Here one major difference
must be taken into account in evaluating the evidence. T-
effector cells, whether helper cells or cytotoxic cells can
be transferred to irradiated syngeneic mice in distinct contrast to the failure to observe transfer of B-effector cells.
'Early T-memory' (12) is probably mostly due to transfer of
active helper cells. Helper cells which have recently divided are functional even if treated with mitmycin-C to prevent further division (7). The transfer of T-memory at later
times after priming is sensitive to mitomycin C and so is not
due to effector cells (7). Generation of helper cells and memory cells within the same clone may occur just as with B-cell
clones; the conversion of effect cells into memory cells is
not yet ruled out however. The generation of cytotoxic T-
cells and memory cells capable of giving rise to cytotoxic
T-cells (27) could also fit within the model shown in Fig. 11.
Here it is very likely that effector cells and memory cells
are two distinct populations (27). The apparent difference
between B-cells and T-cells in the development of memory may
not exist at the level of an individual clone.

ACKNOWLEDGEMENTS

The expert technical assistance of Mr. E.J. Egbuta and
Mrs. D. Millican is gratefully acknowledged. A.J. McM. was
supported by an M.R.C. Junior Research Fellowship and I.M.Z.
by an M.R.C. Scholarship.

REFERENCES

1. J.L. Gowans, and J.W. Uhr, J. Exp. Med., 124, 1017 (1966).
2. G.F. Mitchell, and J.F.A.P. Miller, Proc. Nat. Acad. Sci. U.S.A. 59, 296 (1968).
3. A.J.S. Davies, E. Leuchars, V. Wallis, R. Merchant and E.V. Elliot, Transplantation, 5, 222 (1967).
4. N.A. Mitchison, Eur. J. Immunol., 1, 18 (1971).
5. V. Schirrmacher, and K. Rajewsky, J. Exp. Med., 132, 1019 (1970).
6. N.A. Mitchison, Eur. J. Immunol., 1, 10 (1971).
7. M. Feldman, A. Basten, Eur. J. Immunol., 2, 213 (1972).
8. B.A. Askonas, A.R. Williamson, and B.E.G. Wright, Proc. Nat. Acad. Sci. U.S.A. 67, 1398 (1970).
9. H.W. Kreth and A.R. Williamson, Nature, 234, 454 (1971).
10. B.A. Askonas, and A.R. Williamson, Eur. J. Immunol., 2, 487 (1972).
11. B.A. Askonas, A.J. Cunningham, H.W. Kreth, G.E. Roelants, and A.R. Williamson, Eur. J. Immunol., 2, 494 (1972).
12. A.J. Cunningham, and E.E. Sercarz, Eur. J. Immunol., 1, 413 (1971).
13. J.E. Niederhuber, and E. Moller, Cellular Immunol., 6, 407 (1973).
14. H.W. Kreth, and A.R. Williamson, Eur. J. Immunol., 3, 141 (1973).
15. D.W. Dresser and H. Wortis, Nature,
16. A.R. Williamson, in Hand book of Experimental Immunology (2nd edition) D.M. Weir, editor Blackwell Scientific Publications Oxford (1973).
17. G.F. Mitchell, J.H. Humphrey, and A.R. Williamson, Eur. J. Immunol., 2, 460 (1972).
18. N. Willcox, and A.J. McMichael, manuscript in preparation.
19. A.J. McMichael, and A.R. Williamson, manuscript in preparation.
20. A.J.L. Macario, E. Conway de Macario and F. Celada, Nature New Biol., 241, 22 (1973).
21. P.A. Bretscher, and M. Cohn, Science, 169 1042 (1970).
22. G.G. Klaus, and A.J. McMichael, Manuscript submitted for publication.
23. G.E. Roelants, and B.A. Askonas, Nature, 239 N.B. 63 (1972).
24. I.M. Zitron, Ph.D. Thesis, (1974).
25. A.J. McMichael, this volume.

26. J. Watson, R. Epstein and M. Cohn, <u>Nature</u>, <u>246</u>, 405 (1973).
27. E. Simpson, Personal Communication.
28. V.A. Byers and E.E. Sercarz, J. Exp. Med., <u>127</u>, 307 (1968).

ANTIGEN DEPENDANCE OF CLONAL MEMORY

A.J. McMichael

N.I.M.R. Mill Hill, London NW7 1AA U.K.

ABSTRACT Using a transferable clone of memory cells, S13, the effect of antigen dose on the regeneration of memory was investigated. Both proliferation to antibody forming cells and to memory cells were shown to be strictly antigen dependant.

INTRODUCTION

Proliferation of lymphoid cells and their different-iation into antibody forming cells (AFC) is dependent on antigen, under physiological conditions (1,2). B lymphocytes are precommitted with regard to their specificity (3,4) and exposure to antigen results in selective stimulation of cells able to bind that antigen (3). Normally this trigger has two components, the first provided by the antigen itself and the second by thymus derived (T) cells recognising a separate determinant on the antigen (5).

The events following antigenic stimulation in vivo lead to AFCs and memory cells (6,7). Memory cells themselves may then be stimulated in a similar fashion in secondary respon-ses. In a previous paper we investigated the time course of regeneration of memory cells in the propagation of a single anti DNP clone S13 (8). Like AFC production this pathway was antigen dependant. There is, however, little data on the relationship between antigen dose, AFC and memory cells, except in sheep red cell systems. Cunningham and Sercarz (9), and Niederhuber and Moller (10) showed that high priming doses of sheep red cells favoured B memory production. Using the anti DNP clone S13 we have investigated the effect of antigen dose on antibody production and memory cell regeneration.

MATERIALS AND METHODS

CBA/H mice were used throughout. DNP_4OA[1] was the anti-

---

[1] Abbreviations used in this paper:

DNP: 2:4 dinitrophenyl. OA: Ovalbumen. $DI^{131}P$-DNP-Lys: α-N-(3:5 diiodo-4-hydroxy phenacetyl) -N-(2:4 dinitrophenyl)-L-lysine. IEF: Isoelectric focusing.

gen used. ABCs were determined by Farr assay (15). Isoelectric focusing was used as described by Williamson (11).

Cloning: The origin of the anti DNP clone S13 has been described in detail elsewhere (12). It was maintained by serial
in vivo passage, with antigen, into irradiated recipients
(13). Cells from Ovalbumen primed donors were added in low
numbers (1-2 x 10^6/recipient) at each transfer of the clone.
The experiments described were carried out at the fourth and
fifth transfer generations.

A double transfer system was used to assay memory
(Figure 1). Spleen cells from third generation donors were
pooled for transfer at 2 x 10^6 clonal cells per recipient.
OA primed donor cells were added to the inoculum at 1 x 10^6/
recipient. The cells were split into three groups and DNP OA
added at either 0.1µg, 10µg or 1mg per recipient. The cells
were then transferred to irradiated (660r) recipients. These
mice were bled and titred 10 days later. Two mice from each
group, whose titres were close to the mean of the group, were
used as donors for the second transfer 37 days later. Their
cells were transferred to groups of 6 irradiated mice at 5 x
10^6, 2.5 x 10^6, 1.25 x 10^6 and 0.62 x 10^6 cells per recipient.
Again, cells from OA primed donors were mixed at 1 x 10^6 per
recipient. 100µg DNP OA recipient was also added to the
cells. The recipients were bled at days 10 and 17.

RESULTS

Transfer of the S13 clone, recognisable by its characteristic IEF spectrum, had been shown to be absolutely
dependant on antigen in a previous experiment (8). In this
experiment three antigen doses were investigated, covering
a range that extended beyond the conventional clone transfer
dose of 10-100µg. The antibody produced was nearly all of
the S13 clone type when judged by IEF (8). Several
animals shared a weak second clone pattern; this was present
in some lines of S13 and had been present in the donors for
this experiment. Some of the sera in the 10µg and 1mg groups
were very high titre and their sera did not always focus
clearly on the IEF gels. Farr assay showed that ABCs were
highest in the group given 1mg and lowest in the group given
0.1µg (Fig. 2). The difference in mean titre was significant
(p =< 0.01) between the 1mg and 10µg group, but was not significant between the 10µg and 0.1µg group.

The second transfer was designed to assay for memory
cells in each of these three groups of mice. Cells were
therefore transferred at four different cell doses from donors from each group in order to determine the threshold level

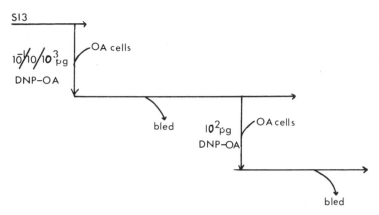

Figure 1. Experimental design. Horizontal lines represent groups of mice and vertical lines cell transfers. Third generation S13 donors were transferred to three groups of eight mice at 2 x 10^6 cells/recipient. Each group received either 0.1µg, 10µg or 1mg DNP$_4$OA per mouse. Recipients were bled and then spleens from two mice in each group were pooled and used for the second transfer. These recipients received 5 x 10^6, 2.5 x 10^6, 1.25 x 10^6 or 0.62 x 10^6 cells each plus 100µg DNP OA.

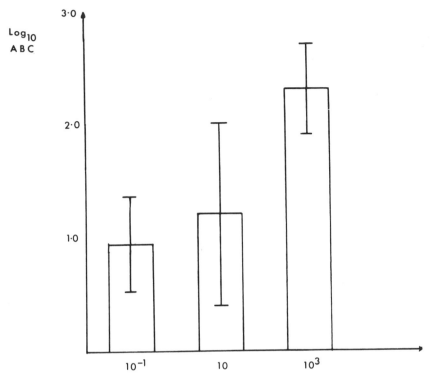

Figure 2. Anti DNP Titres of recipients of the first transfer. Titres are given as $\log_{10}$ ABC, calculated from a standard curve for S13 antibody after Farr test (15), and are
represented by the height of the column. Geometric means
are shown for members of each recipient group, whose donors
received the antigen doses shown in micrograms. The bars
represent standard deviations. The difference in titre
between the $10\mu g$ and $1mg$ group was significant $p < 0.01$;
but that between the $10\mu g$ and $0.1\mu g$ group was not significant.

for successful transfer. A uniform dose of 100μg DNP$_4$OA was given.

Retransfer was scored as positive in an individual if its serum showed the characteristic S13 IEF spectrum. The IEF results are shown in Fig. 3. All responses were of S13 antibody although several were very weak and showed only the major band Fig. 4.

The 5 x 10^6 cell dose from donors that had received 1mg of antigen was supra threshold, although one recipient remained negative. Positives were found at all cell doses from these donors. Transfer from donors that had received 10μg of DNP OA showed only a threshold response at the 5 x 10^6 cell dose. Recipients from donors that had received 0.1μg of antigen were negative apart from a very weak response in one mouse in the 5 x 10^6 cell group 17 days after transfer. Anti DNP Farr titres in the second transfer recipients ranged from 10mM x 10^{-8}/ml to <1.0mM x 10^{-8}/ml which is consistent with transfer of small numbers of memory cells. The lowest titres are probably the result of clonal expansion to AFC from a single memory cell only.

DISCUSSION

This result shows that, for the B memory cell clone S13, proliferation to AFC and further memory cells was strictly antigen dependant. Thus the antibody titre was highest when 1mg of DNP OA was given and was significantly greater than after 10μg or 0.1μg. The difference in titres after 10μg and 0.1μg was not significantly different. Memory cell propagation however was clearly greater in the group receiving 10μg than in the group receiving 0.1μg and was maximal in the group receiving 1mg. At very low doses of antigen therefore it seems that AFC rather than memory cell production is favoured. This result is also consistant with the finding for the same clone that early retransfer was successful (8). At these times antigen levels are presumably still high and could thus initiate memory cell regeneration. There is no evidence that the rate of proliferation would vary at different antigen doses so the effect of high antigen dose is likely to be a combination of favouring the memory cell pathway followed by a sustained series of cell divisions. Another possibility arises from the fact that DNP$_4$OA is not a homogenous antigen. A small fraction may be highly substituted and be of functional importance at very high antigen doses.

These results do not agree entirely with previous reports that memory builds up slowly after the peak of antibody production, at times when antigen concentration is low

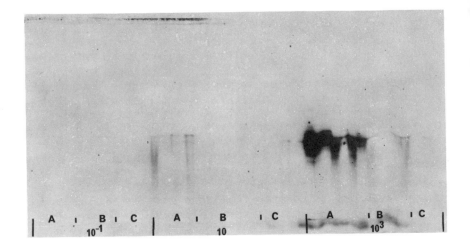

Figure 3. Isoelectric focusing spectrum of recipients of the second transfer. Whole sera, ten days after transfer, were focused on a pH 5-8 gel and developed with DI^{131}P-DNP-Lysine. Recipients of 5 x 10^6 cells (A), 2.5 x 10^6 cells (B) and 1.25 x 10^6 cells (C) are shown for donors that received 10^{-1}, 10 or 10^3 micrograms of antigen. The characteristic spectrum of S13 is clearly seen in recipients of the donors that had received 1mg of DNP OA. Lower titre sera show only the strongest band.

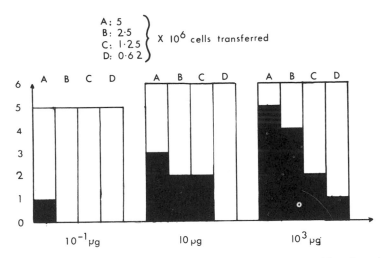

Figure 4. Transfer threshold for S13 memory cells in the second transfer. The height of each column represents the number of mice in the recipient group A-D. The solid area shows the number of mice in each group showing S13 antibody 17 days after transfer, judged by IEF. The antigen dose in micrograms received by the donor of each group is indicated.

(7,9). We have, however, been looking at a single high affinity B cell clone (K_D 3 x 10⁻⁹), with an added sufficiency of T cell help, so that antigen dose is the only variable. In normal primary and secondary immune responses there may be a very complex relationship between antigen, antibody, macrophages and helper cells. Antibody in particular may favour memory cell regeneration by decreasing signal (2) (8). Similarly the result of Feldbush (14), in an anti-hapten transfer system, that a 1mg dose of DNP BGG was suboptimal in memory regeneration may have been affected by the continuing presence of antibody at the time of rechallenge.

ACKNOWLEDGEMENTS

The expert technical assistance of Mr. E.J. Egbuta is gratefully acknowledged. The author was supported by an M.R.C. Junior Research Fellowship.

REFERENCES

1. A.J.S. Davies, E. Leuchars, V. Wallis, R. Marchant, and E.V. Elliot, Transplantation, 5, 222 (1967).
2. G.F. Mitchell and J.F.A.P. Miller, Proc. Nat. Acad. Sci. U.S.A. 59, 296 (1968).
3. F.M. Burnet, The Clonal Selection Theory of Acquired Immunity. Cambridge University Press (1959).
4. G.L. Ada, and P. Byrt, Nature, 222, 1291 (1969).
5. N.A. Mitchison, Eur. J. Immunol., 1, 10 (1971).
6. N.A. Mitchison, Eur. J. Immunol., 1, 18 (1971).
7. V. Schirrmacher, and K. Rajewsky, J. Exp. Med., 132, 1019 (1970).
8. A.R. Williamson, A.J. McMichael and I.M. Zitron, This volume p.
9. A. Cunningham, and E. Sercarz, Eur. J. Immunol., 1, 413 (1971).
10. J.E. Niederhuber, and E. Moller, Cell. Immunol., 6, 407 (1973).
11. A.R. Williamson in D.M. Weir, Editor. Handbook of Experimental Immunology. Blackwell Scientific Publications, Oxford. (1973).
12. N. Willcox, and A.J. McMichael, Manuscript in preparation.
13. B.A. Askonas, A.R. Williamson, and B.E.G. Wright, Proc. Nat. Acad. Sci. U.S.A. 67, 1398 (1970).
14. T.L. Feldbush, Cellular Immunology, 8, 435 (1973).
15. A. Brownstone, N.A. Mitchison, and R. Pitt-Rivers, Immunology, 10, 481 (1966).

REGULATION OF THE ANTIBODY RESPONSE TO TYPE III PNEUMO-
COCCAL POLYSACCHARIDE BY THYMIC-DERIVED CELLS

Phillip J. Baker, Benjamin Prescott, Philip W. Stashak
and Diana F. Amsbaugh

Laboratory of Microbial Immunity
and the Laboratory of Microbiology
National Institute of Allergy and Infectious Diseases
National Institutes of Health
Bethesda, Maryland 20014

ABSTRACT. Thymic-derived suppressor cells were found to influence the magnitude of the antibody response to Type III
pneumococcal polysaccharide (SSS-III), primarily by limiting
the extent to which antibody-forming cells proliferate after
immunization. Such an inhibitory process also appears to
play an important role in the development of low-dose paralysis to this antigen. These findings are discussed within the
framework of a general homeostatic control mechanism in which
the magnitude of the antibody response to SSS-III is governed
by the activities of two functionally distinct types of thymic-derived cells that act in an opposing manner.

INTRODUCTION

Several reports from our laboratory have provided evidence to indicate that the Ab* response to SSS-III is regulated by the activities of two functionally distinct types of
T cells having opposing functions; such regulatory cells have
been referred to as amplifier and suppressor T cells (1-3).
The ability of ALS or ATS to increase the magnitude of the Ab
response to SSS-III is apparently due to the inactivation of
suppressor T cells which, in contrast to amplifier T cells,
exert a negative influence on the Ab response (1-3).
The objective of the present work was to obtain more precise information concerning how suppressor T cells produce
their inhibitory effects. This was accomplished by examining
the effect of treatment with ALS on the kinetics for the ap-

---

*The abbreviations used are: Ab, antibody; SSS-III,
Type III pneumococcal polysaccharide; T cells, thymic-derived
cells; B cells, bone marrow-derived precursors of Ab-forming
cells; ALS, anti-mouse lymphocyte serum; ATS, anti-mouse thymocyte serum; i.p., intraperitoneal; PFC, plaque-forming
cells; LPS, bacterial lipopolysaccharide

pearance of Ab-forming cells. The results obtained indicate
that suppressor T cells act primarily by limiting the extent
to which Ab-forming B cells proliferate after immunization.
Such an inhibitory process plays a role, not only in regulating the magnitude of the Ab response normally produced after
immunization, but also in the development of low-dose paralysis, a phenomenon which appears to be mediated by activated
suppressor T cells.

MATERIALS AND METHODS

Antigen. The immunological properties of the SSS-III
used have been described (4-7). Unless stated otherwise,
mice were given a single i.p. injection of an optimally immunogenic dose (0.5 μg) of SSS-III in saline; the magnitude
of the Ab response produced was assessed at peak, 5 days later.
Immunological procedures. PFC making Ab specific for
SSS-III were detected by a modification of the technique of
localized hemolysis-in-gel (5-8); only values for SSS-III-
specific PFC were considered in this work. Student's t test
was used to evaluate the significance of the differences observed; differences were regarded as being significant when
p values <0.05 were obtained.
Animals. Female BALB/cAnN mice (8 to 12 weeks of age),
obtained from NIH, were used in most experiments to be described. Homozygous athymic nude (nu/nu) mice, as well as
phenotypically normal thymus-bearing littermate controls (nu/+
or +/+ mice) were provided by Dr. Norman Reed, Department of
Microbiology, Montana State University, Bozeman, Montana; pertinent information concerning the lack of normal T cell functions in these mice has been given (2,9-12).
ALS. The horse ALS used in this work, Lot 13162, was
purchased from Microbiological Associates, Bethesda, Md. Details concerning the ability of this preparation of ALS to
prolong mouse skin grafts and to enhance the Ab response to
SSS-III have been reported (2,3). Mice were given a single
i.p. injection of 0.5 ml of ALS at the time of immunization
with SSS-III; such treatment regularly produces maximal enhancement (at least 15 to 20-fold) of the Ab response to this
antigen (2,3).
Mitotic Inhibitor. Velban (vinblastine sulphate), purchased from Eli Lilly and Co., Indianapolis, Ind., was used
as a mitotic inhibitor (13,14). Mice were given a single
(i.p.) injection of either 5 μg or 50 μg of Velban (in saline)
at designated time intervals after immunization with SSS-III

RESULTS

Effect of treatment with ALS on the kinetics for the appearance of PFC. In order to examine the effects of treatment with ALS on the kinetics for the appearance of PFC, mice
were given a single injection of ALS (0.5 ml) at the time of
immunization with 0.5 µg of SSS-III; then, PFC/spleen were
determined at various time intervals (2-6 days) after immunization and the results obtained, which are summarized in Figure 1, were compared to those of immunized mice, not given
ALS.

The kinetics for the appearance of PFC differed strikingly for both groups of mice. For mice not given ALS, the
curve shown could be divided into two phases; a phase during
which PFC increased at a relatively rapid rate (2-3 days after immunization), and a phase during which there was a gradual decline in the rate of appearance of PFC until maximal
numbers were attained on day 5. In contrast, the effects of
treatment with ALS on the kinetics for the appearance of PFC
first became apparent, 3 days after immunization. In this
group of mice, PFC increased at a uniform exponential rate,
throughout the first 5 days of the immune response; this resulted in about a 15 to 20-fold increase in the magnitude of
the PFC response, although there appeared to be no change in
the maximal rate at which PFC appeared. Since these findings
suggested that all additional PFC produced in response to ALS
arose as a result of cell proliferation, the following two
experiments were conducted to test this view:

Mice were given a single injection of 5 µg of Velban, a
mitotic inhibitor, at different time intervals after immunization with SSS-III; no ALS was administered. Then, PFC/
spleen were determined, 5 days after immunization and the
values obtained were compared to those of control mice, i.e.,
mice not given Velban; the data were expressed in terms of
the percent decrease in PFC/spleen, relative to the controls.
The data of Figure 2 show that Velban was most effective in
reducing the magnitude of the PFC response when given during
the first 2-3 days after immunization; thereafter, little or
no reduction in the PFC response was noted. Since the kinetic data of Figure 1 show that the rate of appearance of PFC
was most rapid during the same time interval, these findings
indicate that cell proliferation occurs mainly during the
first 2 days of the Ab response to SSS-III (5,6,15); little
or no proliferation take place thereafter.

In another experiment, both ALS-treated and non-ALS-
treated mice were given a larger dose (50 µg) of Velban, 4
days after immunization with SSS-III; numbers of PFC/spleen

417

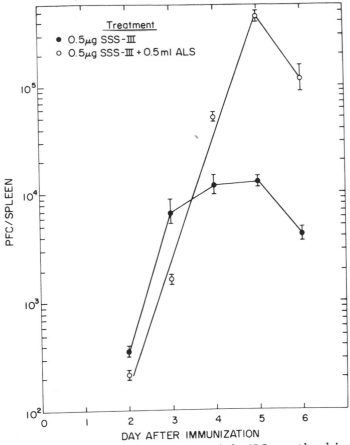

Fig. 1. Effect of treatment with ALS on the kinetics for the appearance of PFC.

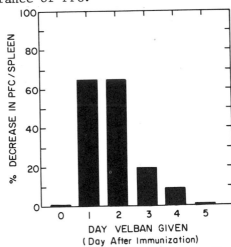

Fig. 2. Effect of treatment with Velban (5 µg) on the magnitude of the 5 day PFC response to 0.5 µg SSS-III.

were determined, 1 day later, i.e., on the 5th day of the immune response. The results of Table 1 show that treatment with Velban had no significant effect on the PFC response of mice not given ALS (Group A vs Group B, p >0.05). Since without ALS treatment, only slight increases in PFC occur, 4-5 days after immunization (Figure 1), this affirms that the dose of Velban used had no adverse effect upon the ability of PFC to synthesize and secrete Ab. In contrast, treatment with Velban produced about a 75% reduction in the PFC response of ALS-treated mice (Group C vs Group D, p <0.001); in fact, the resultant values obtained were no different than those detected on day 4 for ALS-treated mice, not given Velban (Group D vs Group E, p >0.05). Since treatment with Velban completely arrested the further development of PFC, only in the case of ALS-treated mice, these findings provide strong support for the view that the enhancement observed following treatment with ALS is largely due to the continued proliferation, rather than differentiation, of Ab-forming B cells.

Low-dose paralysis to SSS-III. The data of Table 2 illustrate that prior treatment or priming with marginally immunogenic (0.001 µg or 0.005 µg), as well as optimally immunogenic (0.5 µg) doses of SSS-III, greatly reduces the capacity of mice to respond to an optimally immunogenic dose of this antigen, given a few days or weeks later; in comparison to the values obtained for unprimed mice, priming resulted in about a 65-90% reduction in the magnitude of the PFC response to subsequently administered antigen. This form of unresponsiveness, which persists for several weeks or months after priming, was termed low-dose paralysis, in contrast to the longer-lasting high-dose paralysis, regularly obtained with a large dose (50-100 µg) of this antigen (5,16). Low-dose paralysis is not induced spontaneously; rather, it is first demonstrable after a latent or inductive period of 2-3 days, regardless of the dose of antigen used for priming (5, 17). This form of unresponsiveness can be induced with amounts of antigen that give rise to no, or at best extremely small amounts, of serum Ab and PFC; thus, it does not appear to be mediated by Ab, produced as a consequence of priming (17). Other studies have established the fact that paralysis-inducing doses of SSS-III do not reduce the capacity of mice to respond to serologically unrelated antigen (17); low-dose paralysis, therefore, is antigen-specific and cannot be attributed to the phenomenon of competition between antigens. In view of these and other findings, we examined the possibility of whether suppressor T cells play a significant role in the development of this form of unresponsiveness.

419

TABLE 1

Effect of treatment with Velban (50 µg) on the magnitude of the PFC response of ALS-treated (0.5 ml) and non–ALS-treated mice immunized with 0.5 µg SSS-III.

Group	Treatment[a]	PFC/spleen[b]	Day of assay for PFC
A	0.5 µg SSS-III	4.102 + 0.033 (12,600)	5
B	0.5 µg SSS-III + 50 µg Velban	4.014 + 0.062 (10,300)	5
C	0.5 µg SSS-III + 0.5 ml ALS	5.370 + 0.074 (234,000)	5
D	0.5 µg SSS-III + 0.5 ml ALS + 50 µg Velban	4.745 + 0.171 (55,500)	5
E	0.5 µg SSS-III + 0.5 ml ALS	4.717 + 0.019 (52,000)	4

[a]ALS was given at the time of immunization with SSS-III; Velban (50 µg) was given (i.p.), 4 days after immunization.

[b]Log_{10} PFC $\pm$ $s_{\bar{x}}$ for 9-19 mice; geometric means given in parentheses.

TABLE 2

Effect of prior treatment (priming) with a single injection of SSS-III on the ability of mice to respond to subsequent immunization with an optimally immunogenic dose.

Interval between priming and subsequent immunization	Dose of SSS-III used for priming		
	0.001 µg	0.005 µg	0.5 µg
2 days	2.787 ± 0.279[a] (610)	2.698 ± 0.093 (500)	2.376 ± 0.029 (237)
14 days	---	3.511 ± 0.083 (3,200)	3.232 ± 0.052 (1,704)
25 days	3.639 ± 0.040 (4,356)	3.153 ± 0.041 (1,422)	2.508 ± 0.084 (322)
Controls (unprimed mice)	4.083 ± 0.047 (12,100)		

[a]Log_{10} PFC/spleen ± $s_{\bar{x}}$ for 8-10 mice, 5 days after immunization with 0.5 µg SSS-III; geometric means shown in parentheses.

The data of Table 3 summarize the results of an experiment in which we attempted to induce low-dose paralysis in both athymic nude and thymus-bearing littermate control mice. In the case of the thymus-bearing controls, priming with 0.005 µg of SSS-III resulted in about a 70% decrease in the magnitude of the PFC response to an optimally immunogenic dose of antigen, given 3 days later.

Treatment with the same low dose of antigen, however, produced no significant change in the capacity of nude mice to respond to subsequent immunization. It should be noted that nude mice do not differ greatly from thymus-bearing littermate controls in their ability to respond to an optimally immunogenic dose of SSS-III (Table 3; 2,10), and in contrast to thymus-bearing littermate controls, treatment with ALS fails to increase the magnitude of the Ab response to SSS-III in nude mice (2). These findings suggest that functionally active T cells appear to be required in order to elicit low-dose paralysis. If this is so, then one would expect treatment with ALS, which results in the extensive depletion of T cells (18-23), to reduce significantly--if not abolish--low-dose paralysis; the data of Table 4 indicate that this indeed occurs. Mice make a very low PFC response to 0.005 µg of SSS-III (Group F), and priming with this dose of antigen greatly reduces their capacity to respond to an optimally immunogenic dose given, 3 days later (Group A vs Group B, p <0.001). However, if mice previously given this same low dos of antigen are treated with ALS at the time of subsequent immunization, one obtains a response, similar to that of unprimed mice given only 0.5 µg of antigen (Group A vs Group C, p >0.05), but much less than that of unprimed mice given ALS at the time of subsequent immunization (Group C vs Group D, p <0.001). Such an effect cannot be attributed to an enhanced response to the dose of antigen used for priming (Grou E vs Group C, p <0.001). These results illustrate that treat ment with ALS abrogates low-dose paralysis to SSS-III, and that priming with low doses of antigen, besides decreasing the capacity of mice to respond to subsequent immunization, may also reduce the degree of enhancement obtained following treatment with ALS.

DISCUSSION

Treatment with several preparations of ALS or ATS has been shown to produce a significant increase in the magnitude of the Ab response to SSS-III in different strains of inbred mice (24-25). Normal sera from various animal species fail to give enhancement and the ability of ALS to induce enhance-

TABLE 3

Inability to induce low-dose paralysis to SSS-III in athymic nude mice.

Mice	Treatment		PFC/spleen[b]	Value[c]
	Priming (0.005 µg SSS-III)	Immunization (0.5 µg SSS-III)		
Thymus-bearing littermates	−	+	3.534 ± 0.058 (3,400)	
	+	+	2.991 ± 0.124 (970)	<0.01
Athymic nude	−	+	3.354 ± 0.274 (2,260)	
	+	+	3.177 ± 0.177 (1,500)	>0.05

[a] Mice were immunized, 3 days after priming.

[b] Log_{10} PFC/spleen $\pm s_{\bar{x}}$ for 5–6 mice, 5 days after immunization; geometric means are shown in parentheses.

[c] Probability value, Student's t test.

TABLE 4 — Abrogation of low-dose paralysis to SSS--III in mice treated with ALS at the time of immunization.

Group	Treatment given[a] Priming (0.005 µg SSS-III)	Immunization (0.5 µg SSS-III)	ALS (0.5 ml)	PFC/spleen[b]
A	-	+	-	4.107 ± 0.067 (12,800)
B	+	+	-	3.337 ± 0.065 (2,170)
C	+	+	+	4.349 ± 0.126 (22,300)
D	-	+	+	5.554 ± 0.029 (384,000)
E	+	-	+	2.891 ± 0.152 (780)
F	+	-	-	1.488 ± 0.301 (50)[c]

[a] Mice were immunized with SSS-III, with or without ALS treatment, 3 days after priming.

[b] Log_{10} PFC/spleen ± $s_{\bar{x}}$ for 14-16 mice, 5 days after immunization; geometric means shown in parentheses.

[c] No PFC were detected in 7 of 15 mice examined. For the purpose of calculating the mean ± $s_{\bar{x}}$,

ment can be removed by absorption with thymocytes, but not non-lymphoid cells (16). Such enhancement can be abrogated by the infusion of syngeneic thymocytes; however, the infusion of peripheral white blood cells, a population reported to contain 60-90% T cells (26-27), results in further enhancement (1). Subsequent studies conducted in our laboratory established that T cells are required in order to obtain ALS-induced enhancement (2), and that enhancement cannot be attributed to (a) cross reactivity between ALS and SSS-III, (b) a reversal of Ab-mediated feedback inhibition, (c) a stimulatory effect of ALS upon either T cells or B cells, (d) the inactivation solely of T cells that normally have a negative influence upon the magnitude of the Ab response, or (e) the creation of additional "metabolic space" due to T cell depletion (2,28). SSS-III does not require "helper" T cells in order to elicit a normal Ab response (29-31), and ALS-induced enhancement can be demonstrated under conditions in which "helper" T cell activity, essential for a normal Ab response to erythrocyte antigens, is either completely eliminated or substantially reduced (2,24). Since commonly used adjuvants, e.g., LPS, pertussis vaccine, polynucleotides, and Freund's complete adjuvant, as well as X-ray treatment, do not increase the Ab response to SSS-III (unpublished observations), it is unlikely that this form of enhancement can be attributed to an adjuvant effect on the part of ALS. Instead, all of these findings can best be explained by postulating the existence of two functionally distinct types of T cells (amplifier and suppressor cells), which act in an opposing--but not necessarily similar--manner to regulate the magnitude of the Ab response to SSS-III. According to this model, ALS-induced enhancement is due to the inactivation of suppressor T cells that, in contrast to amplifier cells, exert a negative influence on the magnitude of the Ab response, normally produced after immunization (1,2).

The objective of the present work was to obtain more precise information concerning how suppressor T cells produce their inhibitory effects. This was accomplished, first, by examining the influence of ALS treatment on the kinetics for the appearance of PFC, and then determining whether cell proliferation, rather than differentiation, accounted for all additional PFC detected. Without ALS treatment, the kinetics for the appearance of PFC were biphasic. During the first 3 days of the immune response, PFC appeared at a relatively rapid rate; this was followed by a phase during which the rate of appearance of PFC gradually declined until maximal numbers were attained, 5 days after immunization (Figure 1). Since Velban, a mitotic inhibitor, significantly reduced the magnitude of the PFC response, only when given at time intervals when the rate of appearance of PFC was most rapid (Figure 2), cell proliferation appears to take place mainly during the first 2 days of the Ab response to SSS-III; little or no proliferation occurs thereafter (5,6,15).

Different results were obtained in the case of mice given ALS at the time of immunization with SSS-III. The effects of treatment with ALS first became apparent, 3 days after immunization. Instead of observing a gradual decline in the rate of appearance of PFC beyond 3 days, PFC increased at a uniform exponential rate, throughout the first 5 days of the Ab response (Figure 1); this resulted in a 15 to 20-fold increase in the magnitude of the PFC response, and treatment with Velban completely arrested the further development of additional PFC (Table 1). Since the Ab response to SSS-III is almost monoclonal in nature (32), one may conclude from these findings that suppressor T cells, which are activated during the course of an Ab response to SSS-III, first begin to express their inhibitory effects at about 3 days after immunization, and that such cells act primarily by limiting the extent to which clones of Ab-forming B cells proliferate in response to antigen.

Prior treatment with a low dose of SSS-III has been shown to reduce the capacity of mice to respond to an optimally immunogenic dose of antigen given a few days or weeks later (Table 2; 5,17). Such low-dose paralysis, which is antigen-specific (17), appears to be T cell-dependent (Table 3) and is abrogated by treatment with ALS (Table 4). This form of unresponsiveness is demonstrable only after a latent or induction period of 2-3 days; at this time, suppressor T cells first begin to influence the kinetics for the appearance of PFC (Figure 1), and "helper" T cells are maximally activated by low doses of other antigens (33). Furthermore, there is evidence to indicate that T cells are much more efficient than B cells in their ability to recognize antigen (34-36), and T cells have been shown to facilitate the induction of unresponsiveness in B cells to other antigens (37). These observations suggest that suppressor T cells can be activated by low doses of antigen, and that the presence of such cells, at the time of subsequent immunization, imposes additional restraints upon the capacity of B cells to proliferate in response to antigen, thereby causing fewer numbers of PFC to be produced (low-dose paralysis).

Prior treatment with a low dose of antigen, besides further limiting the extent to which B cells proliferate, also appears to reduce greatly, if not eliminate, the ability of ALS to increase the magnitude of the Ab response to SSS-III

(Table 4). Such an inhibitory effect could be the result of the inactivation of amplifier T cells which are required for ALS-induced enhancement (2); this interpretation is consistent with the fact that suppressor T cells have been shown to inhibit the antigen-induced proliferative response and functional activities of other types of T cells (38-39), which could contribute to the development of low-zone paralysis to "helper" T cell-dependent protein antigens (17). Suppressor T cells, therefore, may provide a homeostatic control mechanism for limiting the clone size of all types of lymphoid cells and thus play an important role in preventing the development of lymphoproliferative disorders and autoimmune disease. In this context, lymphoid cell malignancies are often associated with the development of autoimmune disease and as studies conducted with NZB mice appear to indicate, such occurrences are preceded by a progressive decrease or loss of several types of T cell functions, including suppressor T cell activity (3,40-45).

Although suppressor T cells may be activated by low doses of antigen, there is no information to suggest that such cells cannot be activated by large doses of antigen as well. Indeed, the ability of all--including optimally immunogenic--doses of SSS-III to induce paralysis (Table 2; 5) implies that this is the case and that the activation of suppressor T cells may be a natural consequence of immunization. Such a concept is consistent with the dose-response relationships observed in earlier studies and provides a basis for our previously stated views concerning the concomitant development of immunity and paralysis during the course of an Ab response to SSS-III (5,6,16). However, the inability of ALS to abrogate high-dose paralysis to SSS-III (unpublished observations) indicates that other factors may contribute to the development of unresponsiveness following the administration of supra-optimal doses of this antigen. Aside from the effects produced by activated suppressor T cells and treadmill neutralization of Ab by excess circulating antigen (46-47), high-dose paralysis appears to be largely the result of a central failure of the immune mechanism, in which a decrease in the rate of Ab synthesis is an initial step in the development of unresponsiveness by B cells (6,16). Thus, the development of an unresponsive state appears to be an extremely complex process in which, depending on the antigen, dose and experimental procedure employed, several--rather than only one--mechanism may be involved.

REFERENCES

1. Baker, P. J., Stashak, P. W., Amsbaugh, D. F., Prescott, B. and Barth, R. F., J. Immunol. 105, 1581 (1970).
2. Baker, P. J., Reed, N. D., Stashak, P. W., Amsbaugh, D. F. and Prescott, B., J. Exp. Med. 137, 1431 (1973).
3. Baker, P. J., Stashak, P. W., Amsbaugh, D. F. and Prescott, B., J. Immunol. 112, 404 (1974).
4. Baker, P. J. and Stashak, P. W., J. Immunol. 103, 1342, (1969).
5. Baker, P. J., Stashak, P. W., Amsbaugh, D. F. and Prescott, B., Immunol. 20, 469 (1971).
6. Baker, P. J., Stashak, P. W., Amsbaugh, D. F. and Prescott, B., Immunol. 20, 481 (1971).
7. Baker, P. J., Prescott, B., Stashak, P. W. and Amsbaugh, D. F., J. Immunol. 107, 719 (1971).
8. Baker, P. J., Stashak, P. W. and Prescott, B., Appl. Microbiol. 17, 422 (1969).
9. Aden, D. P., Reed, N. D. and Jutila, J. W., Proc. Soc. Exp. Biol. Med. 140, 548 (1972).
10. Manning, J. K., Reed, N. D. and Jutila, J. W., J. Immunol. 108, 1470 (1972).
11. Reed, N. D. and Manning, D. D., Proc. Soc. Exp. Biol. Med. 143, 350 (1973).
12. Manning, D. D., Reed, N. D. and Schaffer, C. F., J. Exp. Med. 138, 488 (1973).
13. Syeklocha, D., Siminovitch, L., Till, J. E. and McCulloch, E. A., J. Immunol. 96, 472 (1966).
14. Perkins, E. H., Sado, T. and Makinodan, T., J. Immunol. 103, 668 (1969).
15. Baker, P. J. and Landy, M., J. Immunol. 99, 687 (1967).
16. Baker, P. J., Prescott, B., Barth, R. F., Stashak, P. W. and Amsbaugh, D. F., Ann. N. Y. Acad. Sci. 181, 34 (1971).
17. Baker, P. J., Stashak, P. W., Amsbaugh, D. F. and Prescott, B., J. Immunol., in press.
18. Tyler, R. W., Everett, N. B. and Schwarz, M. R., J. Immunol. 102, 179 (1969).
19. Leuchars, E., Wallis, V. J. and Davies, A. J. S., Nature (Lond.) 219, 1325 (1968).
20. Schlesinger, M. and Yron, I., Science (Wash., D.C.) 164, 1412 (1969).
21. Denman, A. M. and Frenkel, E. P., Immunol. 14, 115 (1968).
22. Lance, E. M., J. Exp. Med. 130, 49 (1969).
23. Parrott, D. M. V. and deSousa, M., Clin. Exp. Immunol. 8, 663 (1971).
24. Baker, P. J., Barth, R. F., Stashak, P. W. and Amsbaugh, D. F., J. Immunol. 104, 1313 (1970).

25. Barthold, D. R., Stashak, P. W., Amsbaugh, D. F., Prescott, B. and Baker, P. J., Cell. Immunol. 6, 315 (1973).
26. Iverson, J. G., Clin. Exp. Immunol. 6, 101 (1970).
27. Davies, A. J. S., Transplant. Rev. 1, 43 (1969).
28. Barthold, D. R., Presoctt, B., Stashak, P. W., Amsbaugh, D. F. and Baker, P. J., J. Immunol., in press.
29. Humphrey, J. H., Parrott, D. M. V. and East, J., Immunol. 7, 419 (1964).
30. Davies, A. J. S., Carter, R. L., Leuchars, E., Wallis, V. and Detrick, F. M., Immunol. 19, 945 (1970).
31. Howard, J. G., Christie, G. H., Courtenay, B. M., Leuchars, E. and Davies, A. J. S., Cell. Immunol. 2, 614 (1971).
32. Amsbaugh, D. F., Hansen, C. T., Prescott, B., Stashak, P. W., Barthold, D. R. and Baker, P. J., J. Exp. Med. 136, 931 (1972).
33. Kappler, J. W. and Hoffman, M., J. Exp. Med. 137, 1325 (1973).
34. Mitchison, N. A., Cell Interactions and Receptor Antibodies in Immune Responses, O. Mäkelä, A. Cross and T. V. Kosunen (eds.), Academic Press, New York, 1971, p. 249.
35. Mitchison, N. A., Rajewsky, K. and Taylor, R. B., Developmental Aspects of Antibody Formation and Structure, J. Sterzl and J. Riha (eds.), Academic Publ. House, Prague, Czechoslovakia, 1970, p. 547.
36. Müller, E. and Greaves, M. F., Cell Interactions and Receptor Antibodies in Immune Responses, O. Mäkelä, A. Cross and T. V. Kosunen (eds.), Academic Press, New York, 1971, p. 101.
37. Gershon, R. K. and Kondo, K., Immunol. 18, 723 (1970).
38. Gershon, R. K., Cohen, P., Hencin, R. and Liebhaber, S. A., J. Immunol. 108, 586 (1972).
39. Zembala, M. and Asherson, G. L., Nature (Lond.) 244, 227 (1973).
40. Fudenberg, H. H., Arth. Rheum. 9, 464 (1966).
41. Anderson, L. G. and Talal, N., Clin. Exp. Immunol. 9, 199 (1971).
42. Allison, A. C., Denman, A. M. and Barnes, R. D., Lancet 2, 135 (1971).
43. Shirai, T., Yoshiki, T. and Mellors, R. C., Clin. Exp. Immunol. 12, 455 (1972).
44. Gershwin, M. E. and Steinberg, A. D., Lancet 2, 1174 (1973).
45. Barthold, D. R., Kysela, S. and Steinberg, A. D., J. Immunol. 112, 9 (1974).
46. Howard, J. G., Ann. N. Y. Acad. Sci. 181, 18 (1971).
47. Howard, J. G., Transplant. Rev. 8, 50 (1972).

THYMOCYTE SUBPOPULATION WITH SUPPRESSIVE ACTIVITY

Wulf Droege

Basel Institute for Immunology, Basel, Switzerland.

ABSTRACT. In experiments with chickens, a suppressive effect of thymus cells could be demonstrated several weeks after cell transfer if the respective antigen was given repeatedly during the period after the transfer. In such experiments the suppressive effect appeared to be antigen specific, and the ME-sensitive antibody (IgG) was as well or even more suppressed than the total antibody titer (practically IgM). The suppressive effect was found to be better maintained over a period of time by repeated application of high doses of antigen than by low doses. By all these criteria, the suppressive effect of thymus cells appeared to be similar to the suppression ("partial tolerance") that is observed after neonatal application of antigen.

The "fingerprinting" of thymus cells by combination of size distribution analysis, preparative cell electrophoresis and density gradient centrifugation revealed 3 major subpopulations of small lymphocytes in the thymus of mice and chickens. The sequential appearance and disappearance of the 3 cell types in the chicken in relation to functional properties suggests 1) that suppressor activity and G.v.H. reactivity are associated with different cell types, and 2) that the suppressor cells may be the predominant cell population in the thymus in early life.

INTRODUCTION

During the last three years, an enormous number of reports have been accumulating on suppressive effects of thymus cells and thymus-derived cells (1,2). A detailed comparison of all these reports forces the conclusion that various reports are probably dealing with different phenomena. All observations, however, seem to be explained by a minimum of two different phenomena, which may be in some experimental situations operating simultaneously:
1. Antigen specific suppression by a cell type different from G.v.H. reactive T cells and probably also different from helper T cells.
2. Non-specific suppression by a cell type indistinguishable from "classical T cells" and, e.g. present in the hydro-

cortisone resistant pool of thymocytes.

The first 4 reports on suppressive effects of thymus cells, namely the reports by Baker (3), Gershon (4), Okumura and Tada (5) and by Droege (6), all seem to be dealing with the first type of suppression, despite the fact, that these data were obtained with very different experimental systems.

Our own work was mainly concerned with the identification and characterization of the suppressor cell. The present report will mainly be dealing with this aspect. At first, a brief characterization will be given, simply as a basis to compare our suppressive effect with the effects in other reports. The effect in our system is antigen-specific, and some experimental details suggest that we are dealing essentially with the same phenomenon that was found in mice by R. Gershon and was described in his paper on "Infectious Immunological Tolerance" (4). The suppressive effect of thymus cells will also be compared with the phenomenon of "partial tolerance" that is obtained by neonatal application of antigen. It is hoped that this comparison will help to evaluate the biological or technical significance of the suppressive effect. Finally, some data will be presented on subpopulations of thymus cells, and on the identity of the suppressor cell.

COMPARISON OF THE SUPPRESSIVE EFFECT OF THYMUS CELLS WITH THE SUPPRESSION BY NEONATAL APPLICATION OF ANTIGEN

Fig. 1 shows the experimental design, which we used to test for specificity (7). A control group of animals (white Leghorn chickens line 96 from Hy-line, Iowa) received Antigen A on day 10 and then repeatedly 3 times weekly until day 22. Another Antigen B was given on day 30, and then both antigens together or either antigen alone on day 34. The antigens were rabbit erythrocytes (RRBC) and brucella abortus. At various times after challenge, usually 8 days later, the agglutinin titers against both antigens were determined.

Table 1 shows the inhibition of the agglutinin titers against brucella abortus after repeated application of either high or low doses of the antigen. With high doses, it can be seen that the titers are suppressed both after neonatal application of antigen and after transfer of thymus cells. Both the ME-resistant antibody (IgG), as well as the total titers (mainly IgM) are suppressed. In contrast to the 5 to

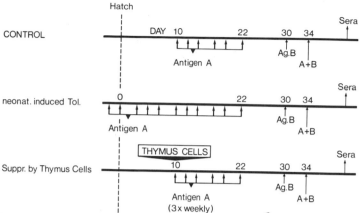

Fig. 1: Schedule for the experiments in Tables 1-3. Br. abortus and RRBC were used as Antigen A and Antigen B, or vice versa. The first immunization of AgB was omitted in some experiments (see footnotes of Tables 2 and 3). (from Droege (7)).

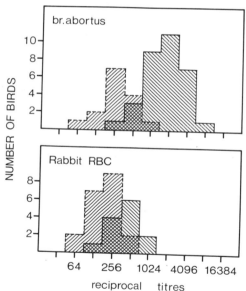

Fig. 2: Frequency histogramms of the observed titres after transfer of thymus cells (---) or in the controls (——). Br. abortus or RRBC were used as Antigen A according to the schedule of Fig. 1. (from Droege (7)).

TABLE 1: Effects of neonatal application of antigen and of thymus cell transfer on the total and ME-resistant antibody titres against <u>brucella abortus</u>[a]

Inject. started at day	Cells given (day 10)	No. of animals tested	Total titres[c]	ME-resistant titres[c]
A	Repeated injections of high doses of Br. abortus[b]			
6-14[e]	-	32	5620	1660
0	-	31	2290	382
10	10d T[d]	15	1120	281
B	Repeated injections of low doses of Br. abortus[b]			
6-10[e]	-	37	2090	603
0	-	21	2050	512
10	10d T[d]	34	1390	267

a) Experimental schedule . See Fig. 1.

b) <u>Br. abortus</u> antigen was given in doses of 1×10^{10} organisms (high dose) or 5×10^7 organisms (low dose).

c) Geometric mean.

d) Thymus cell preparations from 10 day old normal donors were injected into 10 day old recipients (2×10^8 cells i.p.).

e) Pooled data from different experiments.

(from Droege (7)).

6-fold reduction after high doses of antigen, we observed only little suppression after repeated application of low doses of antigen. This suppression was low, both after neonatal application of antigen and after transfer of thymus cells.

Table 2 shows the specificity of suppression. As already seen in the previous Table, the ME-resistant titers for the Antigen A are suppressed both after neonatal application of antigen and after thymus cell transfer. This effect is statistically highly significant because of the large number of animals tested. The response to the RRBC (Antigen B), however, is not significantly different in the 3 experimental groups. This was found regardless of whether the animals were challenged with both antigens simultaneously or separately, indicating that the suppression is not due to release of a non-specific factor. The specificity in these experiments seem to parallel the situation in the earlier experiments by Gershon. Gershon found that spleen cells from mice, several weeks after transfer of thymus cells and after repeated application of antigen, were able to suppress specifically the response to this antigen in a secondary recipient (4). When RRBC are given as Antigen A and brucella abortus as Antigen B, the RRBC response is suppressed and the brucella abortus response unaffected (data not shown).

Table 3 shows the effect after low doses of brucella abortus as Antigen A. In this case, the suppression is very small, but because of the large number of animals still statistically significant. Again, the response to the unrelated antigen is unaffected.

The methodology of these experiments was carefully checked. We tested the reproducibility of our titrations on different days and tested also the biological variation, which is seen in Fig. 2. The frequency distribution of the titers in the control group is quite significantly different from the distribution after thymus cell transfer. In the meantime, a suppressive effect was also observed on the number of plaque-forming cells in the spleen, using SRBC as antigen (data not shown).

In summary, the suppressive effect of thymus cells seems to be identical to the suppression by neonatal application of antigen by all of the following criteria:
1. Both serum titers and numbers of antibody-forming cells

TABLE 2: ME-resistant antibody response of chickens after repeated injections of high doses of brucella abortus

Group	Inject.[a] started at day	Cells given	Anti-RRBC titres[c]	Anti-Br. abortus titres[c]	P values[f]
I	6 – 14[e]	–	759 (7)	1660 (32)	–
II	–5 – 0[e]	–	641 (9)	382 (31)	<.00001
III	10	10d T[d]	n.t.	281 (15)	<.00001
IV	10	9wk T[d]	658 (14)	610 (8)	<.005

a) All animals received repeated injections of 1×10^{10} Br. abortus organisms as Antigen A and one injection of 5×10^8 RRBC as Antigen B before final challenge with 5×10^8 Br. abortus plus 5×10^8 RRBC according to the schedule in Fig. 1 (exception see b).

b) The first immunization with Antigen B was omitted in these animals.

c) Geometric mean; (number of animals tested).

d – e) See notes on Table 1.

f) P-values for differences to group I were computed by Student's t test.

(from Droege (7)).

436

TABLE 3: ME-resistant antibody response of chickens after repeated injections of <u>low</u> doses of <u>brucella abortus</u>.

Group	Injections started at day[a]	Cells given	Anti-RRBC titres[c]	Anti-Br. abortus titres[c]	P values[f]
I	$6 - 10$[e]	-	121 (24)	603 (37)	-
II	-5 or 0[e]	-	n.t.	512 (21	n.s.
III	10	10d T[d]	133 (17)	267 (34)	<.0005
IV	10	7wk T[d]	157 (34)	299 (43)	<.001

a) All animals received repeated injections of 5×10^7 <u>Br. abortus</u> organisms as Antigen A and a final challenge with 5×10^8 <u>Br. abortus</u> plus 5×10^8 RRBC (Antigen B) according to the schedule in Fig. 2. The first immunization with Antigen B was omitted in these experiments.

b-f) See Table 2.   (from Droege (7)).

TABLE 4: Agglutinin (IgM) response to 5×10^7 <u>brucella abortus</u> organisms in 10 day old chickens after transfer of thymus cells from normal (TN) or bursectomized (TBx) Donors.

	Proportion of responders
10d N	(0/12)
TN → 10d N	(7/19)
TN → 10d Bx	(0/12)
TBx → 10d N	(5/12)

(from Droege (6)).

in the spleen are suppressed.

2. The suppression by neonatal application of antigen and by thymus cell transfer are both antigen specific under the test situation described.

3. ME-resistant antibody titers (IgG) are as well or even more suppressed than the total titers (mainly IgM), both after neonatal application of antigen and after thymus cell transfer.

4. In both cases, after neonatal application of antigen and after thymus cell transfer, suppression is better maintained by repeated application of high doses of antigen than by low doses.

5. Neonatal application of antigen and the transfer of thymus cells result in similar degrees of suppression.

6. Both neonatal application of antigen (SRBC) and transfer of thymus cells result in a decreased accumulation of antigen in the spleen, as tested by ^{125}I-labelled anti-SRBC-Fab-fragments (W. Droege and G.F. Mitchell, unpublished).

The data suggest that the two phenomena may be identical : the neonatally induced partial "tolerance" may be mediated by suppressor cells through an active process. The thymus is experimentally a convenient source for suppressor cells. The experiments show that an antigen specific suppression (partial tolerance) can be obtained, when the antigen is given right after hatching or earlier. At a later time, the same dose of antigen does not produce suppression any more. However, apparently the same effect can still be obtained at such a later time, if thymus cells are given together with the first dose of antigen.

CHARACTERIZATION OF THE "SUPPRESSOR CELL"

Now I want to discuss briefly the identity of the "suppressor cell". Our first report on the suppressive effect of thymus cells in the chicken in 1971 contained already one interesting observation: thymus cells of normal chickens were suppressive, thymus cells of neonatally bursectomized birds of the same age did not suppress. One of these experiments is shown in Fig. 3. The primary response of 6 week old chickens to brucella abortus was determined in the sera 6,8 and 13d after immunization. Transfer of thymus cells from normal chickens of the same strain suppressed the response substantially, while the same number of thymus cells from neonatally bursectomized donors had practically

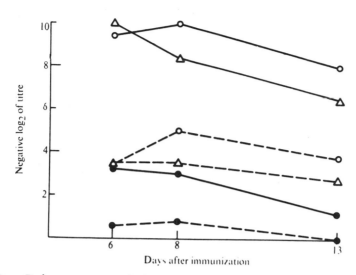

Fig. 3: Primary agglutinin response against <u>Br. abortus</u> in 6 week old chickens after transfer of thymus cells from normal donors (●), from neonatally bursectomized donors (o), or without thymus cells (Δ), ——— = total titres, --- = ME-resistant titres.   (from Droege(6))

439

no effect. Thymus cells from bursectomized donors were also less effective in suppressing the secondary response when tested by the schedule in Fig. 1 (7). By the bursa dependency, the suppressive effect was partially separated from an amplifying effect of thymus cells, that was seen under different experimental conditions and was given both by thymus cells from normal and from bursectomized donors (6) (Table 4). The normal 10 day old chicken does not give detectable agglutinin titers in response to low doses of brucella abortus. After transfer of thymus cells, a significant propo -rtion of animals can produce a detectable IgM response, but the same number of thymus cells, when transferred into neonatally bursectomized recipients cannot induce a detectable response. Apparently, the thymus cells cannot provide the antibody by themselves, but need in addition a component, which is bursa dependent, and which in this case is provided by the host. Thymus cells from bursectomized donors, are just as good in providing this effect as normal thymus cells. If one accepts this as a cooperation between T- and B-cells, one would conclude that cooperative T-cells are not bursa dependent and therefore probably different from the "suppressor cells".

There is good evidence now that the "suppressor cell" is also different from G.v.H. reactive cells. Moreover, using a combination of 3 different physical methods we have identified three different types of small lymphocytes in the thymus of chickens (8,9) as well as mice (10). The data strongly suggest that the suppressive activity in the chicken thymus and the G.v.H. reactivity are associated with different cell types.

Fig. 4 shows first the principle of the "fingerprinting technique" (10). In this case, mouse thymocytes were first fractionated by preparative cell electrophoresis, and the cell fractions then analysed for their cell volume distribution. From the data, contour lines of equal cell number were constructed, and plotted in this two dimensional fingerprint. One can see one cell type with a relative constant size 1.0 in the low electrophoretic mobility region, then another cell type II with a size 1.1, and finally a cell type III with a size 1.4 and electrophoretic mobility 1.15. The thymus of hydrocortisone treated mice contains only the larger cell type III. A series of studies has proven that size plus electrophoretic mobility are perfect markers to describe individual cell types.

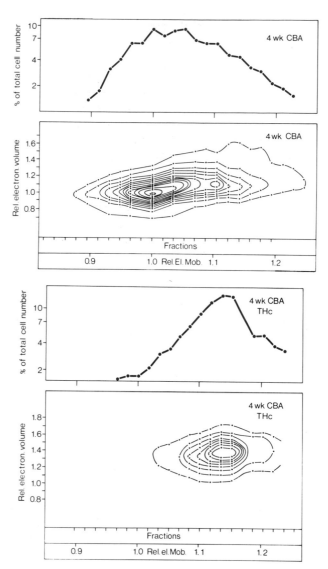

Fig. 4: Top: Electrophoretic distribution profile of thymus cells from normal 4 week-old CBA (left side) and from 4 week-old hydrocortisone treated CBA mice (right side). Bottom: Successive contour lines of constant cell numbers in a two dimensional graph of size versus electrophoretic mobility (finger print). The outer contour line represents 0.05% of the total cell number, the inner lines multiples of 0.05%. Cell type I appears with a volume of 1.0, cell type II has a relative volume of about 1.1, and cell type III a relative volume of about 1.4.
(from Droege, Zucker and Jauker (10)).

441

Fig. 5 shows schematically the 3 cell types in the mouse and the chicken thymus in fingerprints of electrophoretic mobility versus size or buoyant density versus size. This analysis allows choice of the optimal fractionation technique according to the special question under test. The analysis also gives an estimate of how well a given pair of cell types can be distinguished. The cell types I and III in the chicken thymus, e.g. are quite different by all 3 parameters, while other cell types are not well distinguished.

Table 5 shows the sequential appearance and disappearance of the three cell types in the chicken thymus at different ages. Only cells of the smallest type I are seen shortly after hatching (8). All three types of small lymphocytes are seen between 8 and 16 weeks after hatching, and in the adult animal, after strong involution of the thymus, cell type III is the only type left (8). This adult chicken thymus has strong G.v.H. reactivity, and this activity is also found in the 8-16 week old thymus but poorly in the very young thymus (11,12). The suppressive activity, on the other hand, seems to be associated with the early predominant cell type I. It is undetectable in the strongly involuted thymus of the adult bird. At certain times the adult chicken thymus regains size, and suppressive activity is then occasionally found again.

Neonatal bursectomy has a quite dramatic effect on the cellular composition of the chicken thymus in particular on the cell type I (9,13,14). In the normal 4 month old bird, cell type I is found equally well in the heavy as well as light fractions of the gradient. In bursectomized animals, cell type I is greatly depleted in the heavy fractions. This phenomenon is paralleled by the deficiency in suppressive activity in these bursectomized birds, as mentioned before. This subfraction (Ih) is, therefore, a candidate for the "suppressor cell".

These cells, despite being bursa dependent should be different from typical B cells, since the B cells are found in the light fractions of the density gradient (15) and also since B cells are serologically detectable in relatively large numbers in the strongly involuted adult thymus (16,17) which lacks cell type I and also lacks suppressive activity.

In any case, the suppressive activity is detectable relatively early in life, and may in fact be the early pre-

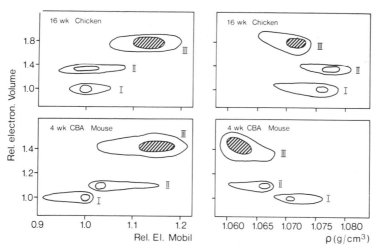

Fig. 5: Schematic illustration of the 3 cell types of the chicken thymus (top) and mouse thymus (bottom) in the "fingerprints" of electrophoretic mobility versus size (left) and density versus size (right). The largest cell types III (with strong shading) are presumably the medullary lymphocytes (see ref. 8 and 10).

TABLE 5: Cell types and reactivities in the chicken thymus

Age	Cell Types		Reactivities	
		B-cells*		
0-2 wks	I	+	poor GvH,	Suppr.
8-16 wks	I, II, III	++	GvH,	Suppr.
8 mnths	III	+++	GvH,	no Suppr.
16 wk Normal	I_1, I_h, II III		GvH,	Suppr.
16 wk Bursect.	I_1, II, III		GvH,	poor Suppr.

* by serological tests (specific antisera)

dominant function in the thymus. This, finally, raises the question of its biological significance. Despite the statistical significance of the suppressive effect in all our experiments, we do not believe, that the 6-fold reduction in antibody titer we observe, has much biological meaning by itself. The probability, however, that these suppressor cells are responsible for the suppression by neonatal application of antigen, and that this phenomenon in turn is principally identical to the neonatally induced allograft tolerance, seems to me quite high. The obvious predictions would be that suppressor cells could be used to induce allograft tolerance, and that suppressor cells are – at least in part – responsible for self tolerance. The early predominance of this cell type could be taken as support for this concept. If this is so, these relatively small effects would have served the purpose not only of getting preliminary information about the suppressive phenomenon, but more important, to identify and purify the cell type responsible for this effect.

REFERENCES

1. R.K. Gershon, Contemporary Topics in Immunology, in press.
2. W. Droege, Current Titles in Immunology, Transplantation and Allergy, 1, 95 and 131 (1973).
3. P.J. Baker, P.W. Stashak, D.F. Amsbaugh, B. Prescott and R.F. Barth, J. Immunol. 105, 1581 (1970).
4. R.K. Gershon and K. Kondo, Immunology 21, 903 (1971).
5. K. Okumura and T. Tada, J. Immunol. 107, 1682 (1971).
6. W. Droege, Nature 234, 549 (1971).
7. W. Droege, Eur. J. Immunol. in press.
8. W. Droege, R. Zucker and K. Hannig, Cell. Immunol. in press.
9. R. Zucker, U. Jauker and W. Droege, Eur. J. Immunol. in press.
10. W. Droege, R. Zucker and U. Jauker, Cell. Immunol. in press.
11. N.L. Warner, Aust. J. Exp. Biol. Med. Sci. 42, 401 (1964).
12. W. Droege, D. Malchow, J.L. Strominger and T.J. Linna, Proc. Soc. Exp. Biol. Med. 143, 249 (1973).
13. W. Droege, D. Malchow and J.L. Strominger, Eur. J. Immunol. 2, 156 (1972).

14. W. Droege, D. Malchow and J.L. Strominger, Eur. J. Immunol. $\underline{2}$, 161 (1972).
15. P. Tamminen, A. Toivanen and P. Toivanen, Eur. J. Immunol. $\underline{3}$, 521 (1973).
16. L. Hudson, personal communication.
17. B. Albini and G. Wick, in Adv. Exp. Med. Biol.,B.D. Jaukovic and K. Isakovic, Ed., Plenum Press, New York-London $\underline{29}$ (1973).

SUPPRESSOR T CELLS IN LOW ZONE TOLERANCE

E. Kölsch, R. Mengersen and G. Weber

Heinrich-Pette-Institut für experimentelle
Virologie und Immunologie
an der Universität Hamburg
2 Hamburg 20, Martinistrasse 52, Germany

One of the major issues concerning the role of
suppressor T cells is whether or not they are involved in the induction and maintenance of immunological tolerance or whether they act only regulatory in preventing overshooting of certain immune
responses.

There are two ways by which suppressor T cells
could induce and maintain immunological tolerance
in humoral responses; either by recognizing an
antigen-binding syngeneic cell or by reacting
against the idiotypes of collaborating cells or
antibody-forming cell precursors. We have been
studying two types of low zone tolerance, both
being identical in an operational sense as they are
induced by subimmunogenic doses of antigen. The
first example concerns low zone tolerance in the
humoral immune response to the bacteriophage fd and
is mainly unresponsiveness of IgG antibodies (1).
The second type concerns tumor immunity. It is
characterized by a preferential take of tumors and
a lack of in vivo cytotoxicity in mice pretreated
with small subimmunogenic doses of irradiated
tumor cells (2). We will discuss here whether
these operationally identical types of low zone
tolerance can be seen within the same conceptual
framework.

The humoral immune response to the bacteriophage fd will be described first, especially the
conditions under which low zone tolerance by subimmunogenic doses of antigen is induced and maintained. The observation which led us into a
detailed study of the role of suppressor T cells

was the fact that we were unable to restore with
normal spleen cells the immunological capacity of
animals made tolerant by low doses of antigen.
This suggested dominance of unresponsiveness in our
system. The key experiment showing that this low
zone tolerance is maintained or at least accompanied by the activation of suppressor T cells (3) is
outlined in the following scheme (Fig. 1): 1 x 10^7
thymocytes taken from normal CBA/J mice were transferred into syngeneic recipients which were thymectomized, lethally irradiated and reconstituted with
fetal liver. The next day these recipients were
subdivided into 4 groups and, together with 4
groups of normal mice, on 5 consecutive days injected with saline, 5 x 10^2, 5 x 10^3 or 5 x 10^8
phages/g body weight, respectively. On the sixth
day the recipients' spleens were removed. One half
of the cells of the animals of each group were
treated with anti-θ serum and C', the other half
with C' alone. The washed cells (2 x 10^7/mouse)
were transferred into normal mice which had never
seen the antigen before. Four days later (day 10)
all mice were challenged with an immunogenic dose
of 5 x 10^8 fd/g body weight. Two and three weeks
later (day 24 and 35) the antibody titers were
measured. The results of such a transfer experiment
are shown in Figure 2. The dashed columns show the
antibody titers three weeks after an immunogenic
dose of antigen of normal mice which received educated T cells pretreated with saline, either
5 x 10^2, 5 x 10^3 or 5 x 10^8 fd/g body weight. T
cells educated with 5 x 10^3 suppress the immune
response in normal mice. The black columns demonstrate how anti-θ treatment before transfer of the
spleen cells into normal mice abolishes this suppressive effect. The open bars show the response
of the mice in the tolerance control. They exhibit
the usual picture of low zone tolerance to phage fd
It is clear from the data in Figure 2 that T cells
educated in the recipients with a dose of antigen,
which in an intact animal induces low zone tolerance, can upon transfer suppress the antibody
production in normal mice which had not been exposed to the antigen before.

The suppressive capacity of transferred T cells
in completely normal animals shown in this experiment is specific for the antigen (3). The main

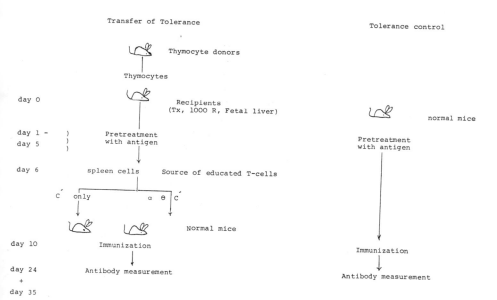

Figure 1

Experimental design of the transfer of low zone tolerance into normal mice by educated T cells.

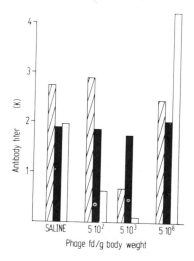

Fig. 2

Transfer of low zone tolerance into normal mice by educated T cells.

(See text for explanation.)

449

point to be made is that it can be induced only
with an antigen dose known to induce low zone
tolerance. This suggests an intimate association
between low zone tolerance and the activity of
suppressor T cells. However, one has to be cautious
about the conclusions which can be drawn. There are
still two major possibilities to explain the data:
suppressor T cells could indeed be responsible for
the induction and maintenance of low zone tolerance
in the way described above. Alternatively, tolerogenic doses of antigen might block collaborating
cells and activate suppressor cells. In this situation activation of the suppressor cell might not be
the actual mechanism of tolerance induction but
merely a safeguard for maintaining tolerance once
it is established by suppressing newly arising
clones.

It might be worthwhile to consider the possible
mode of action of suppressor cells maintaining low
zone tolerance. In this connection the second system is of interest. It deals with low zone tolerance in tumor immunity. In short, pretreatment of
Balb/c mice with 10^4 - 10^7 lethally irradiated
Balb/c mastocytoma cells leads to immunity of these
animals to the tumor (Fig. 3). Previous injection
of 10^1 - 10^3 irradiated tumor cells leads upon
challenge with living tumor cells to a preferential
take of tumors (Table 1) and to the inability to
mount a cytotoxic response in the pretreated animals as compared to the controls (2). This type of
tolerance is different from enhancement on several
grounds (2). So far, we have been unable to demonstrate T cell suppressor activity in the tolerant
animals, which still could be due to technical
difficulties. However, the experiments already put
some restrictuion on the possible mechanisms operating in low zone tolerance. Generation of cytotoxic
T cells recognizing the antigen, as considered
above to be one possible mechanism for tolerance in
the humoral response to fd, would result in cytotoxicity (immunity) against the mastocytoma cells.
Therefore, we are left with two alternatives:
maintaining a unifying concept of low zone tolerance in both types of responses, it would mean that
not recognition of the antigen but recognition of
an idiotypic determinant is the mechanism by which

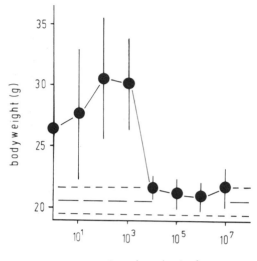

pretreatment of mice

Figure 3

Tumor growth in Balb/c Str. mice pretreated with subimmunogenic and immunogenic doses of killed mastocytoma cells.

Groups of 10 animals each were injected with graded doses (10^0 - 10^7) of killed (1400 r) tumor cells 3 times at weekly intervals and challenged with 1×10^5 living mastocytoma cells. Animals were weighed 15 days later. Mean body weight (●) and standard deviations (vertical bars) are given. Mean body weight (—— ——) and standard deviations (----) of control animals, which received neither killed or living tumor cells, are indicated.

Table 1. Tumor incidence in Balb/c mice pretreated with killed mastocytoma cells

Group	Pretreatment (killed cells)	Challenge (3 x 10^4 living cells)	Increase in body weight (g)										
			0	1	2	3	4	5	6	7	8	9	10
1	10^0	+	9	2	1								
2	10^1	+	10	1				1[a]			1[a]		1[a]
3	10^2	+	6	4									3[a]
4	10^3	+	11	2							1[b]		
5	10^4	+	10	4									
6	10^5	+	12	2									
7	10^6	+	9	4									
8	–	+	21	7	1	1[c]							
			No tumors				Tumors						

[a] On day 18, all dead by day 22. [b] On day 28, dead by day 32. [c] This animal was definitely tumor-free; it started with a low weight at the beginning of the experiment and weighed 22.6 g on day 28 and remained at this weight. All other weights determined on day 28. The animals were pretreated by weekly injections for 7 weeks. They were uniformly challenged with 3 x 10^4 living mastocytoma cells. Groups 2, 3 and 4 are significantly different from group 8 at p < 0.03 (χ^2-test).

452

suppressor T cells operate. It is possible, however, that suppression of immune responses by low doses of antigen, which we call in both cases low zone tolerance, is based on different mechanisms, depending on the antigen used. Blockade of induction of cytotoxic T cells could operate in the tumor system. Blockade of collaborating with concomitant activation of cytotoxic suppressor T cells would then be the mechanism working in the humoral response.

This work was supported by the Deutsche Forschungsgemeinschaft.

References

1. Weber, G., and Kölsch, E. (1972): Eur. J. Immunol. 2, 191.

2. Kölsch, E., Mengersen, R., and Diller, E. (1974): Eur. J. Cancer, in press.

3. Weber, G., and Kölsch, E. (1973): Eur. J. Immunol. 3, 767.

ANTIBODY INDUCED SUPPRESSOR T-CELLS

Leonore A. Herzenberg and Charles M. Metzler

Department of Genetics
Stanford University School of Medicine
Stanford, California 94305

ABSTRACT. Perinatal exposure of SJL male x BALB/c female hybrids to antibody to the paternal (Ig-1b) immunoglobulin allotype specifically suppresses Ig-1b production as the animals age. A suppressor T-cell found in all lymphoid tissues including bone marrow, is responsible for the suppression. About half the exposed animals become completely suppressed (chronically suppressed). Many others are partially suppressed.

Chronically suppressed mice, by definition, have no Ig-1b in circulation and no Ig-1b producing cells in spleen. Nevertheless, many have normal numbers of splenic lymphocytes with membrane bound Ig-1b (committed precursors).

When spleen from normal (SJL x BALB/c)F1 donors is mixed with lymphoid cells from chronically suppressed syngeneic donors and transferred to irradiated (600R) BALB/c mice, production of total serum Ig-1b is suppressed. In similar mixture-transfers with DNP-primed normal donors the Ig-1b anti DNP PFC response is suppressed.

There is an apparent antagonism between suppressor T-cells and cooperator T-cells in the anti DNP response. In a three cell system in which a constant number of hapten (DNP-KLH) primed normal spleen cells is transferred together with both carrier (ovalbumin) primed normal spleen and unprimed suppressed spleen, suppression is reversed either by lowering the number of cooperators or increasing the number of suppressors.

The relationship of this antagonism with respect to the extent of suppression in animals exposed to maternal anti-allotype serum is discussed.

** ** ** ** **

Although the cells which produce antibody in response to antigenic stimulation are the progeny of antigen binding B-cells (1-3), in many cases it is actually the T-cell population which determines how much, and perhaps what class of antibody is produced (cf. 4). This regulation is a complex phenomenon which can involve one or more opposing T-cell functions. T-cells have now been shown both to increase the antibody response by "cooperating" with B-cells to initiate differentiation and maturation to antibody production and to decrease the response by actively suppressing formation of antibody-producing cells (5, 6).

Neither of these T-cell functions or the interaction between them is well understood on a mechanistic level. It is not even clear at present whether cooperator T-cells and suppressor T-cells are different cells or simply the same cell able to function in different modes. Nevertheless, evidence is now accumulating which suggests that the immune response to many antigens evoked by a given immunization regime depends in large part on the balance between the synergistic and antergistic activity of T-cells rather than the availability of B-cell precursors (7).

Our studies involve a suppressor T-cell population in mice which regulates the overall immunoglobulin production (hence, antibody production) of one of the parental allotypes in an allotype heterozygote. This population is induced (or expanded) when the heterozygote is exposed perinatally to anti allotype antibody. Once induced, its activity is maintained for the life of the animal and often completely suppresses production of the allotype as the animal ages (8, 9).

The suppressor cell is found in all lymphoid tissues of completely suppressed animals. It is active when transferred to young normal syngeneic mice (i.e., mice never exposed to anti allotype antibody) and may be repeatedly passaged in such mice. When mixed with spleen cells from normal mice and transferred to irradiated recipients, it specifically suppresses production of the target allotype whether measured as reduction of the total serum level of the allotype or reduction of an allotype marked antibody produced in response to specific antigenic stimulation.

The evidence that the suppressor is a T-cell may be summarized as follows: 1) anti Thy 1.2 (θ) treatment removes suppressor cell activity from suspensions of lymphoid tissues; 2) suppressor activity is recovered in effluents of lymphoid cells passed through nylon wool columns (these columns retain B-cells, but not T-cells [10]); and 3) neonatal thymectomy prevents development of suppression (6).

Thus far we have demonstrated suppressor T-cells in only one hybrid (SJL x BALB/c) and long term ("chronic") allotype suppression in these hybrids for only one H-chain class of immunoglobulins (γ G_{2a} which carries the Ig-la and Ig-lb allotypes). We have looked for "chronic" Ig-lb suppression in other BALB/c hybrids, and for suppression of γG_1 allotypes in the same hybrid, but have found little or no evidence for "chronic" suppression except for this one case (6). Perhaps this is because suppressor cells exist only in this restricted situation, but we should point out that we have by no means searched exhaustively for conditions to establish "chronic" suppression in other cases. The ease of obtaining large numbers of completely suppressed animals has tended to channel the major part of our efforts into studying this system as a potential model for regulation of immunoglobulin synthesis by T-cells in the hope that information gained here might be useful in less obvious systems.

The reasons for this qualification become apparent when the quantitative aspects of the suppressor activity are considered. The SJL x BALB/c hybrid is similar to all other hybrids between Ig^b carrying males and BALB/c females in that after exposure to maternal anti Ig-1b it shows a short delay ($\sim$3 weeks) in onset of Ig-1b production. But unlike the other hybrids, the SJL x BALB/c recover poorly from this short-term suppression. Instead, they continue to show varying degrees of impairment of Ig-1b production throughout life. By six months of age, less than half the exposed animals in this cross are able to produce detectable Ig-1b levels in circulation. The rest are completely suppressed (8).

The serum Ig-1b levels for a litter of SJL x BALB/c hybrids exposed to maternal anti Ig-1b are shown as a function of age in Table 1 (modified from 8). There is considerable variability in the degree of suppression seen, from animals who are completely suppressed through-out life to those who show little or no decrease in serum Ig-1b whenever tested. This litter has a larger propor-tion of completely suppressed mice than is observed when data from many litters is pooled. The usual partition is about 10% completely suppressed, 50% producing some Ig-1b before six months of age but little or none there-after, and the remainder producing Ig-1b throughout life though often at reduced levels (8).

In general, those animals whose Ig-1b levels have dropped below detectability (<.01 mg/ml) by 6 months of age will remain completely suppressed for life. Some will go through periods when Ig-1b is detectable in their serum, but these episodes are usually brief.

We have adopted the term "chronically" suppressed to describe those animals without detectable Ig-1b in serum even though nearly all exposed animals show some degree of long term (or chronic) suppression. This

Table 1

Ig-1b Production in a Litter of (SJL × BALB/c)F_1 Offspring Born to a BALB/c Female Immune to Ig-1b

Mouse	Age (wk)											
	4	5	6	7	8	9	10	13	19	22	40	48
1-3*	-¶	-	-	-	-	-	-	-	-	-	-	-
4	-	-	-	-	-	-	.01	-	.01	-	-	-
5	-	.05	-	-	-	-	-	-	··	··	-	··
6	-	-	-	-	-	-	-	-	>.5	Dead		
7	-	-	-	-	-	>.5	-	.05	-	-	-	-
8	-	-	-	-	>.5	>.5	.05	.05	>.5	-	-	-
9	.05	.05	.01	-	>.5	>.5	.05	.05	-	.05	-	-
10	.01	.01	.01	.01	>.5	>.5	.14	.14	··	>.5	>.5	>.5
11	-	-	-	-	>.5	>.5	.14	>.5	>.5	>.5	.14	>.5
12	.14	>.5	.14	.05	>.5	>.5	.14	.01	>.5	>.5	>.5	>.5
13	-	-	-	-	>.5	>.5	>.5	-	.05	>.5	>.5	>.5

* These mice, phenotypically negative for the paternal allotype (Ig-1b), were back-crossed to the maternal (Ig^a) strain, and the presence of the paternal (Ig^b) allele was confirmed.

¶ Levels determined by immunodiffusion.   - = <.01;   ·· = not tested.

74.12

458

hairsplitting definition was required for practical reasons, since we tend to use only "chronically" suppressed animals for cell transfer studies. These are always tested for Ig-1b just prior to transfer to be sure that no donors are in remission.

The non "chronically suppressed" animals have received much less analytical attention thus far although they may prove to be quite useful for regulatory studies. Experience has shown that if their allotype levels have not dipped below detectability by 6 months of age, the serum Ig-1b will generally be maintained at roughly the 6 month level for the rest of the animal's life, even if that level is only 1/10 the level in normal hybrids.

This curious ability to maintain relatively constant low allotype levels was the first indication that allotype suppression might represent a regulatory mechanism which is stimulated to a greater or lesser degree in various animals. Further evidence along the same line comes from cell transfer experiments which show that recipients of low doses of suppressor cells often show a similar partial suppression of allotype production over a long period of time.

Transfer of lymphoid tissue from "chronically suppressed" donors into young, normal syngeneic recipients (2 week) results in long term suppression of the recipients. The pattern of suppression is shown as a function of cell dose in Table 2. At the highest cell dose, no Ig-1b becomes detectable in the serum. At intermediate cell doses, Ig-1b synthesis begins at the normal time (there is no short-term suppression in these animals) but soon falls off. By 6 months of age, no allotype is detectable in circulation. At the lowest cell doses, none of the animals become completely suppressed but many show significant suppression of production, especially after 6 months of age.

A similar dose dependance occurs in irradiatedrecipients of mixtures of normal spleen cells with spleen or other lymphoid cells from suppressed donors. Recipients of intermediate doses frequently maintain low level allotype production over long periods of time (see Table 3).

These experiments provide reasonably good evidence to support the hypothesis that allotype levels in those animals not completely suppressed by perinatal exposure to maternal anti-allotype antibody (i.e., non-chronically suppressed mice) are regulated by smaller numbers of suppressor cells otherwise similar to those found in

459

Table 2

Transfer of Spleen Cells from Suppressed Donors
to 2 Week Old Syngeneic Normal Recipients

Suppressed[1] Spleen Cells Transferred ($\times 10^6$)	No. of[2] Recip.	Mean Ig-1b in Serum (mg/ml)[3] Age (Weeks)					
		8	10	12	16	20	24
15	30	0	··	··	0	··	··
5	10	<.06	.2	.4	<.09	<.09	<.08
1	10	.14	.4	>.5	>.5	>.5	>.5

[1] Donors were SJL x BALB/c exposed to maternal anti Ig-1b over 6 months of age with <.01 mg/ml Ig-1b in circulation.

[2] Estimated by immunodiffusion. (0) = <0.01 mg/ml. ·· = Not tested.

[3] Recipients were 2 week old normal (SJL x BALB/c) hybrids.

74.11

460

Table 3

Titration of Suppressor Activity in Spleen
of Chronically Suppressed SJL x BALB/c Mice

Spleen Cells Transferred[1]			Mean Ig-1b in serum (mg/ml)[2] Weeks After Transfer				
Normal (x 10⁶)	Suppressed (x 10⁶)	No. of Recip.[3]	1	2	3	4	6
12	10	4	>.23	.03	0	0	0
12	3	4	>.41	.1	.12	.07	.01
12	1	4	>.5	>.5	>.5	>.41	>.17
12	-	4	>.5	>.5	>.5	>.5	>.5

[1] Suppressed Donors: see legend, Table 1
Normal Donors: SJL x BALB/c, 4 months of age.

[3] Recipients: Irradiated (600R) BALB/c, transferred i.v. ~18 hours
post irradiation.

[2] Estimated by immunodiffusion. (0) = <0.01 mg/ml.

74.13

461

"chronically" suppressed mice. In both kinds of mice, the size (or activity) of the suppressor population might well be determined early in life (as in the case of the young recipients of suppressor lymphoid cells) although it reaches its full expression only as the animal ages.

To look for suppressor cells in partially suppressed mice we tried using them as donors in a mixture-transfer experiment (i.e., suppressed spleen plus normal spleen transferred to irradiated recipients). The marginal suppression which resulted was consistent with there being fewer or less active suppressor cells in the donors, but because we were somewhat limited as to the maximum number of cells we could transfer, (and because we didn't work on these experiments exhaustively) we were unable to state how many cells might have been present.

Determining suppressor activity in these animals, however, may tell only part of the story. We have now obtained evidence from experiments on suppression of an adoptive hapten-carrier secondary response which suggests that the level of T-cell cooperator activity in suppressed animals may also play an important role in regulating the production of Ig-1b. In these studies, there appears to be an antagonism between allotype suppressors and carrier primed cooperators when transferred together such that, at least within limits, either increasing the number of cooperators or decreasing the number of suppressors will increase the allotype marked antibody response.

For these experiments we used formation of anti-DNP plaque forming cells (DNP-PFC) developed with anti Ig-1b as an index of suppression. The data in Table 4 show that the Ig-1b adoptive secondary response to DNP-KLH in irradiated recipients of long-term DNP-KLH primed normal hybrid spleen cells is suppressed by the concurrent transfer of spleen cells from "chronically suppressed" animals. As with suppression of total serum Ig-1b, the extent of suppression is dependent on the number of suppressor cells added. Suppression is specific in that only the Ig-1b DNP-PFC are suppressed.

To study the relationship between the suppressors and cooperators, we switched to a "heterologous" hapten carrier response where the same DNP-KLH primed normal spleen cells were used as the source of hapten primed B-cells but ovalbumin primed normal spleen cells were used as the source of carrier primed T-cells. DNP-ovalbumin was the stimulating antigen. With this system we could hold

Table 4

Suppression of Ig-1b anti DNP Response

| DNP-KLH 1° Normal Spleen x10^6 | Unprimed Spleen | | PFC/10^6 | | |
	Normal x10^6	Suppressed x10^6	Direct	Ig-1a +Ig-4a	Ig-1b
12	10	-	34	3800	400
12		1.1	29	4300	410
12		3.3	40	3300	170
12		6.7	40	2300	120
12		10	42	3300	17

100 ug alum pptd DNP-KLH + 2 x 10^9 B. pertussis injected i.p. 1-3 months prior to transfer.

10 ug aqueous DNP-KLH boost i.v. 1 day after transfer.

Donors: (SJL x BALB/c)F$_1$; recipients BALB/c irradiated (600R) ~18 hours prior to transfer.

74.10

B-cells constant while varying both cooperator and suppressor cell dose.

The data from these experiments indicate a clear antagonism between the two types of T-cells in that suppression is relieved either by increasing the cooperators or decreasing the suppressors (see Table 5). There is complete suppression of Ig-1b PFC at all suppressor cell and cooperator doses except when the largest number of cooperators and the fewest number of suppressors are transferred. Going down three-fold in cooperators or up three-fold in suppressors is enough to totally suppress the response. Thus the number of PFC produced is determined essentially by a balance between cooperator and suppressor activities, at least within limits.

These experiments have some relevance to the one cell-two cell suppressor-cooperator question. The fact that suppressor cells in these experiments were taken from unprimed animals is a prima facia argument for suppressors being different from cooperators. Unfortunately, though, this conclusion is restricted to allotype suppressors. It cannot be generalized to antigen specific suppressors described earlier in this session until these, too, can be separated physically from cooperators.

It is interesting to speculate on the mechanism of the antagonism between suppressors and cooperators, however there are still too many unknowns to make such speculation fruitful. I would like to underscore this by pointing out that although the suppressors behave like competitive inhibitors of cooperators, the data presented is insufficient to differentiate between a direct suppressor-cooperator interaction model and a model which supposes that more suppressors are needed to suppress the larger number of B-cells activated by increasing the number of cooperators.

The demonstration of antagonism does, however, provide a useful framework within which to consider the overall picture of allotype suppression in SJL x BALB/c hybrids and its potential relationship to suppression in other strains. Let us suppose that the allotype levels in any given mouse are determined by positive vectors (e.g., cooperator activity, antigenic stimulation and negative vectors (e.g., suppressor activity, catabolism). Then the "chronic" allotype suppression seen in SJL x BALB/c hybrids exposed perinatally to maternal anti-allotype antibody could be due to an excessive imbalance of the

Table 5

Antagonism Between Suppressor and Cooperator T-Cells

Unprimed Suppressed Spleen $(x\ 10^6)$	Ovalbumin (Carrier) 1° Normal Spleen * $(x\ 10^6)$		
	1	3	10
Expt. 1 0	23	72	246
1	0**	0	64
3	0	0	0
	2.7	8	24
Expt. 2 0	80	290	330
1.6	0	45	50
4	0	0	0

* All animals received 12 x 10^6 hapten primed (DNP-KLH) spleen cells together with carrier primed spleen, and were boosted with 10 ug DNP-ovalbumin 1 day after transfer.

** 0 means <5 ppm.

74.14

465

positive and negative vectors (e.g., over-induction of
suppressors, general debilitation of suppressors, or both).
Similarly, the increase in the number of "chronically"
suppressed animals as the animals age could be due to a
shift in the balance between the vectors.

The failure to see "chronic" suppression in other
hybrids, as well as in a number of the anti-allotype
exposed SJL x BALB/c mice, might then represent our inability to find conditions to induce sufficient suppressor
activity to counteract the forces favoring allotype production in these mice.

It is somewhat arrogant to suggest that induction of
allotype suppressors by early exposure to anti-allotype
antibody may be a general phenomenon since by our own
admission we haven't been able to find them. However, if
I may be permitted to delve into ancient history, there is
some data in our first publication on allotype suppression
which we might now interpret as evidence that a population
of allotype suppressor cells similar to those found in
SJL x BALB/c but less active is inducible in C57BL/10 x
BALB/c mice (10).

C57BL/10 x BALB/c mice exposed to maternal anti-
allotype antibody show a delay of about three weeks in
onset of allotype production. After that the serum allotype levels increase rapidly. But although the serum
levels in these animals climb at roughly the same rate as
the controls and eventually reach normal range, calculation of the actual rate of allotype production in these
animals suggests an impairment of production as late as
fifteen weeks of age.

In Figure 1, the two solid curves show the Ig-1b
levels in serum averaged for three litters of controls and
three litters of mice exposed to maternal antibody (11).
The dashed curve (which joins the controls at 10 weeks)
shows the estimated allotype levels for the suppressed
mice if production of allotype proceeded at the same rate
as controls once the maternal antibody had removed as
much allotype as it could absorb. The point of the figure
was to demonstrate that "mopping up" by maternal antibody
could not explain allotype suppression. But the method
used to estimate theoretical allotype levels also allowed
estimation of the parameters which would approximate the
observed data, and thereby allowed us to recognize a persistent difference in the rate of allotype synthesis
between control and suppressed mice.

Figure 1.

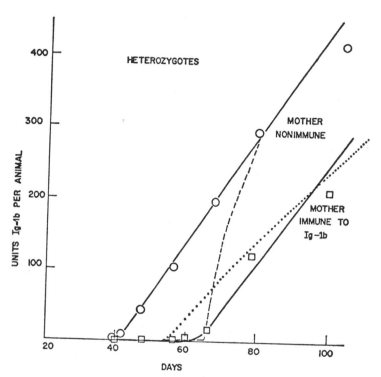

FIG. 1. Calculated increase in Ig-1b level in heterozygotes. Solid curves reproduced from Fig. 3. Dashed curve (---) was calculated on the basis of 500 units of Ig-1b removed but no change from the rate of production of Ig-1b found for the controls. Dotted curve (···) was calculated on the basis of 150 units of Ig-1b removed and the rate of production of Ig-1b equal to one-half the control rate. A half-life of 6 days was used for both curves. Corrections for the amount of Ig-1b withdrawn in serum sampling were made. For $t = 0, 1, 2, \ldots 179$, the rate of production of Ig-1b at time t (PRO$_t$) was found by equation (1) and substituted in equation (2) to determine the amount of Ig-1b expected at time t (Calc Ig$_t$).

$$(1) \quad PRO_{(t+1)} = (Ig_{(t+1)} - Ig_t) + \left(\frac{\ln 2}{T} + k\right) Ig_t \text{ and}$$

$$(2) \quad \text{Calc } Ig_{(t+1)} = \text{Calc } Ig_t + q \cdot PRO_t - \left(\frac{\ln 2}{T} + k\right) \text{Calc } Ig_t - \vartheta$$

where Ig$_t$ is the observed Ig-1b level in control at time t; T, the half-life in days (6, in curves in figure); k, the fraction of total Ig-1b present in the animal removed by sampling averaged per day (0.1/7 in curves in figure); q, the fraction by which the rate of production (PRO) is altered; and ϑ, the amount of Ig-1b withdrawn at $t = 0$.

Reprinted from (11).

To make this comparison, we set up an equation (see legend for Figure 1) which expressed the rate of allotype production as a function of the observed total allotype level (corrected for the fluid space of the animal) and the amount of allotype lost because of catabolism and test bleeding. Assuming a 6 day half life (which was consistent with observed values) and a fluid space of 8.8% body weight, we determined the rate of synthesis in the controls. Then by including another variable, i.e. loss due to maternal antibody, we tried various combinations of loss and rates of synthesis to approximate the curve for the suppressed animals.

We found that in order to account for the continued lag between the suppressed animals and the controls, it was necessary to postulate that the suppressed animals produced the allotype at 1/2 the rate determined for the controls. In no way could we approximate the suppressed curve by assuming the normal rate of production in suppressed mice after the release of suppression.

Clearly there are more direct methods, especially with modern techniques, to test whether suppressor cells are induced in this strain combination. And there are other ways to interpret the reduction in allotype synthesis (e.g., decrease in available B-cell precursors). But it is worth considering this data because it suggests that induction of suppressors in response to maternal anti-allotype antibody may be a more general phenomenon than our gross screening procedures have allowed us to recognize thus far.

General phenomenon or not, however, there still remain the questions as to whether allotype suppressor cells bear any similarity to cells which suppress antibody formation to particular antigens and whether suppressors are involved in regulation of antibody production. Hopefully continued work on the SJL x BALB/c system will yield some insights into these problems.

REFERENCES

1. Wigzell, H. Transplant. Rev. 5, 76 (1970).
2. Julius, M. H., T. Masuda and L. A. Herzenberg, Proc. Nat. Acad. Sci. 69, 1934-1938 (1972).
3. Julius, M. H., R. G. Sweet, C. G. Fathman and L. A. Herzenberg, AEC Symposium Series (C.O.N.S. 73-1007) (1974).

4. Claman, H. N. and E. A. Chaperon, Transplant. Rev. 1, 92 (1969).
5. Miller, J.F.A.P., Ann. Immunol. (Inst. Pasteur) 125C, 213 (1974).
6. Herzenberg, L. A. and L. A. Herzenberg, Contemp. Top. Immunobiol. 3 (1974). In press.
7. Gershon, R. V. Ibid.
8. Jacobson, E. B., L. A. Herzenberg, R. Riblet and L. A. Herzenberg, J. Exper. Med. 135, 1163 (1972).
9. Herzenberg, L. A., E. C. Chan, M. M. Ravitch, R. J. Riblet and L. A. Herzenberg, J. Exper. Med. 137, 1311 (1973).
10. Julius, M. H., E. Simpson and L. A. Herzenberg, Eur. J. of Immunol. 3, 645-649 (1973).
11. Herzenberg, L. A., L. A. Herzenberg, R. C. Goodlin and E. C. Rivera, J. Exper. Med. 126, 701 (1967).

T CELL REGULATION: THE "SECOND LAW OF THYMODYNAMICS."

Richard K. Gershon

Department of Pathology
Yale University School of Medicine
New Haven, Connecticut 06510

ABSTRACT. Five examples in which T cells act as "thymostats" are presented. In all instances a regulatory T cell population has been shown to alter the response of another T cell population. When the responding T cell population is highly active, the regulator acts to suppress the response; when the activity of the responding cells is low, the regulatory cells act to augment it.

INTRODUCTION

The concept that T cells act as regulatory cells rather than as cells which simply amplify the immune response is rapidly gaining wide acceptance. The evidence on which this concept is based has recently been reviewed by several authors (1-3). In addition, most of the workers responsible for the original discoveries in this area (with the notable exception of Tada's group (see 1-3)) will be discussing their work at this meeting. Therefore, it will not be my purpose to review the evidence for the existence of suppressor T cell activity. Rather I will discuss one particular aspect of the factors which determine whether regulatory T cells will act to suppress immunologic activity. If the reader accepts the fact that during the reading of this paper at the conference, there was a slight protrusion of the author's cheek produced by his tongue, he can then think of the concept being put forth as the "second law of thymodynamics"; that is to say for every T cell dependent augmentation there is an equal and opposite T cell suppression. Put in another way I suggest that there is a continuous spectrum of interaction effects between T cells and their target cell populations. These interactions may have either amplifying or suppressive end results. One of the factors determining the direction of the net result is the activity of the responding cell (ie:the regulatee). When it is quite active, a regulatory T cell acts to suppress it; when its activity is low, the regulating cell boosts it. Thus, the regulating cell acts (tongue returning to cheek) as a "thymostat."

Before I present the evidence on which this concept is based a qualifying statement is in order. The so-called suppressor T cell can have both specific and non-specific effects (1-3). Thus in some circumstances the suppressor T cell suppresses only the response to the antigen which activated it. Under other conditions it suppresses the response to unrelated antigens. Whether the same rules apply to the activation of these two types of effects is unknown. Nor is it known whether or not the two are interrelated. The specificity of the effects I will be discussing below is unknown. It seems most likely that they fit the category of non-specificity, although it is possible that there is hidden within, a specific effect as well.

RESULTS AND DISCUSSION

The concept of the thymostatic T cell stems from an incisive observation made by a medical student who had come to do some research in my lab. At that time we were looking into the possible role of interaction effects between different cell populations in the production of graft vs. host splenomegaly. We had done a rather large number of experiments mixing cell populations together and were getting intriguing but irreproducible results. Liebhaber took the experimental book home with him one night and came back the next day with a straight line (4) which is reproduced in Figure 1. The data analyzed in this fashion showed that when parental thymic T cells, inoculated into sub-lethally irradiated F_1 hosts, produce a relatively large spleen body weight ratio the addition of a constant number of F_1 spleen cells to them decreases the spleen size. Conversely, when they produce a relatively low spleen-body weight ratio the addition of F_1 spleen cells increases the splenomegaly. Thus the effects the F_1 spleen cells have on the splenomegaly produced by the parental T cells, is dependent on what the parental T cells themselves are doing.

Analysis of the mechanism by which the F_1 cells produced these bi-directional effects was hampered by the fact that the assay used for measuring parental cell activity required the proliferation of the F_1 cells (5,6). To simplify the system somewhat we developed a new assay that could measure the activity of the cells responding to the host antigens directly (7,8). The assay consists of injecting lethally irradiated F_1 mice with parental thymocytes and quantitating the amount of DNA the injected cells synthesize, as a measure of their activity. We used uptake of the thymidine analog 5-iodo-2-deoxyuridine (IUDR) labelled with ^{125}I as a measure of DNA synthesis, as 24 hours after its inoculation all IUDR not intimately associated with DNA is cleared from the lymph-

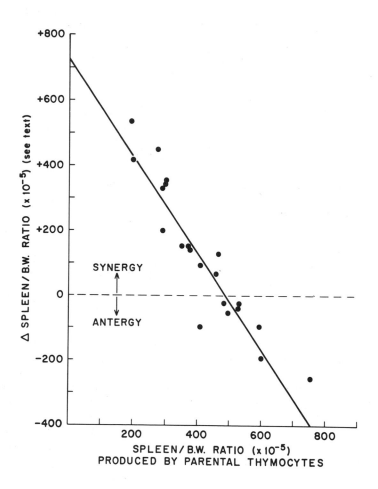

Figure 1. Relationship of the spleen/B.W. ratio produced
parental thymocytes alone, inoculated into sub-lethally
radiated F_1 hosts, to the change ($\triangle$) produced by the incor-
ration of F_1 spleen cells with the thymocyte inoculum.

oid tissue (9). At this time the spleens and lymph nodes of test mice can be harvested and the number of gamma emissions they produce indicates how much DNA they have synthesized. Using this system we have made the following observations:

1. <u>Regulation of parental T cell activity by F_1 thymocytes</u>. (10,11)(Figures 2 & 3). The addition of a constant number of F_1 thymocytes to varying numbers of parental T cells produces a constant effect. At the higher end of the parental T cell dose, the F_1 cells suppress the response. At the lower end of the dose they augment it. There is a great deal of variation in activity of different batches of T cells. Despite this variation one can get a consistent result if one studies enough points on the dose-response curve. Thus, one can find in one experiment the high dose effect at 9×10^7 cells (Figure 2) and in the next experiment at 3×10^7 cells (Figure 3). In both cases one finds however that as the number of parental cells is reduced the suppressive effect of the F_1 T cells disappears and augmentation takes its place. One can rule out DNA synthesis by the F_1 cells as a contributory factor, as they can produce their regulatory effects even after being given 900R, which totally abolishes their ability to synthesize DNA (11).

2. <u>Regulation of parental T cell activity by lethally irradiated parental thymocytes</u> (11)(Figure 4). In the above experiments, the F_1 thymocytes used as a regulatory cell population had no antigen to respond to in the F_1 mice. They were able to act as a source of antigen for the parental cell. However it is possible (but unlikely) that they may have affected the parental cell response by virtue of that attribute. We have been able to show, however, that parental thymocytes rendered incapable of DNA synthesis by 900R of irradiation can produce the same effects on DNA synthesizing parental cells, as can F_1 cells. In this case the regulating cell population does not act as a source of antigen. Thus, in dose response studies it can be shown that at high doses of responding cells a constant number of 900R irradiated parental cells act to suppress the response while at lower doses they act to augment it.

3. <u>Interactions between cortisone resistant and cortisone sensitive T cell sub-populations</u> (12,13)(Figure 5, Table 1). These studies were performed by giving a given number of parental T cell donors an injection of 2.5 mg. of cortisone acetate, 48 hours before harvesting their cells. An equal number were untreated. The recovered thymocytes from

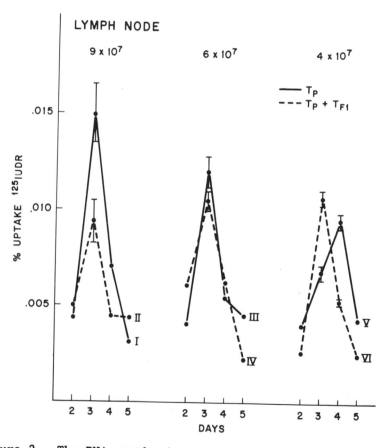

Figure 2. The DNA synthetic responses of 3 doses of parenal thymocytes (9,6 and 4 x 10⁷) in the inguinal lymph nodes f lethally irradiated recipient F₁ mice in the absence (Tp) r presence (Tp + TF₁) of a constant number of F₁ thymocytes 2.5 x 10⁷). Each point is the mean response ±S.E. of 3 test ice.

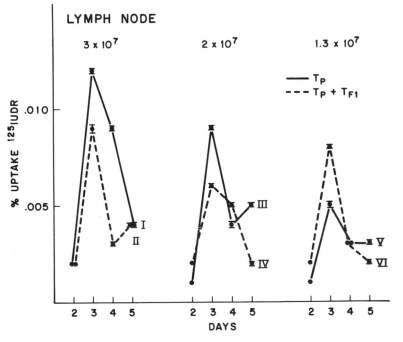

Figure 3. The DNA synthetic responses of 3 doses of parental thymocytes (3,2 and 1.3 x 10⁷) in the inguinal lymph nodes of lethally irradiated recipient F_1 mice in the absence (Tp) or presence (Tp + TF$_1$) of a constant number of F_1 thymocytes (7.5 x 10⁶). Each point is the mean response ± S.E. of 3 test mice.

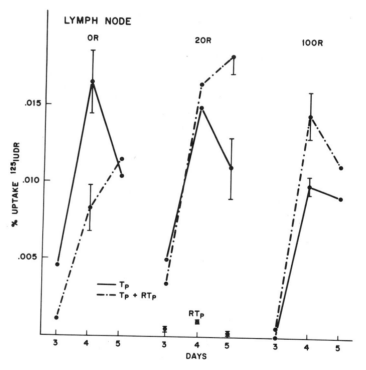

Figure 4.   The DNA synthetic response of 4 x 10⁷ parental
thymocytes in the inguinal lymph nodes of lethally irradiated
mice.   Some of the responding thymocytes were reduced in
number and activity by treatment with 20R or 100R or were
untreated (OR) prior to inoculation.   Their response in the
absence (Tp) or in the presence of 4 x 10⁷ 900R irradiated
parental thymocytes (Tp + RTp) is presented.   In addition
the responses of the 900R irradiated cells is also presented
(RTp).   Each point is the mean response ± S.E. of 4 test mice.

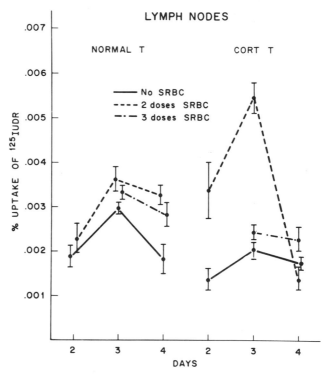

Figure 5. The DNA synthetic response of a normal unfractionated thymocyte inoculum (Normal T) and the isolated cortisone resistant fraction contained in that inoculum (Cort T)
in a GVHR, with or without additional daily stimulation with
SRBC. Each point is the mean response ± S.E. in the inguinal lymph nodes of 3 test mice.

Table 1

THE EFFECT OF CORTISONE SENSITIVE THYMIC T CELLS ON THE
ABILITY OF CORTISONE RESISTANT T CELLS TO SUPPRESS TUMOR
GROWTH.[1]

Dosage of Thymic T Cells $(\times 10^6)$[2]	Treatment	Results	P <
30	Untreated (Cortisone Resistant and Cortisone Sensitive)	9.9 + 5.5	0.01
30	Cortisone Resistant fraction	92.6 + 7.5	0.001
60	Untreated (Cortisone Resistant and Cortisone Sensitive)	12.5 + 2.1	0.01
60	Cortisone Resistant fraction	2.6 + 0.49	

[1]
Each number represents the mean number of tumor cells
(+S.E.) remaining in the abdominal cavity of C_3H mice 4
days after tumor inoculation. The mice also received
different doses of sensitized T cells. The results are
presented as a percentage of tumor cells present in normal
C_3H controls inoculated with the same number of tumor
cells. (There were 4-6 mice in each experimental group).

[2]
1 spleen equivalent was transferred to each test mouse.

both groups of donors were sub-divided so that each recipient
received the same percent of cells from a donor's thymus.
Thus, in theory, all recipient mice got the same number of
cortisone resistant cells; those mice which received the untreated thymocyte population got in addition a large number
of cortisone sensitive cells. By this technique we were able
to determine what effect the cortisone sensitive cells have
on the highly reactive resistant population. We found that,
under high degrees of stimulation, the cortisone sensitive
cells acted to suppress the response; under lesser degrees of
stimulation they acted to augment the response. This was tru
using DNA synthesis as the assay (Figure 5) and also true
when we used the cells immunized to the F_1 antigens as a
source of tumor killer cells (Table 1).

4. Interactions between spleen seeking and lymph node
seeking T cell sub-populations (14)(Figures 6 & 7). We
inoculated parental thymocytes into lethally irradiated F_1
mice and at intervals thereafter removed the cells that had
localized in the spleens,by splenectomy. We then measured
the subsequent DNA synthetic response of the cells which had
localized in the recipient's lymph nodes. When we removed th
spleen in the first 24 hours after inoculation we found that
the subsequent response of the cells in the lymph nodes was
markedly augmented. Studies with chromium 51 labelled cells
showed that after 3 hours post inoculation, removal of the
spleen did not lead to increased localization of cells in the
lymph nodes. Thus, the observed increase was not due to a
simple diversion of cell traffic. When splenectomy caused an
increase in the nodal response, reinoculation of the cells
removed at the time of splenectomy suppressed the response.
As with the other systems described above the augmentation
only occurred when high doses of parental cells were studied.
When low doses of parental thymocytes were used, splenectomy
led to a decrease in the nodal response. We have recently
extended the studies to parental lymph node cells and
parental spleen cells (Figure 7).(The studies mentioned above
used parental thymocytes as the source of reactive cells).
Interestingly, we have found, in confirmation of similar find
ings by Wu and Lance (15),that splenectomy after the inoculation of parental spleen cells produces the same effects as
does splenectomy after the inoculation of parental thymocytes
On the other hand, splenectomy after the inoculation of paren
tal lymph node cells does not affect the subsequent response
of the cells which localize in the lymph nodes. These exper-
ments suggest that the cell which regulates the lymph node
response is present in the thymus and in the spleen but not

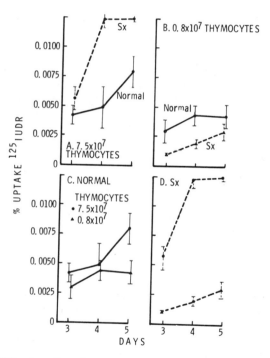

Figure 6. Effect of splenectomy 3 hr after the inoculation of different doses of parental thymocytes on the DNA synthetic response of these cells in the lymph nodes of lethally irradiated F_1 mice. In A & B the test groups are compared at the 2 doses studied. In C & D the thymocyte doses are compared to one another in the 2 different groups.

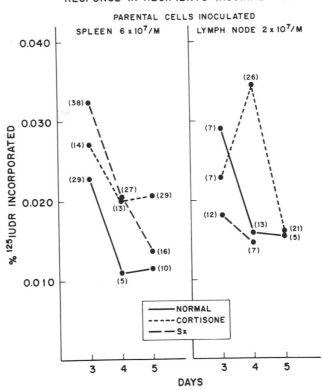

Figure 7. The DNA synthetic response of parental spleen and lymph node cells in the inguinal lymph nodes of lethally irradiated F_1 mice. Three hours after the parental cells were inoculated some recipient mice were inoculated with 2.5 mg. of cortisone and others were splenectomized. Each deter mination is the mean of 3 test mice and the numbers in paren theses are the coefficients of variation. (Parental thymocytes and their cortisone resistant fraction, both react in a fashion similar to the spleen cells and therfore quite different from the lymph node cells ; that is to say both splenectomy and cortisone treatment at 3 hours post inoculation can increase their response.)

in the lymph node. It does not appear that the splenic micro-environment per se causes the cells to produce their regulatory effects.

5. Augmentation of T cell responses by drugs. When a high dose of parental T cells is inoculated into lethally irradiated F_1 mice, and the recipient mice are inoculated 3 hours later with cortisone, the subsequent response of the cells which localize in the lymph nodes is markedly augmented (Figure 7). No consistent effect is produced on the response in the spleen. This holds true even when the inoculated T cells have been pre-selected for cortisone resistance. When a low number of T cells are inoculated the injection of cortisone may reduce the response. These results, along with similar studies performed with a number of different cytotoxic agents,which will be published in detail shortly,suggest that a regulatory cell is activated early in the response to antigen; that its activation makes it sensitive to some cytotoxic agents such as cortisone; and that the regulatory effect it has depends on the strength of the reaction. When the reaction is high it dampens the response; when it is low it tends to augment it.

In summary, I have presented 5 different instances of regulatory interactions between T cell sub-populations which have bi-directional effects. In all cases, when the responding cell (regulatee) is highly active the net interaction effect is suppressive. When the responding cell is relatively inactive the net interaction effect is augmentative. I suggest that these results can be best understood by thinking of a T cell, perhaps with attributes similar to the F_1 cell of Asofsky, Cantor and Tigelaar (16), as a "thymostat". It receives signals from responding cells. When it receives a high level of signal it acts to suppress the response. When the signals it receives are faint, it acts to augment it. Such circular interactions between T cell sub-populations may play an important role in immunologic homeostasis.

ACKNOWLEDGMENTS

The experimental work reported herein was supported by grants CA-08593 and AI 10497 and the experimentor by an RCDA CA-10,316 from the N.I.H. Kazunari Kondo and Ellen Searle rendered expert technical assistance. I am most grateful to my colleagues who participated in the collaborative studies. The data presented in Figures 1 (from ref. 4), 2-4 (from ref.

11) and 6 (from ref. 14) are reprinted by permission of the respective publishers.

REFERENCES

1. Katz, D.H. and Benacerraf, B. Adv. Immunol. 15, 1 (1972)
2. Droege, W. Current Titles in Immunology, Transplantation and Allergy. 1, 95 and 131 (1973).
3. Gershon, R.K. Contemporary Topics in Immunobiol. 3, 1 (1974).
4. Liebhaber, S.A., Barchilon, J., and Gershon, R.K. J. Immunol. 109, 238 (1972).
5. Simonsen, M. Prog. Allergy. 6, 349 (1962).
6. Elkins, W.L. Progr. Allergy. 15, 78 (1972).
7. Gershon, R.K. and Hencin, R.J. Immunol. 107, 1723 (1971)
8. Gershon, R.K. and Liebhaber, S.A. J. Exp. Med. 136, 112 (1972).
9. Fox, B.W. and Prusoff, W.H. Cancer Res. 25, 234 (1965)
10. Gershon, R.K., Cohen, P., Hencin, R., and Liebhaber, S.A. J. Immunol. 108, 586,(1972).
11. Gershon, R.K., Liebhaber, S. and Ryu, S. Immunol. (In Press).
12. Gershon, R.K. and Cohen, P. Ann. N.Y. Acad. Sci. (In Press).
13. Frank, G., Freedman, L. and Gershon, R.K. J. Immunol. (Submitted).
14. Gershon, R.K., Lance, E.M. and Kondo, K. J. Immunol. 11 546 (1974).
15. Wu, C.W. and Lance, E. Cell.Immunol. (In Press).
16. Asofsky, R., Cantor, H. and Tigelaar, R.E. In Progress in Immunology, B. Amos, ed., Academic Press, New York, p. 369 (1971).

T CELL FACTORS IN THE REGULATION OF THE B CELL RESPONSE

Richard W. Dutton

Department of Biology
University of California, San Diego
La Jolla, California 92037

ABSTRACT. Allogeneic culture supernatants contain a soluble factor that will replace T cells in the respone of Nude spleen cell suspensions to erythrocyte antigens. The presence of the factor increases the frequency of B cells that respond and the burst size of antibody-forming cells per responding unit. The addition of the factor can be delayed up to 48 hours after the addition of antigen and the same effect still be observed. These and other experiments suggest that the factor may be involved in maturation of the B cell rather than the initiation of the proliferation phase of the response.

INTRODUCTION

The immune response to all but certain antigens requires some "helper" activity of antigen specific T cells or some appropriate substitute for this activity. The mechanism of this helper activity has been the subject of intensive research by a number of investigators (1,2,3). Three major possibilities have emerged: 1. A cell surface interaction between T and B cells is required. Katz and his colleagues (4) have provided evidence that there may be a rigorous requirement for genetic compatibility for success-ful interaction to occur. 2. Helper activity is mediated via an antigen specific soluble mediator. Feldmann and his colleagues (5) have presented evidence that the soluble mediator is an immunoglobulin molecule, IgT, which has special affinity for the surface of a macrophage. Antigen-IgT complexes presented to B cells by macrophages are immunogenic while free antigen-IgT complexes are tolerogenic. 3. We have proposed that helper activity is effected by a non-antigen specific soluble mediator synthesized by the T cell on interaction with carrier antigen (3). The require-ment for associated recognition of hapten and carrier deter-minants by B and T cells is assured since only B cells in the immediate vicinity of a stimulated T cell and which are also interacting with antigen receive a sufficient stimulus to respond.

There is now a considerable body of evidence in support of all three models (see this volume). It is not the purpose here to discuss their relative merits except insofar as to make two points. First, it is possible and indeed likely that there are different requirements and different mechanisms involved in responses to differing antigens in the differing experimental models. Second, the models are not mutually exclusive. To illustrate this, it is not impossible, although perhaps unlikely, that cell surface interactions between genetically compatible T and B cells are required to generate IgT which then binds antigen, fixes to the macrophage surface and causes the macrophage to release a non-antigen specific mediator that allows the B cell response to antigen.

The present paper concerns only the third experimental model in which the ability of T depleted mouse spleen cell populations to respond to burro erythrocytes is restored by a soluble non-antigen specific mediator present in the 24 hr culture supernatant of allogeneic mouse spleen cell cultures or by Con A activated irradiated normal spleen.

The question being asked is not the nature of such a factor but merely the time at which this activity must be made available to the B cells relative to the time that the response is _initiated_ by the addition of antigen.

A number of speculations as to the nature of the T cell-B cell collaboration have seen the T cell or some product as providing a second signal for the _initiation_ of the B cell response to signal 1, i.e., the antigen (6). Tacitly assumed in this model is the idea that signal 2 must be present at the start of the response since signal 1 alone, it is suggested, leads on to tolerance. The question whether the second signal must be present throughout the response or only at the start has not been discussed.

It was, thus, somewhat surprising when Schimpl and Wecker in 1972 (7) showed that the response of spleen cell suspensions from the congenitally a-thymic Nude mouse to SRBC was more efficiently restored when allogeneic culture supernatants were added at 48 hrs rather than at the start of culture.

We repeated and confirmed these studies using an experimental model that allows the measurement of both the frequency of the B cells that respond and the average number of PFC produced per responding B cell (8,9). The experiments described will show that the kinetics of the response, the frequency of responding B cell and the average burst size are just the same if the T cell help is added at 24 or 48 hrs instead of time zero. It will also be shown that the

responding B cells start to proliferate prior to the addition
of T cell help, that the initiation of proliferation
requires the presence of antigen and treatment of the Nude
spleen cell suspensions with rabbit anti-mouse brain serum
and complement prior to incubation does not prevent these
effects. Factors in fetal bovine serum are also not necessary for initiation of the response.

RESULTS AND DISCUSSION

When varying numbers of spleen cells are cultured in
the presence of excess, carrier primed, T cells the frequency
of cultures that respond at various cell numbers shows a
Poisson distribution from which the frequency of the responding unit can be calculated. This frequency has been taken
as the frequency of B cells able to respond to the antigen
in question (8).

In T depleted cultures the frequency of responding cells
is much depressed (Figure 1). The response can be restored
either by the addition of carrier specific T cells (irradiated carrier primed spleen) or by allogenic culture supernatants (Figure 1 and Table 1). The characterization of the
factors in allogenic culture supernatants has been described
elsewhere (8). In brief, they have been shown to contain at
least two active factors. One, a dialysable factor,
increases only the burst size of the response, and does not
affect the frequency of responses. The other, molecular
weight, 28,000, increases the frequency of responses and the
burst size.

Figure 2 and Table 2 show the effect of the time of
addition of T help on the frequency and the size of the
response (see also 9). We have experienced some variability
in the effectiveness of restoration of the response by allogeneic culture supernatants when Nude spleen cell suspensions
are used as a source of T depleted populations. We have,
therefore, added irradiated normal spleens (BDF$_1$) plus
concanavalin A (2 µg/ml) as a more reliable source of T
help. (It should be pointed out that for these experiments
in which we are interested in events that take place prior
to the addition of T help, the form that the T help takes is
irrelevant.)

It can be seen that restoration of both the frequency
and the burst size of the response is equally good whether
help is added at t=0 or t=24 hrs. If T help is added at
=48 hrs, variable results are obtained. In roughly half of
some 30 experiments the responses are the same or better
than at t=0. In the other half, smaller or no responses

Figure 1. Restoration of the anti-SRBC response of spleen cells from ATxBM mice with allogeneic culture supernatants or irradiated SRBC-primed spleen cells. ATxBM spleen cells were cultured at different concentrations for 4 days with SRBC alone, o, or in the presence of irradiated spleen cells from SRBC primed mice, Δ, or allogeneic culture supernatant, □. The number of anti-SRBC PFC per culture were determined and scored as negative, if there were less than 2 PFC, or positive, if there were two or more PFC per culture. The percent negative cultures is plotted on a logarithmic scale against the number of spleen cells per culture on a linear scale (data from Hunter and Kettman, 8). *

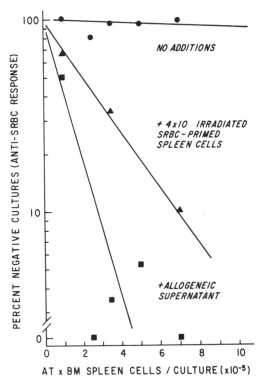

* The effects of mitogen-stimulated T cells on the response of B cell to antigen and the mechanism of T cell stimulation of the B cell response. R.W. Dutton and P. Hunter. in Cellular Selection and Regulation in the Immune Response. Edited by Gerald M. Edelman. Raven Press, New York © 1974

Table 1

RESPONSES OF ATxBM CELLS AT LIMITING DILUTIONS[a]

Culture medium and additions	Antigen	No. of cells containing one anti-SRBC responding unit x 10^{-5}	Anti-SRBC PFC per responding unit
Normal	SRBC	93.9 (45.3-195)[b]	5.2 (2.5-10.7)
Normal + 2 x 10^6 irradiated SRBC-primed cells	SRBC	2.97 (2.22-3.99)	33.7 (25.2-45.3)
Allogeneic culture supernatant	SRBC	1.21 (0.91-1.62)	47.6 (35.8-63.8)

[a] Data from Hunter and Kettman (8).

[b] Bracketed figures are the 95% confidence limits of each value.

Table 2

RESPONSE OF NUDE SPLEEN CELLS AT LIMITING DILUTION

T help[a] added at	No. cells with one anti-BRBC unit x 10^{-5}	Anti-BRBC per responding unit
0 hr	3.9	50
40 hr	3.9	55

[a] T help was provided by the addition of 10^6 irradiated BDF$_1$ spleen plus 2 μg/ml Con A.

See footnote on page 488.

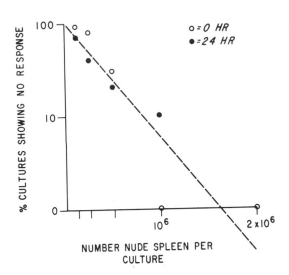

NUMBER NUDE SPLEEN PER
CULTURE

Figure 2. The effect of time of addition of T cells on
the response of spleen cells from Nude mice. Nude spleen
cells were cultured at various cell numbers with burro
erythrocytes (BRBC) and the number of anti-BRBC PFC measured at day 4. T cells were added either at time zero, o,
or at 24 hr, ●. The percent negative cultures were plotted
against spleen cell number per culture as indicated in the
legend to Figure 1. The source of T cell activity was
irradiated spleen cells from BDF_1 mice plus 2 µg/ml Con A
(data from Dutton and Hunter, 9).

ASSAY ON	PFC PER CULTURE		
	ZERO	10	100
DAY 2			
DAY 3			
DAY 4			

Figure 3. The kinetics of the response of spleens from
Nude mice. T help (10^6 irradiated BDF_1 + Con A, 2 µg/ml)
added at t=0 or t=40 hrs -●-●-●-. The antigen, burro
erythrocytes was added at t=0. (#274). See footnote on p. 488.

were obtained.

The kinetics of the response are illustrated in Figure 3. It can be seen that the number of PFC in cultures where T help was added at 40 hrs the response lags a little behind that of cultures where T help was added at t=0 when measured at day 3 but overtakes by day 4. It is clear that the rate of increase of the number of PFC between day 3 and day 4 cannot be accounted for by anything short of a frantic burst of proliferation. It would, therefore, seem more likely that proliferation was initiated prior to the addition of T help. That this is, indeed, the case is shown by the data in Table 3. Here antigen was added at t=0 and any cells proliferating in response to antigen were killed by a "hot pulse" of high specific activity H^3 thymidine present only between 24 and 48 hrs. In another experiment (Figure 4) it can be seen that no response is obtained if the addition of antigen is delayed until 48 hrs. The initiation of proliferation is thus dependent on the addition of antigen.

Two hypotheses have occurred to us to explain these results. First, antigen alone is sufficient to start the immune response and the proliferation of the responding B cells. The T cell factor or help is not needed for this phase of the response. The T cell factor, however, is required for some maturation process which allows the B cells to switch from inserting IgM monomer into their membranes to secretion of polymeric IgM from the cell (10).

Alternatively, it is possible that there is a small amount of T help available at time zero in the cultures of Nude spleen. On this explanation, the amount of help would be adequate for the first 48 hrs but then further T help would have to be added at that time. The early T help could be provided either by small numbers of T cells present in the spleens of Nude mice or by a factor present in the 5% fetal bovine serum contained in the medium.

The kinetics of the response when T help is delayed speaks against this explanation since these cultures are seen to be behind at day 3 as far as numbers of antibody-forming cells are concerned and they then catch up by day 4 (Figure 3). This argues in favor of a maturation role for T help but the arguement is admittedly somewhat weak.

A more direct test was therefore attempted. In the experiment illustrated in Figure 5, the Nude spleen cell suspensions were treated with rabbit anti-mouse brain antiserum plus complement prior to the culture incubation. The concentration of antiserum used was at least twice that required to completely abolish the response of BDF_1 mice to antigen and the proliferation response to T cell mitogens.

491

ADDITION, TIME			RESPONSE		
A G	S N	PULSE			
0	—	—			
0	0	—			
0	48	—			
0	48	24-48			
48	48	—			
PFC/CULTURE		ZERO	I	10	100

Figure 4. Antigen requirement for the initiation of proliferation. Spleen cell suspensions from Nude mice were incubated with additions added at the times indicated. The hot pulse was given by the addition of 10 µc H^3 thymidine added at 24 hrs and terminated by the addition of 100 µg cold thymidine at 48 hrs. 3×10^6 Nude spleen cells were incubated in 1 ml cultures. The antigen was burro erythrocytes. (#230).

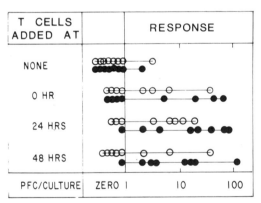

T CELLS ADDED AT	RESPONSE		
NONE			
0 HR			
24 HRS			
48 HRS			
PFC/CULTURE	ZERO I	10	100

Figure 5. The effect of rabbit anti-mouse brain plus complement treatment on the response of spleen cell suspensions from Nude mice. T help (10^6 irradiated BDF_1 spleen $\pm$ Con A, 2 µg/ml) was added at 0, 24, or 48 hrs. 10^6 Nude spleen cells (treated -•-•-•- or untreated -o-o-o-) were incubated with burro erythrocytes added at t=0. (#330)

Table 3

CELL DIVISION IN NUDE SPLEEN BEFORE ADDITION OF T CELLS
ANTIGEN (BRBC) ADDED AT t=0

Culture Conditions	Anti-BRBC PFC Per Culture			Expt. No.
	Time of T Cell Addition			
	Not Added	0 Hr	48 Hr	
Control	5	260	190	257
Pulse	-	45	30	
Block	-	290	155	
Control	10	165	185	258
Pulse	-	30	5	
Block	-	165	95	
Control	0	-	-	261
Pulse	-	95	10	
Block	-	275	165	

8×10^6 Nude spleen cells/culture. T cells = 2×10^6 irradiated BDF_1 spleen + 2 µg/ml Con A. Pulse = 10 µc H^3 thymidine at 30 c/mM at 24 hrs. The pulse was terminated by the
addition of 100 µg cold thymidine per 1 ml culture at 48 hrs.
Block = 10 µc H^3 thymidine at 30 c/mM plus 100 µg cold thymidine, both at 24 hrs. (Data from Dutton and Hunter, 9).
See footnote on page 488.

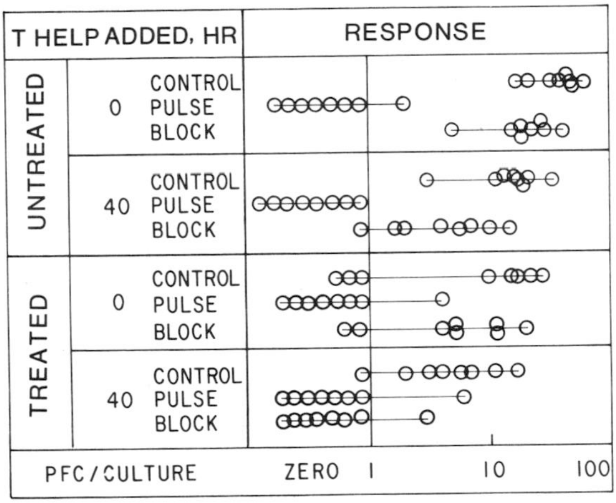

T HELP ADDED, HR			RESPONSE

Figure 6. The response of anti-mouse brain treated spleen cell suspensions from Nude mice incubated in serum-free medium. 0.1 ml cultures containing 10^6 treated or untreated Nude spleen cells were incubated in a serum-free medium and T help (10^6 irradiated BDF_1 + 2 µg/ml Con A + 5% fetal bovine serum) was added at 0 or 40 hrs. Burro erythrocytes were added at t=0. Control cultures had no further additions. The pulse cultures had 1 µc H^3 thymidine (per 0.1 ml) added at t=24 and 10 µg of cold thymidine added at t=40. Block cultures had both hot and cold thymidine added at t=24. The assay was on day 4.

It can be seen that the treated cells did at least as well as the untreated cells when T cell help was added at 0, 24, or 48 hrs.

In a second experiment Nude spleen cells were incubated in serum-free medium with antigen for 0, or 24 hrs prior to the addition of T help. The cells still responded as well when T help was added late. In a final preliminary experiment this effect was again observed with untreated Nude spleen cells in serum-free medium (upper panel of Figure 6). The mean response size was 37 PFC/culture when T help was added at zero time and 17 PFC/culture when added at 40 hours. The entire response was knocked out when hot pulsed with tritiated thymidine during the period 24-40 hours. Finally, in the bottom panel, it can be seen that even anti-mouse brain antigen and complement-treated cells still responded in serum-free medium when T help was added at 40 hours. When T help was added at zero time, the mean PFC per culture was 1 and it dropped to 6 when help was added at 40 hours. It should be noted, however, that the blocked pulse was not effective possibly because the 100 μg cold thymidine was inhibitory to these "maltreated" cells. Whatever the reason it prevents one from demonstrating in this case that division took place prior to the addition of T help. A further experiment in deficient serum (i.e., serum that does not support a primary immune response) gave almost identical results. Although it is not possible to exclude totally the possibility that some T cell help is still present in the 0-48 hour period even under these conditions, the results would seem to favor the hypothesis that proliferation can be initiated by antigen alone and that T cell help is needed later for some maturation process.

ACKNOWLEDGEMENTS

This work was supported by USPHS grant AI-08795 and American Cancer Society grant IM-1G. Dr. R. W. Dutton is supported by American Cancer Society Career Development Award PRA-73

The skilled technical assistance of Sara Albanil is gratefully acknowledged.

REFERENCES

1. Katz, D. H. and Benacerraf, B. (1972) Adv. Immunol. 15, 1.

2. Feldmann, M. and Nossal, G. J. V. (1972) Transplant. Review 13, 3.

3. Dutton, R. W., Falkoff, R., Hirst, J. A., Hoffmann, M., Kappler, J. W., Kettman, J. R., Lesley, J. R. and Vann, D. (1971) Progr. Immunol. 1, 355.
4. Katz, D. H., Hamaoka, M. E., Dorf, P. H., Maurer, P. H. and Benacerraf, B. (1973) J. Exp. Med. 138, 734.
5. Feldmann, M., Cone, R. E. and Marchalonis, J. J. (1973) Cell. Immunol. 9. 1.
6. Bretscher, P. and Cohn, M. (1970) Science 169, 1042.
7. Schimpl, A. and Wecker, E. (1972) Nature New Biol. 237, 15.
8. Hunter, P. and Kettman, J. R. (1974) Proc. Nat. Acad. Sci. 71, (in press).
9. Dutton, R. W. and Hunter, P. (1974) in Cellular Selection and Regulation. Raven Press, (in press).
10. Melchers, F. and Andersson, J. (1973) Transplant. Review 14, 76.

ANTIGEN SPECIFIC T CELL FACTORS AND THEIR
ROLE IN THE REGULATION OF T-B INTERACTION

Marc Feldmann

ICRF Tumour Immunology Unit,
Department of Zoology, University College
London, WC1E 6BT, England

ABSTRACT. The mechanism of T-B lymphocyte cooperation in the
response to hapten protein conjugates in vitro was investigated. It was found that populations of activated T cells
(ATC)[1] cultured with antigen released a specific factor
which, when bound to the surface of macrophages permits them
to trigger cells. This factor was identified as a complex
of antigen and an immunoglobulin which was termed IgT. IgT
was also found to participate in the regulation of the antibody response. In the absence of macrophages, or if present
in high concentration, IgT complexes suppressed lymphocyte
function, causing specific T cell suppression. IgT complexes
present on the surface of macrophages induced a non-specific
suppression of cooperative responses by blocking receptor
sites for IgT. This nonspecific suppression strongly
resembles that of 'antigenic competition'. This communication reviews the evidence supporting this mechanism of T-B
cooperation and its regulation, and also discusses the
aspects of this scheme which need further clarification.

---

[1] The abbreviations used are: Anti MIg: Antimouse Ig antiserum; Anti K: Antimouse K antibody; Anti μ: Antimouse μ
antibody; Anti T: heterologous (sheep) antimouse T cell
antiserum; ATC: activated T cells; DNP: dinitrophenyl
determinant; DNPPOL: dinitrophenyl polymeric flagellin;
FγG: Fowl gamma globulin; IgT: Immunoblobulin released by
T cells: Ig: Immunoglobulin; NIP: 4-hydroxy-3-iodo-5-
nitrophenylacetyl determinant; NIP SIII: Type III pneumococcal polysaccharide conjugated with NIP; KLH: Keyhole
limpet hemocyanin; S/N: Supernatant; TNP: Trinitrophenyl
determinant

INTRODUCTION

Recent in vitro studies of the mechanism of T-B co-operation in the antibody response to hapten protein conjugates have indicated that populations of activated T cells (ATC) release, in the presence of antigen, a specific factor which binds to macrophages, permitting them to stimulate B cells to synthesize antibody (reviewed in 2,3). By absorption of ATC supernatant with sepharose beads conjugated with antimouse Ig antibody it was found that the specific factor contained Ig determinants (1,2,3). Since it was only released by viable T cells, this immunoglobulin factor was termed IgT. A diagramatic representation of this scheme of cooperation is shown in Fig 1. Subsequent studies have implicated IgT in two other immunological phenomena which depend on T cells, namely specific T cell suppression, and antigenic competition. This communication briefly reviews the evidence for the three cell model of T-B inter-action involving IgT as a specific medicator, and some of the evidence relating the mechanism of specific T cell suppression and antigenic competition to this model of cell cooperation. The multiple functions of IgT suggest that it plays an important role in immune induction and homeostasis.

METHODS

These have all been published elsewhere (see, for example, 4,5).

SPECIFIC COOPERATION MEDIATED BY SUBCELLULAR SUPERNATANTS OF ACTIVATED T CELLS

While the initial experiments to demonstrate that co-operation between T and B cells did not involve direct T/B contact were performed in double chamber flasks (4), sub-sequent experiments have been performed using supernatants of T cells activated (in irradiated mice) to protein carriers (Fowl gamma globulin, FγG or Keyhole limpet hemocyanin, KLH) which were cultured for 2 days in the presence of the dinitrophenylated carrier. Such super-natants were filtered through a 0.22μ millipore filter and were either used immediately, or could be kept at -20° for some months. The assays for the helper capacity of these supernatants was to add serial dilutions of S/N to populat-ions of mouse spleen cells containing B cells and macro-phages. Both hapten primed and unprimed B cells responded to ATC supernatants, at the appropriate dilution.

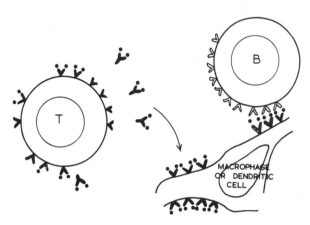

INTERACTION   VIA Ig T ANTIGEN   BOUND   TO
MACROPHAGES

Figure 1

Schematic model of cooperation between T and B cells, after
T cells have been activated by antigen.
IgT complexed with antigen is released from ATC, and binds
to the surface of 'macrophages'.

With excess concentrations of supernatant immunogenicity
was reduced (6). The results of a typical experiment of this
sort, using normal mouse spleen cells depleted of T cells by
antiserum, are shown in Table 1. Specificity of the response
is indicated and by the lack of response to NIPKLH, incorporated in the same cultures (NIP and DNP, despite both being
nitrophenyl haptens cross react weakly.)
     The use of T cell supernatants to provide helper
function facilitates an analysis of its chemical basis. The
role of the immunoglobulin (Ig) in the mediation of specific
help was evaluated by the use of antimouse Ig (anti MIg)
antibody coupled to sepharose beads. Absorption of ATC
supernatants with sepharose conjugated polyvalent antiMIg,
or specific antiK chain or anti μ chain antibodies removed
the specific helper activity from these supernatants, as
shown in Table 2. This experiment indicated that the
specific helper factor is an immunoglobulin; and that its
heavy chain possesses μ-like determinants, confirming prior
results (7). The importance of adherent cells in cooperation is shown in Table 3. Thus these results support
the 3 cell concept of T-B cooperation, involving macrophage
like cells as the third cell in the cooperation (1,2,3,7).
     Antibody responses in vitro such as those described in
Tables 1,2 and 3 and others published previously (e.g. 4,7)
are mainly IgM in nature. Since the mechanisms of T-B cooperation for IgM responses may differ from those for IgG
responses, it was thus important to verify the major
conclusions for IgG responses also, i.e. specific role of
ATC supernatants, and of adherent cells in specific cooperation. Using B cells from mice multiply primed with
trinitrophenylated Keyhole limpet hemocyanin (TNP-KLH), by
the method of Bullock and Rittenberg (8) good IgG responses
may be obtained in vitro. The results in Tables 2 and 3
indicate that ATC supernatants may induce optimal IgG
responses, but only in the prefence of adherent cells, in
close analogy to the results obtained with IgM responses
(5,7).

REGULATION OF THE ANTIBODY
RESPONSE BY T CELL SUPERNATANTS

     Specific cooperation, as envisaged in Fig 1, takes
place on the membrane of a non-lymphoid third party adherent
cell, presumbaly a macrophage or a dendritic reticulum cell.
Thus, as expected no responses were obtained in the
absence of adherent cells (5,7). Furthermore a state of
partial tolerance has been induced by incubation of lymphoid

cells, depleted of macrophages with T cell supernatants in immunogenic concentrations (9), or by incubating whole spleen cell populations with supraimmunogenic concentrations of ATC supernatant (6). The nature of the factor in ATC supernatant inducing partial tolerance was investigated by absorbing ATC supernatants with anti Ig antibodies coupled to sepharose beads. As shown in Table 4, polyvalent anti Ig, or specific anti K or anti μ antibodies removed the specific inhibitory factor from the ATC supernatant; indicating a close resemblance of the suppressive factor to the specific IgT mediator of cooperation (1,2,3,7).

A nonspecific form of suppression may also be induced by supernatants of ATC. Experiments designed to analyse, in vitro, the mechanism of antigenic competition induced by the injection of red cells in vivo had revealed a reversible lesion at the macrophage surface (10). It was thus possible, because of the central and nonspecific role of the macrophage in T-B cooperation that antigenic competition was due to competition for the binding of IgT-antigen complexes to the appropriate receptors on the surface of macrophages. This concept was supported by demonstrating the incapacity of macrophages, which had been incubated with a T cell supernatant of one specifically to bind a second supernatant, of different antigenic specificity, in an immunogenic way.

By incubating ATC supernatants with sepharose beads coupled with anti Ig antibodies, the nature of the 'nonspecific blocker' i.e. the inducer of a state analogous to antigenic competition, was also found to be a molecule possessing Ig determinants (Table 5).

CELLULAR SOURCE OF IgT

The results presented above suggest that T cell released Ig (IgT) has an important role in cell cooperation and its regulation. The cellular source of IgT thus becomes an important issue; which is at present unresolved. While it is possible to demonstrate that the cell releasing IgT is a T cell, by the use of anti θ, anti T and anti Ig antiserum on populations of helper cells obtained from immunized or irradiated mice (11), it is not possible to use these cell populations to determine the cell source of IgT, because of the problems of antibody cytophilic for T cells which could have been adsorbed in vivo (12,13). Thus a system was developed, in collaboration with Dr Sirkka Kontiainen which permits virgin T cells to be immunized in vitro into highly effective helper cells (14). Using this system (Table 6) it was possible to induce helper cells from highly purified

population of T cells, e.g. cortisone resistant thymus cells
which had been further depleted of B cells by treatment with
anti Ig serum (15) and by passage through a nylon wool
column (16). These results suggest, but by no means prove
the T cell origin of IgT. Proof will require further
purifications, and incorporation studies.

Another approach to this problem is by the use of
lymphoid cell lines which bear both the θ antigen, taken to
be a marker of T and not B lymphocytes, and membrane Ig.
Since these tumours have been cloned, and grow _in vitro_,
there can be no question as to the synthesis of their Ig by
these cells. Ig produced by these cells does have some of
the characteristics expected of IgT, namely that it blocks
cooperative responses, but not thymus independent antibody
responses (17).

AN INTEGRATED MODEL OF CELL COOPERATION AND ITS REGULATION

The model of cell cooperation (Fig 1) illustrates the
specific events after the activation of T cells into helper
cells. These studies emphasize the role of IgT and its
interaction with a non-lymphoid macrophage like cell, not
only in the induction of the response, but also in its
regulation. Induction of responses involves the binding of
IgT to the membrane of these macrophages. Specific suppression of lymphocyte function occurs as a consequence of the
binding of complexes of IgT and antigen to the surface of
lymphocytes (T or B). This latter situation closely
resembles the mechanism of antibody-mediated suppression
induced by complexes of antigen and humoral antibody
(reviewed 1,18). Non-specific suppression was caused by IgT
complexes blocking the receptors for IgT on macrophages.

Macrophages have an important function in the regulation
of the nature of IgT action, in determining whether it is
'positive' or 'negative'. The maximal levels of cooperative capacity are set by the number of macrophage
surface IgT complexes. Since IgT is highly cytophilic for
these macrophages, which are much more common than antigen
specific lymphocytes, the bulk of IgT would rapidly become
membrane bound, and could act in a cooperative way. Only
when there is local excess, and many of the IgT receptors
are saturated, would significant concentrations of IgT be
present in the microenvironment, capacle of reacting with
antigen specific lymphocytes. This action of IgT complexes
explain the triphasic T cell/immune response curves usually
found, with an incremental phase, a plateau, and a

diminution (e.g. ref. 1). Clearly IgT complexes would act in a local fashion preventing the overstimulation of antigen specific lymphocytes. Whether these complexes can also act in a more diffuse fashion, to induce T cell mediated tolerance or 'infectious tolerance' (19) remains to be established. The functional blockage of macrophage IgT receptors by these complexes has been reported to be the lesion in a model of antigenic competition induced in vivo (10,20). The consequences of antigenic competition in immune homeostasis have been adequately described elsewhere (21,22). Many problems remain in the evaluation of the relevance of these in vitro findings to in vivo immune physiology. First, it is now known that IgT complexes function equally well in vivo as in vitro, inducing considerable responses in T cell deprived rats, as shown by Tada et al (23), or mice as shown by Rieber and Riethmuller (24). The importance of adherent cells for the induction of antibody responses has been confirmed by Gisler et al (25) in vitro, by Cone et al (26), and by Rieber and Riethmuller (24) who found these complexes bind to macrophage like cells, but not to lymphocytes. Thus it is known that binding of IgT complexes to macrophages is of importance in inducing cooperative responses. Not yet known however, is the mechanism by which IgT complexes, once bound to macrophages actually triggers B cells. On theoretical grounds, it was suggested that if IgT complexes induce the formation, on the macrophage membrane of a matrix antigenic determinants, these could, by resembling the surface of thymus independent antigens, trigger B cells. Two lines of evidence support the concept of IgT induced antigen-matrices - firstly, autoradiographs of surface IgT bound to macrophages always indicated a patchy distribution (26). Secondly, macrophages incubated with a mixture of two T cell supernatants were unable to induce a response to either antigen (20) despite significant binding of each to macrophages. These results clearly do not exclude the possibility that macrophages, after binding IgT complexes, become activated to release various mediators, as suggested by Waldman and Munro (27) and by Schrader (28).

Similarly the mechanism of IgT complex induced suppression is not understood in detail. A major point of uncertainty is the duration of suppression, and of its reversibility - is it a long lasting tolerance, or a reversible block? Preliminary studies have indicated that T cells are more sensitive to this form of suppression, than B cells. Whether this indicates a difference in the mechanism of tolerance induction in T and B cells remains to be established. In vivo, there are now several reported examples of T cell mediated tolerance, described in diverse experimental models e.g. by Gershon and Kondo (19) using red cells, by Ada and Cooper (29) and Basten et al (30) using protein antigens. The mechanisms of these are compatible with the concept of 'excess help', i.e. with the same class of IgT as the helper molecule (see discussion in ref. 2). However, using rat thymocytes, Tada and his colleagues (23) have been able to separate by column chromography an IgT molecule which participates in cooperation, from a non-immunoglobulin, lower MW molecule which suppressed IgE responses. Whether there are different T cell suppressor molecules in different species, or in the IgE vs. IgG responses is not yet known.

The results already obtained in a combination of in vitro/in vivo systems have indicated that the macrophage surface block of cooperative responses produced by the injection of red cells in vivo (10) may be mimicked by the addition of ATC supernatant to macrophages (20). Since this block can also be relieved by trypsinization, and because both cooperative and competition inducing activities are removed by incubation with anti MIg antibody coupled to sepharose, it was deduced that the blocking factor was IgT complexes, presumably those involved in the cooperative response to the first (competing) antigen.

However, these experiments do not formally exclude the possibility that the IgT involved in antigenic competition is different from that involved in cell cooperation. Thus there currently is much uncertainty about the diversity of classes of IgT molecules, in view of the diversity of their function. I prefer the simpler hypothesis of only one class of IgT, based on the fact that it is conceivable to propose mechanisms by which one molecule could exert such different effects.

Quite a separate issue from the above, the effector functions of IgT, is the cellular source of IgT. This issue has relevance to the T cell receptors for antigen. At the moment it is not yet proven that IgT is biosynthesized by T cells. Certain lines of evidence indicate that certain T cells may adsorb Ig of B cell origin (e.g. 12,13). But none of these studies have yet investigated whether this Ig has any of the properties of IgT (see above). Other lines of evidence suggest that T cells may synthesize IgT. For example Rieber et al (31) trypsinized mouse thymus cells, and demonstrated that treated cells took up much less ^{125}I labelled Fab anti Ig (<35%) than before. After 8 hours incubation at 37°, these cells took up more Fab anti Ig than immediately after trypsinization, approximately 70% as much as cultured untreated thymus cells.

Another approach, which may prove fruitful, is the analysis of θ positive, Ig positive lymphomas (e.g. 32,33). If it can be proved that these tumours are indeed T cell derived; it will be established that T cells synthesize Ig. Such studies are in progress.

ACKNOWLEDGEMENTS

This work was supported by the Imperial Cancer Research Fund. Marc Feldmann was supported by a C.J. Martin Fellowship of the National Health and Medical Research Council, Australia. The generous gifts of reagents by Drs. M.F. Greaves, M.D. Cooper, R. Mage, O. Makela and I. McConnell, and the technical assistance of Mr B. de Sousa and Miss L. Auty in these studies, was much appreciated.

REFERENCES

1. M. Feldmann and G.J.V. Nossal, Transplant. Rev. 13 3 (1972).
2. M. Feldmann, Series Hematologica (in press).
3. M. Feldmann, In, Lymphocytes - structures and function, (Ed.) J.J. Marchalonis, Marcel Dekker Inc, New York
4. M. Feldmann and A. Basten, J. Exp. Med. 136, 49 (1972).
5. M. Feldmann, J. Exp. Med. 135, 1049 (1972).
6. M. Feldmann, Eur. J. Immunol. (submitted).
7. M. Feldmann, J. Exp. Med. 136, 737 (1972).
8. W.W. Bullock and M.B. Rittenberg, Immunochemistry 8, 310 (1970).
9. M. Feldmann, Nature New Biology 242, 82 (1973).
10. J.W. Schrader and M. Feldmann, Eur. J. Immunol. 3, 711 (1973).
11. M. Feldmann, J. Sprent and L. Hudson, Eur. J. Immunol. (in press).
12. B. Pernis, J F.A.P. Miller, L. Forni and J. Sprent, Cell. Immunol. (in press).
13. A.F. Williams and S. Hunt, unpublished data (1973).
14. S. Kontiainen and M. Feldmann, Nature New Biology 245, 285 (1973).
15. T. Takahashi, L.J. Old, K.R. McIntire and E.A. Boyse, J. Exp. Med. 134, 815 (1971).
16. M. Julius, E. Simpson, and L.A. Herzenberg, Eur. J. Immunol. 3, 645 (1973).
17. M. Feldmann and A. Boyslton, Nature (in press).
18. E. Diener and M. Feldmann, Transplant. Rev. 8, 76 (1972).
19. R.K. Gershon and K. Kondo, Immunology 21, 903 (1971).

20. M. Feldmann and J.W. Schrader, Cell. Immunology (in press)
21. M.J. Taussig, Current Topics in Microbiology and
    Immunology 60, 125 (1973).
22. P. Liacopoulos and S. Ben Efraim, Prog. Allergy (in press)
23. T. Tada, K. Okamura and M. Taniguchi, Proc. VIII
    Int. Congress Allergology, Excerpta Medica (in press).
24. E.P. Rieber and G. Riethmuller, Eur. J. Immunol. (in
    press).
25. R.H. Gisler, F. Staber, E. Rude and P. Dukor, Eur. J.
    Immunol. 3, 650 (1973).
26. R.E. Cone, M. Feldmann, J.J. Marchalonis and G.J.V.
    Nossal, Immunology 26, 49 (1974).
27. H. Waldmann and A. Munro, Nature 243, 356 (1973).
28. J.W. Schrader, J. Exp. Med. 138, 1466 (1973).
29. G.L. Ada and M. Cooper, unpublished data (1973).
30. A. Basten, J.F.A.P. Miller, C. Cheers and J. Sprent,
    manuscript submitted
31. E.P. Rieber, G. Riethmuller and M. Hadam, Protides
    Biol. Fluids 21, 311 (1974).
32. A.W. Harris, A. Bankhurst, S. Mason and N.L. Warner,
    J. Immunol. 110, 431 (1973).
33. A. Boylston, Immunology 24, 851 (1973).
34. K. Shortman, N. Williams, H. Jackson, P. Russell, P.
    Byrt and E. Diener, J. Cell. Biol. 48, 566 (1971).

Table 1

Specific Cooperation with ATC supernatants in vitro

Cells Cultured	Stimulus	IgM Response (AFC/Culture ± SE)	
		Anti DNP	Anti NIP
Anti T treated normal Spleen	NIL	30 ± 21	27 ± 18
"	DNP POL	1100 ± 106	33 ± 25
"	NIP SIII	20 ± 8	360 ± 55
"	S/N of ATC$_{F\gamma G}$	713 ± 54	40 ± 26
	& DNP FγG	713 ±, 54	40 ± 26
"	"		
	& NIP KLH	680 ± 120	37 ± 32
"	NIP KLH	33 ± 23	27 ± 8
"	DNP FγG	47 ± 12	13 ± 9

Normal spleen cells were depleted of T cells by sheep anti T
cell antiserum. Concentrations of antigens used were DNPPOL
NIP KLH, DNP$_{F\gamma G}$ 10^{-1} μg/ml, NIP SIII 10^{-2} μg/ml. Optimal

egend to Table 1 cont.,
oncentrations of S/N were used. Response measured at 4 days.

Table 2

Immunoglobulin nature of cooperative factor

| Cells Cultured | Stimulus | Response Anti DNP (AFC/Culture ± SE) | |
		IgM	IgG
NP KLH primed spleen	NIL	110 ± 86	0
" "	TNP KLH	3820 ± 271	2670 ± 361
nti T treated TNP KLH primed spleen	NIL	50 ± 32	0
" "	TNP KLH	175 ± 54	0
" "	S/N of ATC$_{F\gamma G}$ +DNPFγG	1625 ± 285	1920 ± 392
" "	S/N Seph-anti MIg	210 ± 122	0
" "	S/N Seph-anti K	160 ± 86	115 ± 85
" "	S/N Seph-anti μ	365 ± 205	85 ± 37

pleen cells from mice primed three times with TNP KLH
dsorbed onto bentonite, were used 6 weeks after the last
njection. TNP KLH was used at $10^{-2}\mu g/ml$. Optimal con-
entration of S/N ATC$_{F\gamma G}$ + DNPFγG used. Similar dilution
nown of anti Ig absorbed SEN. No significant responses were
btained with absorbed S/N even if used at 100 greater
oncentrations.
ata from M. Feldmann and M.F. Greaves, unpublished, 1973)

507

Table 3

Macrophage requirement for collaboration
with cell free supernatant

Cells cultured	Stimulus	Anti DNP Response (AFC/Culture ± SE)	
		IgM	IgG
TNP KLH primed spleen	NIL	53 ± 47	0
" "	TNP KLH	2620 ± 412	1120 ± 366
" "	S/N of ATC$_{F\gamma G}$ & FγG	100 ± 22	10 ± 7
" "	S/N of ATC$_{F\gamma G}$ & DNPFγG	1930 ± 313	860 ± 192
Adherent cell depleted	NIL	30 ± 22	0
TNP KLH primed spleen	TNP KLH	80 ± 67	0
" "	S/N of ATC$_{F\gamma G}$ & FγG	47 ± 18	0
" "	S/N of ATC$_{F\gamma G}$ & DNPFγG	20 ± 15	0

Spleen cells from mice primed three times with TNP KLH, last time four weeks
previously. Adherent cell depletion performed by the technique of Shortman
et al (34).

Table 4

Immunoglobulin nature of T cell suppression

Cells Cultured	Supernatant	Challenge	Anti DNP Response (AFC/Culture ± SE)	
			IgM	IgG
TNPKLH spleen depleted	–	TNPKLH	255± 20	0
of adherent cells	–	NIL	50± 40	0
"	–	DNPPOL	950±155	610±41
"	S/N of ATC$_{F\gamma G}$&DNPFγG	"	110± 80	0
"	" abs Seph-anti MIG	"	1150±155	580±21
"	" abs Seph-anti K	"	1210±210	1650±36
"	" abs Seph-anti μ	"	995±110	910±11
"	" abs Seph-anti NRG	"	155±100	0

TNPKLH primed spleen cells were depleted of adherent cells by the technique of
Shortman et al (34). They were incubated with S/N for 6 hours and then washed and
challenged as shown, with either 10 ng/ml TNPKLH or DNPPOL. Equivalent concentratic
of S/N or absorbed supernatants were used.
(Data from M. Feldmann, submitted for publication, 1974, ref. 29)

Table 5

Ig nature of helper and competitive material from ATC

Macrophages[1] incubated with supernatants from:	Antibody[2] response (AFC/Culture ± SE)	
	DNP	NIP
I ATC$_{KLH}$ & DNP KLH[2]	720 ± 90	10 ± 10
II ATC$_{F\gamma G}$ & NIP FγG[4]	25 ± 20	440 ± 105
III I and then II[5]	655 ± 105	40 ± 25
IV I and II simultaneously[6]	65 ± 40	55 ± 30
V I incubated with sepharose anti Ig beads[7]	0	25 ± 10
VI V and then II	0	375 ± 60
VII I incubated with sepharose NRG beads, then II	575 ± 30	42 ± 20

[1] 10^5 purified adherent cells added to 1.5 x 10^7 normal CBA spleen cells. Four cultures per group. Analogous results obtained with up to 5 x 10^5 macrophages per culture.

[2] IgM response. There was no IgG response.

[3] 100 ng/ml DNP KLH.

[4] 1 μg/ml NIP FγG.

[5,6] One population of macrophages incubated with two supernatants. In group III, the macrophages were washed to remove excess supernatant I.

[7] 2 ml of supernatant incubated with 1 ml of packed sepharose - anti Ig or NRG.

(Data from M. Feldmann and J.W. Schrader, submitted for publication 1974, ref. 19)

Table 6

Induction of helper cells from purified
non-immune T cell populations

Helper Cells	% B	Challenge	Anti DNP Response (AFC/Culture)
NIL		NIL	30
NIL		TNP KLH	23
NIL		DNP POL	1020
LN (10^5)	28	TNP KLH	780
CRT (10^5)	0.2	"	595
CRT, anti Ig (10^5)	0.03	"	610
CRT, anti Ig nylon wool (10^5)	0.002	"	560

Helper cells were induced by 4 day culture of LN (pooled
mesenteric and peripheral) with 1μg/KLH, or CRT (and deri-
vations) with 10^{-1} μg/ml KLH. Percentage of B cells was
established by staining with a fluoresceinated anti Ig and a
heterologous anti B serum. Anti DNP responses of normal
spleen after 4 days culture in response to 10^{-1}μg/ml TNPKLH
and 10^5 cultured 'helper cells', or 1 μg/ml DNPPOL.
(Data from Feldmann, Kontiainen and Greaves, unpublished
1974)

THE NATURE OF THE SIGNALS REQUIRED FOR THE INDUCTION OF ANTIBODY SYNTHESIS

James Watson

The Salk Institute for Biological Studies
P.O. Box 1809
San Diego, California   92112

ABSTRACT: The interaction of antigen with precursors of antibody-forming cells regulates the further development of these cells. Antigen induces precursor cells to proliferate and mature to antibody-forming cells or can lead to the inactivation of precursor cells resulting in tolerance. The phenotype expressed by precursor cells may be determined by changes in the intracellular levels of cyclic AMP and cyclic GMP. Increasing intracellular levels of cyclic AMP leads to the inactivation of precursor cells whereas increasing intracellular levels of cyclic GMP leads to the proliferation and maturation of precursor cells to antibody-forming cells. It is suggested that the interaction of antigen with surface immunoglobulin receptors activates an adenyl cyclase system in precursor cells and that the cooperating cell system has the function of stimulating guanyl cyclase activity in precursor cells. The induction of antibody synthesis requires the delivery of two independent, membrane-mediated signals to precursor cells, which activate each of these enzyme systems. It appears the ratio of cyclic AMP: cyclic GMP rather than the absolute level of a cyclic nucleotide determines the phenotypic expression.

INTRODUCTION

The interaction of antigen with surface immunoglobulin receptors on precursors of antibody-forming cells regulates the phenotypic expression of these cells. Precursor cells* appear to be programmed to develop in either of two pathways. The first may be considered an inductive pathway which is expressed when cells are stimulated by antigen to proliferate and mature to antibody-forming cells. The second is the tolerogenic pathway which is expressed when cells are rendered noninducible, or inactivated by antigen (1-4). The question considered here concerns how the interaction of a

---

*The term precursor cells used here refers specifically to precursor antibody-forming cells.

511

specific molecule (antigen) with precursor cells leads to
biochemical changes that determine which phenotype the cell
will express. The small number of specific antigen-binding
cells in any given lymphoid population imposes restrictions
on how biochemical changes that result from the interaction
with antigen can be measured. In addition to binding specific
antigen, lymphoid cells bind a number of agents such as
plant lectins (5-8) bacterial lipopolysaccharides (9-11) and
various catecholamines (12,13). The interaction of these
agents with lymphoid cells elicit a variety of distinctive
changes (5-13). The rationale for the experiments described
here was based upon observations that in many mammalian
cells, membrane-mediated events which result in the intracellular initiation of pleiotypic responses giving rise to
the expression of new morphological or functional characteristics can often be induced by the addition of high concentrations of adenosine 3',5'-cyclic monophosphate (cyclic AMP)
to cells (14,15). Since the enzymes required for the intracellular synthesis of cyclic AMP are membrane-bound possibly
linked to surface receptors, and, agents that stimulate
intracellular cyclic AMP synthesis also influence phenotypic
changes in cells, cyclic AMP has long been considered to be
involved as an intracellular mediator of programmed cell
functions (14-18). In contrast, guanosine 3',5'-cyclic monophosphate (cyclic GMP) may be involved as an intracellular
mediator of events that lead to cell proliferation (18,19).
If antigen induces the expression of predetermined pathways
in precursor cells, these cyclic nucleotides may perform a
role as intracellular mediators of the expression of these
pathways. Since precursor cells have the ability to express
more than one phenotype it is important to distinguish how
intracellular mediators determine which phenotype the cell
is to express.

The work presented here describes the involvement of
cyclic AMP and cyclic GMP in the determination of the developmental pathway a precursor cell follows. First, the
effects of exogenous cyclic AMP and cyclic GMP on the induction of *in vitro* immune responses to heterologous erythrocyte antigens will be considered. The effects of these
exogenous cyclic nucleotides have been compared to those of
two types of catecholamines: isoproterenol, a beta-adrener-
gic agonist which activates adenyl cyclase (12,13,15,16) and
carbamyl choline chloride (carbachol), a cholinergic agonist
which activates guanyl cyclase (13). Second, the effect of
cyclic nucleotides on the mitogenic and immunogenic activities of LPS will be considered. Third, the effect of LPS

and allogeneic supernatant factors on intracellular cyclic AMP and cyclic GMP levels in lymphoid cells will be analyzed. This will be related to the ability of LPS and allogeneic factors to stimulate immune responses in mouse spleen cultures. The results of these investigations lead to the suggestion that the exogenous signals delivered to precursor cells that constitute the inductive stimulus may function via the activators of both adenyl and guanyl cyclase systems in precursor cells.

EFFECT OF CYCLIC NUCLEOTIDES ON PRECURSOR CELL ACTIVITY

The induction of *in vitro* immune responses to SRBC requires the interaction of cooperating cell types (thymus-derived and adherent) with precursor antibody-forming cells (20,21). The addition of agents to spleen cultures could affect any one of these three cell types to inhibit or enhance the production of immune responses. The protocol outlined in Table 1 was used to analyze the effects of cyclic nucleotides specifically on precursor cell activity.

Nude spleen cells as a source of precursor cells were first pretreated with various agents, washed and recultured with activated T cells (T_{SRBC}) which provide a source of both T cells and adherent cells. Sheep erythrocytes (SRBC) were used as antigen.

1. *Raising intracellular levels of cyclic AMP leads to precursor cell inactivation.* The data shown in Figure 1 show the effects of different concentrations of dibutyryl cyclic AMP, isoproterenol, cyclic GMP and carbachol on the induction of immune responses in nude spleen cultures supplemented with T_{SRBC} and SRBC when present during the entire culture period. High concentrations of dibutyryl cyclic AMP ($>10^{-3}\underline{M}$) and isoproterenol ($>10^{-4}\underline{M}$) completely inhibit the inductive process whereas high concentrations of cyclic GMP ($10^{-3}\underline{M}$) and carbachol ($10^{-3}\underline{M}$) show little effect. At lower concentrations both dibutyryl cyclic AMP and isoproterenol show consistent 2- to 6-fold enhancements of immune responses (Fig. 1). The experiment shown in Figure 2 is designed to show the effects of dibutyryl cyclic AMP and isoproterenol just on precursor cells. Pretreatment of nude spleen cells with inactivating concentrations of dibutyryl cyclic AMP ($2\times10^{-3}\underline{M}$) or isoproterenol ($5\times10^{-4}\underline{M}$) for periods up to 12 hours in the absence of SRBC results in marked stimulations (2- to 4-fold) of immune responses upon subsequent challenge with T_{SRBC} and SRBC (Fig. 2). The presence of

513

Table 1

PROTOCOL FOR PRECURSOR CELL ANALYSIS

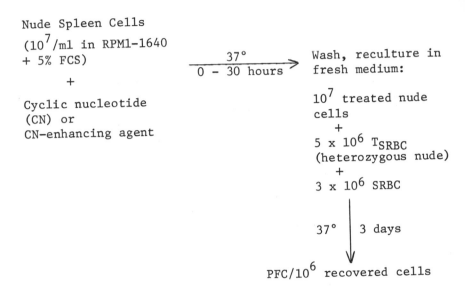

Nude Spleen Cells
(10^7/ml in RPM1-1640
+ 5% FCS)

+

Cyclic nucleotide
(CN) or
CN-enhancing agent

$\xrightarrow[\text{0 - 30 hours}]{37°}$

Wash, reculture in
fresh medium:

10^7 treated nude
cells
+
5 x 10^6 T_{SRBC}
(heterozygous nude)
+
3 x 10^6 SRBC

37° | 3 days

PFC/10^6 recovered cells

Homozygous nude mice were bred as described elsewhere
(8). Heterozygous nude littermates were used to prepare
thymus cells immunized to SRBC (8). *In vitro* immune responses were studied using mouse spleen cultures exactly as
described by Mishell and Dutton (20). Cultures were fed
daily with a nutritional mixture, and hemolytic plague-
forming cells (PFC) were measured using a microscope slide
assay (20). Cyclic nucleotides or cyclic nucleotide-
enhancing agents were dissolved in a balanced salt solution
(20) and added to cultures in 0.1 ml volumes.

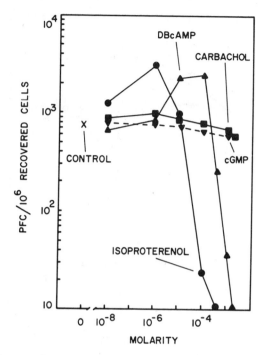

Fig. 1. Effect of cyclic nucleotides on *in vitro* immune responses to SRBC. Nude spleen cells were cultured at a density of 10^7 cells/ml with 5×10^6 T_{SRBC}, 3×10^6 SRBC and the concentrations of the agents indicated. Four days later PFC directed against SRBC were determined. The control value represents the PFC in cultures lacking cyclic nucleotides, isoproterenol or carbachol. All points represent the mean determined from duplicate cultures.

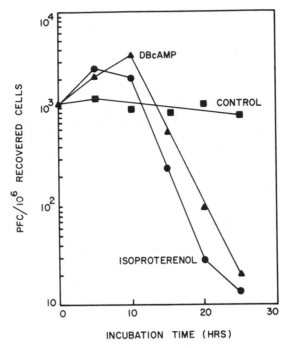

Fig. 2. The kinetics of precursor cell inactivation. Nude
spleen cells were cultured as described in Table 1 with
$2x10^{-3}\underline{M}$ dibutyryl cyclic AMP or $5x10^{-4}\underline{M}$ isoproterenol. At
the times indicated, individual cultures were collected,
centrifuged and recultured in 1 ml fresh medium with $5x10^6$
T_{SRBC} and $3x10^6$ SRBC. Three days after the time of washing,
cultures were assayed for PFC. The control cultures were
treated exactly the same way except that dibutyryl cyclic
AMP and isoproterenol were lacking. All points represent
the mean of duplicate cultures.

SRBC in nude spleen cultures does not affect the results (18). However, when the pretreatment period is extended there follows an exponential decrease in precursor cell activity. Treatment of precursor cells for 20 to 30 hours results in a complete and irreversible inactivation of precursor cells (Fig. 2).

2. *Cyclic AMP-induced inactivation reversed by cyclic GMP.* The data presented in Table 2 demonstrate that the simultaneous presence of cyclic GMP or carbachol can partially or completely reverse the inactivating effects of high concentrations of dibutyryl cyclic AMP or isoproterenol on precursor cells.

The finding that cyclic GMP reverses the inactivating effects of dibutyryl cyclic AMP may be explained by competition between these cyclic nucleotides for entry to precursor cells. However, since cyclic GMP also tends to reverse the inhibitory effects of isoproterenol, and carbachol reverses the inhibitory effects of both dibutyryl cyclic AMP and isoproterenol, the reversal effects appear to be due directly to intracellular changes in cyclic nucleotide levels (Table 2).

3. *Cyclic GMP stimulates DNA synthesis.* The data presented in Table 3 examines the effects of raising intracellular levels of cyclic AMP and cyclic GMP on the initiation of DNA synthesis in nude spleen cells. In the concentration range between $10^{-3}M$ and $10^{-4}M$ cyclic GMP shows marked enhancement (4- to 6-fold) of DNA synthetic activity. In contrast, carbachol generally shows mitogenic activity. Dibutyryl cyclic AMP and isoproterenol inhibit markedly the background incorporation of radioactive thymidine into DNA (Table 3).

4. *Cyclic GMP stimulates immune responses in T cell-depleted cultures.* Cyclic GMP has two effects on immune responses in T cell-depleted cultures. In the absence of added antigen (SRBC) cyclic GMP stimulates small background or polyclonal responses (Table 4). In the presence of SRBC there is a synergistic effect resulting in 5- to 8-fold enhancements of the immune response to SRBC above the background. Carbachol shows a weak polyclonal response, but in the presence of SRBC shows a strong synergistic effect resulting in the stimulation SRBC-specific immune responses (Table 4).

517

Table 2

THE REVERSAL OF THE INACTIVATING EFFECTS
OF CYCLIC AMP BY CYCLIC GMP

Pretreatment of Precursor Cells (24 hours)				$PFC/10^6$ Recovered Cells (Day 3)
cAMP	Isoproterenol	cGMP	Carbachol	
-	-	-	-	767
$2x10^{-3}\underline{M}$	-	-	-	<10
$2x10^{-3}\underline{M}$	-	$1x10^{-3}\underline{M}$	-	130
$2x10^{-3}\underline{M}$	-	-	$1x10^{-3}\underline{M}$	112
$1x10^{-3}\underline{M}$	-	-	-	160
$1x10^{-3}\underline{M}$	-	$1x10^{-3}\underline{M}$	-	305
$1x10^{-3}\underline{M}$	-	-	$1x10^{-3}\underline{M}$	880
-	$5x10^{-4}\underline{M}$	-	-	<10
-	$5x10^{-4}\underline{M}$	$1x10^{-3}\underline{M}$	-	306
-	$5x10^{-4}\underline{M}$	-	$1x10^{-3}\underline{M}$	617
-	$1x10^{-4}\underline{M}$	-	-	250
-	$1x10^{-4}\underline{M}$	$1x10^{-3}\underline{M}$	-	752
-	$1x10^{-4}\underline{M}$	-	$1x10^{-3}\underline{M}$	1050

Nude spleen cells were incubated for 24 hours with the
agents described above, washed and recultured with $5x10^6$
T_{SRBC} and SRBC. Three days later the number of $PFC/10^6$
recovered cells was determined.

Table 3

THE STIMULATION OF DNA SYNTHESIS BY CYCLIC GMP

Concentra- tion (M)	cGMP	Carbachol	cAMP	Isoproterenol
1×10^{-3}	12,714	3,892	513	<100
5×10^{-4}	14,979	3,711	724	<100
2×10^{-4}	11,476	3,530	1,087	545
1×10^{-4}	9,935	3,102	2,114	1208

Nude spleen cells were cultured at a density of 5×10^6 cells/ ml with concentrations of the agents described above. After 24 hours cells were incubated for 6 hours with radioactive thymidine as described elsewhere (11). The data represents the acid-precipitable counts/min of radioactive thymidine. Control cultures lacking the above agents incorporated 3020 counts/min.

Table 4

CYCLIC GMP STIMULATES IMMUNE RESPONSES
IN T CELL-DEPLETED CULTURES

| Concentration | PFC/10^6 Recovered Cells | | | |
| | cGMP | | Carbachol | |
	No SRBC	SRBC	No SRBC	SRBC
$1x10^{-3}$	55	455	27	115
$5x10^{-4}$	68	530	<10	152
$2x10^{-4}$	85	485	14	146
$1x10^{-4}$	50	255	52	97
	cAMP		Isoproterenol	
	No SRBC	SRBC	No SRBC	SRBC
$1x10^{-3}$	<10	<10	<10	<10
$5x10^{-4}$	33	26	<10	<10
$2x10^{-4}$	<10	<10	<10	<10
$1x10^{-4}$	14	48	<10	<10

Nude spleen cells were cultured at a density of 10^7 cells/ml
with the agents indicated. After 2 days cultures were supplemented a second time with the concentrations of the
agents indicated. On day 4 the hemolytic PFC were determined. In control cultures containing SRBC but none of the
above agents there were less than 20 PFC/10^6 recovered cells

EFFECT OF CYCLIC NUCLEOTIDES ON
BACTERIAL LIPOPOLYSACCHARIDE ACTIVITY

LPS exerts three major effects in mouse spleen cultures: First, LPS induces DNA synthesis in most B lympocytes (9-11). Second, high concentrations of LPS increase background immune responses to a wide variety of determinants (10,11,23). This increase in background antibody-forming cells is independent of added antigen and has been termed the polyclonal response (23). Third, lower concentrations of LPS stimulate immune responses to a variety of antigenic determinants presented in nonimmunogenic forms. This can be done by using heterologous erythrocyte antigens in T cell-depleted cultures (10,11) or by using determinants which because of their size (monovalent haptens) or structure (coupled to self components) cannot participate in cell cooperative events (11).

1. *Inhibition of LPS responses by cyclic AMP and enhancement by cyclic GMP.* The data presented in Table 5 show the effects of isoproterenol and carbachol on the mitogenic, polyclonal and synergistic activities of LPS in spleen cultures. Concentrations of isoproterenol greater than $1 \times 10^{-4}\underline{M}$ inhibited LPS-induced responses whereas carbachol at concentrations between $10^{-3}\underline{M}$ and $10^{-5}\underline{M}$ tended to enhance LPS activity.

Since LPS induced DNA synthesis in 23 to 30% of spleen cells in the initial 24 hours of stimulation (11), the effect of LPS on cyclic AMP and cyclic GMP levels in these cells was examined. The data presented in Figure 3 show that following the addition of LPS to mouse spleen cultures there occur rapid, transient increases in intracellular levels of cyclic GMP. This increase is generally 5- to 8- fold above background and reaches a maximum by 15 minutes. Cyclic GMP levels then decrease so that 60 to 120 minutes later they appear less than 2-fold above background levels. In contrast, intracellular levels of cyclic AMP do not show the same rapid and transient changes as observed for cyclic GMP. There is a 2-fold increase in cyclic AMP levels that remain until the onset of DNA synthesis which can be detected 12 to 14 hours after the addition of LPS (Fig. 3).

When higher concentrations of LPS are used the level of cyclic GMP does not vary significantly, however, the intracellular level of cyclic AMP increases (Table 6). This means that the concentration of LPS affects the intracellular ratio

Table 5

EFFECT OF ISOPROTERENOL AND CARBACHOL ON LPS ACTIVITY

Treatment	Counts/ Min (Day 3)	Polyclonal Response TNP-PFC/10^6 (Day 3)	Induced (Clonal) Response (Day 4) No SRBC	SRBC
-	1,924	<10	<10	<10
10 μg LPS	75,172	544	98	440
Isoproterenol				
10 μg LPS + 5x10^{-4}M	174	<10	<10	<10
10 μg LPS + 1x10-4M	30,716	454	47	220
10 μg LPS + 1x10^{-5}M	76,179	468	68	520
Carbachol				
10 μg LPS + 1x10^{-3}M	93,730	647	90	560
10 μg LPS + 1x10^{-4}M	98,887	670	84	620
10 μg LPS + 1x10^{-5}M	79,673	614	104	490

E. coli 0127:B8 LPS was used in nude spleen cultures seeded at an initial density of 10^7 cells/ml.

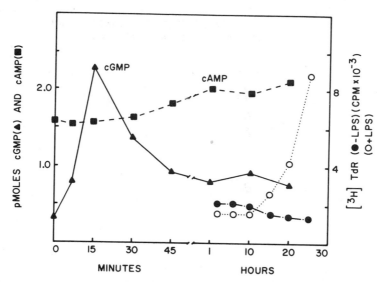

Fig. 3. Effect of LPS on intracellular levels of cyclic AMP and cyclic GMP and the initiation of DNA synthesis. Spleen cells from heterozygous nude mice were cultured at a density of 10^7 cells/ml in Eagle's medium supplemented with 5% FBS. Cultures were left 16 hr after preparation and then 20 μg E. coli 0127:B8 LPS added for the periods described. Both cyclic AMP and cyclic GMP were measured by the radioimmune assay of Steiner et al (25) purchased as assay kits from Collaborative Research, Boston, Mass. as described elsewhere (22). Cyclic nucleotide concentrations have been expressed as picomoles/10^7 cells. For DNA synthetic responses, cultures were incubated with [^{3}H] thymidine for 4 hour periods as described elsewhere (11).

523

CYCLIC AMP AND CYCLIC GMP AS INTRACELLULAR
MEDIATORS OF PHENOTYPIC EXPRESSION

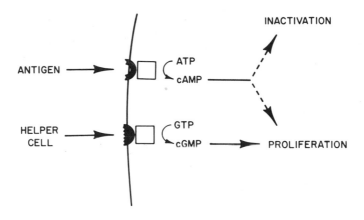

Fig. 4. Cyclic AMP and cyclic GMP as intracellular mediators of phenotypic expression. The interaction of antigen with surface immunoglobulin receptors on precursor cells leads to the activation of adenyl cyclase. Increasing intracellular levels of cyclic AMP initiates events that are required for both inactivation and proliferation pathways. The interaction of the thymus-derived helper cell system with precursor cells leads to the activation of guanyl cyclase. Increasing intracellular levels of cyclic GMP leads to a series of events that combine with cyclic AMP-induced events to lead to cell proliferation. In the absence of helper activity, the cyclic AMP-induced events terminate in precursor cell inactivation.

Table 6

INTRACELLULAR LEVELS OF CYCLIC AMP AND CYCLIC GMP

Treatment	pMoles/10^6 cells (15 min)		cAMP/cGMP
	cAMP	cGMP	
Control	0.68	0.06	11.3
$10^{-3}\underline{M}$ carbachol	0.74	0.16	4.6
$10^{-4}\underline{M}$ isoproterenol	4.8	0.14	34.2
20 µg LPS	0.96	0.32	3.0
100 µg LPS	1.84	0.28	6.5
Allogeneic supernatant			
0.1ml	0.76	0.12	6.3
0.5ml	0.78	0.18	4.3

Cyclic nucleotides were measured by a radioimmune assay (25) as described in the legend to Figure 3. Allogeneic supernatants prepared from C57BL/6 thymus cells activated to BALB/c alloantigens were prepared as described elsewhere (24).

of cyclic AMP: cyclic GMP either by enhancing cyclic GMP levels or by enhancing cyclic AMP levels (22).

ALLOGENEIC SUPERNATANT FACTORS

Thymus cells immunized to alloantigens by the injection of parental thymus cells into irradiated F_1 recipients have been used as a source of cells for the production of humoral factors in culture that stimulate immune responses in T cell-depleted cultures (24). These supernatants are weakly mitogenic and stimulate small polyclonal responses in mouse spleen cultures (24). However, such supernatants stimulate immune responses to a variety of heterologous erythrocyte antigens in anti-theta treated and nude mouse spleen cultures (24). The effects of allogeneic supernatants on cyclic AMP and cyclic GMP in mouse spleen cells are described in Table 6. Such supernatants cause rapid 3- to 5-fold increases in cyclic GMP levels with slight increases in cyclic AMP levels. For comparative purposes, the effects of isoproterenol and carbachol on intracellular cyclic nucleotide levels are also shown (Table 6). Isoproterenol raises intracellular levels of cyclic AMP and carbachol exhibits exactly the reverse effects.

CYCLIC NUCLEOTIDES AS MEDIATORS OF PHENOTYPIC EXPRESSION

Intracellular levels of cyclic nucleotides. The experiments discussed here show four effects: a) Treatment of precursor antibody-forming cells with agents that raise intracellular levels of cyclic AMP lead to inactivation; b) Agents that simultaneously raise cyclic GMP levels partially or completely prevent the inactivation process; c) Cyclic GMP stimulates DNA synthesis in mouse spleen cultures; d) Agents that raise intracellular levels of cyclic GMP stimulate immune responses to SRBC in T cell-depleted spleen cultures.

Agents that interact with precursor cells to raise intracellular levels of cyclic GMP fall into two classes: a) cyclic GMP and LPS show mitogenic activity and stimulate immune responses to erythrocyte antigens in T cell-depleted cultures, and b) carbachol and allogeneic supernatant factors that are only weakly mitogenic but which stimulate immune responses to erythrocyte antigens in T cell-depleted cultures. While LPS shows strong polyclonal effects, cyclic GMP, carbachol and allogeneic supernatant factors show only weak or no polyclonal effects. The most important finding appears to be that agents that raise intracellular levels of cyclic GMP are not necessarily mitogenic. However antigen converts the nonmitogens carbachol and allogeneic factors to selective mitogens in the sense that antigen-specific precursor cells are now induced to proliferate. Antigen also stimulates this clonal expansion of antigen-specific cells in the presence of low concentrations of LPS (11) and cyclic GMP (Table 4). The conclusion is that the proliferation and maturation of clones of antibody-forming cells require signals in addition to raising intracellular levels of cyclic GMP.

The question arises as to whether these effects of cyclic AMP and cyclic GMP are due to their physiological participation as intracellular mediators of exogenous signals that regulate the phenotypic expression of precursor cells. A number of findings favor such a role. First, precursor cells have been programmed to follow inductive and tolerogenic pathways (1-4). There is evidence that the establishment of tolerance results from an irreversible inactivation of precursor cells (26-31). Since high concentrations of cyclic AMP have been shown to be growth inhibiting but not generally toxic in other mammalian systems (32-34) and further, cyclic AMP often switches on programmed cell functions (14-18), the inactivation of precursor cells by cyclic AMP may reflect the triggering of the tolerogenic pathway. If the cyclic AMP-induced inactivation process is due to a non-specific toxic process, there appears to be no reason why cyclic GMP and carbachol should prevent inactivation since these agents do not affect the level of intracellular cyclic AMP resulting from treatment with exogenous cyclic AMP and isoproterenol (22). Finally, LPS stimulates intracellular cyclic GMP synthesis (Fig. 3). Since cyclic GMP mimics the mitogenic effects of LPS, cyclic GMP may participate as an intracellular mediator of LPS activity.

Inductive and tolerogenic pathways. Models that are aimed at describing the inductive stimulus fall into two categories. There are the *one signal* models that postulate the inductive signal delivered to precursor cells arises solely from immunoglobulin receptor activation (35) or from the helper T cells (36). *Two signal* models require the independent delivery of two signals to precursor cells, one via antigen-receptor recognition, and the other via the helper cell-precursor cell interaction (4,11,18,29,37). The best evidence that a two signal system exists is derived from experiments concerning the establishment and breaking

527

of tolerance to different antigens. The injection of DNP-D-glutamic acid-D-lysine (DNP-DGL) into mice rapidly inactivates DNP-specific precursor cells. There are apparently no T cells that bind the copolymer DGL, thus the establishment of tolerance appears to result directly from the interaction of DNP-DGL with precursor cells (27-29). The establishment of tolerance then requires only the interaction of antigen with surface immunoglobulin receptors on precursor cells, therefore, the antigen-receptor interaction must result in the delivery of a signal to cells. The simultaneous delivery of a signal from allogeneic lymphoid cells to precursor cells interacting with DNP-DGL results in the induction of antibody synthesis (27-29). In this experimental situation the delivery of a signal to precursor cells that have interacted with tolerogen diverts cells from a tolerogenic to an inductive pathway. In support of this contention are experiments that show LPS reverses the tolerogenic effects of deaggregated human gamma globulin (d-HGG) (30,31). If LPS mimics or increases the efficiency of delivery of a T cell signal to precursor cells (11), it may divert precursor cells that have bound d-HGG from a tolerogenic to an inductive pathway by completing an inductive stimulus (30,31).

What then is the relationship of cyclic AMP and cyclic GMP to the exogenous signals that normally activate the inductive or tolerogenic pathways. Since LPS,carbachol and allogeneic supernatant factors all stimulate cyclic GMP synthesis in lymphoid cells, and also stimulate immune responses in T cell-depleted cultures, it is a reasonable assumption that cooperating cells may function to stimulate guanyl cyclase activity in precursor cells. It is important to note that synergistic effects in the immune response have been demonstrated between antigen and LPS, antigen and allogeneic supernatant factors, antigen and cyclic GMP, and antigen and carbachol. This implies that clonal proliferation of each precursor cell requires an additional signal. Since the cooperating cell signal may be delivered to precursor cells by a membrane-mediated event, it is interesting to note that guanyl cyclase activity appears to be membrane-associated and can be activated in fibroblasts by a purified growth factor (38).

If the cyclic AMP-induced inactivation of precursor cells is the expression of the tolerogenic pathway, then the interaction of antigen with surface immunoglobulin receptors on precursor cells may normally activate the adenyl cyclase system to raise intracellular levels of cyclic AMP. The reversal of the cyclic AMP-inactivation process by cyclic GMP and carbachol may represent the diversion of precursor cells from a tolerogenic to an inductive pathway. Since the simultaneous raising of intracellular levels of cyclic GMP prevents the inactivation process it is likely that the precursor cell is reacting to the intracellular ratio of cyclic AMP to cyclic GMP, rather than the absolute level of cyclic AMP. The cyclic AMP-induced inactivation process takes 20 to 30 hours to complete. This is approximately the same length of time preceding the initiation of DNA synthesis in the inductive pathway. Increasing cyclic GMP levels leads to the proliferative pathway. However, since LPS raises cyclic GMP levels, and, cyclic AMP and isoproterenol inhibit LPS activity, it is apparently not the absolute level of cyclic GMP that the cell responds to as a proliferation signal, rather it is the ratio of cyclic AMP to cyclic GMP (Fig. 4).

Is the antigenic signal shared by inductive and tolerogenic pathways. There are two ways to consider the biochemical consequences of the delivery of the antigenic signal to precursor cells: a) raising cyclic AMP levels initiates biochemical changes that are *unique* to the tolerogenic pathway, and b) the resulting biochemical changes are required for *both* inductive and tolerogenic pathways. These events proceed to a certain critical point where the delivery of a second signal via the stimulation of guanyl cyclase activity initiates new biochemical changes that *complement* those initiated by antigen to trigger cell proliferation. In the absence of the second signal, the cyclic AMP-induced events terminate in cell inactivation or death. The observations showing that synergy exists between the activity of antigen and cyclic GMP-enhancing agents, indicates this latter consideration is the most likely.

Clonal and polyclonal development. The interaction of antigen and cooperating cells with precursor cells induces the clonal proliferation of specific precursor cells. Estimates for the number of cell division cycles involved generally exceed four. The interaction of high concentrations of LPS with precursor cells leads to the maturation of most precursor cells (4,23). This polyclonal development is apparently independent of added antigen (4,11) and involves only one or two divisions of each precursor cell (22). None of the cyclic GMP-enhancing agents stimulate strong polyclonal responses. The question arises as to whether the signals that drive polyclonal development are the same as those responsible for clonal expansion (11). It may be significant that the intracellular ratio of cyclic AMP: cyclic GMP following LPS treatment varies with LPS concentrations. As the LPS concentration increases, so does the ratio (Table 6). Polyclonal development is seen generally using higher concentrations of LPS (4,11,22,23). An important feature of LPS activity may be its ability at low concentrations to stimulate cyclic GMP synthesis and, at high concentrations to stimulate both cyclic GMP and cyclic AMP synthesis. How a rapid, transient increase in cyclic GMP levels triggers DNA synthetic events some 12 to 14 hrs later is unclear (Fig. 3). What may be important is not this early elevation of cyclic GMP, rather the prolonged change in the intracellular ratio of cyclic AMP to cyclic GMP. A precursor cell may respond to a wide range of cyclic AMP: cyclic GMP ratios to proceed through a division cycle and mature to an antibody-forming cell (polyclonal expression). However, the continued proliferation of antibody-forming cells (clonal expansion) may require that this ratio remain low (Table 6), which does not occur when high LPS concentrations are present. A high concentration of intracellular cyclic AMP may limit continued proliferation.

Phenotypic expression. These interactions have been summarized in Figure 4. It is suggested that the interaction of antigen with immunoglobulin receptors on precursor cells stimulates adenyl cyclase activity and results in the raising of intracellular levels of cyclic AMP. This signals the initiation of metabolic events shared by both inactivation and proliferation pathways. If cells receive a second signal within a period of some 12 to 20 hours resulting in the elevation of intracellular levels of cyclic GMP, they initiate events that complement the cyclic AMP-induced events resulting in proliferation and maturation to antibody-forming cells. However, if the cyclic GMP-activated sequences do not begin, the cyclic AMP-activated pathway results in the inactivation of precursor cells.

ACKNOWLEDGEMENTS

This work was supported by Grant No. AI-11092 to J. W. and Grant No. A-105875 and AI-00430 to Dr. M. Cohn, all from The National Institutes of Health.

REFERENCES

1. J. Lederberg, *Science* *129*, 1649 (1959).
2. K. Rajewsky and E. Rottlander, *Cold Spring Harb. Symp. Quant. Biol.* *547* (1967).
3. D. W. Dresser and N. A. Mitchison, *Adv. Immunol.* *8*, 129 (1968).
4. P. A. Bretscher and M. Cohn, *Nature* *220*, 444 (1968).
5. M. F. Greaves and S. Bauminger, *Nature New Biol.* *235*, 67 (1972).
6. J. Andersson, G. Moller and O. Sjoberg, *Europ. J. Immunol.* *2*, 99 (1972).
7. R. W. Dutton, *J. Expt. Med.* *136*, 1445 (1972).
8. J. Watson, R. Epstein, I. Nakoinz and P. Ralph, *J. Immunol.* *110*, 43 (1973).
9. D. L. Peavy, W. H. Adler and R. T. Smith, *J. Immunol.* *105*, 1453 (1970).
10. J. Andersson, G. Moller and O. Sjoberg, *Cellular Immunol.* *4*, 381 (1972).
11. J. Watson, E. Trenkner and M. Cohn, *J. Expt. Med.* *138*, 699 (1973).
12. J. W. Hadden, E. M. Hadden and E. Middleton, *Cellular Immunol.* *1*, 583 (1970).
13. T. B. Strom, C. B. Carpenter, M. R. Garvoy, K. F. Austen, J. P. Merrill and M. Kaliner, *J. Expt. Med.* *138*, 381 (1973).
14. A. Hershko, P. Mamont, R. Shields and G. M. Tomkins, *Nature New Biol.* *232*, 206 (1971).
15. J. P. Perkins, *Adv. Cyclic Nucleotide Research* *3*, 1 (1973).
16. M. P. Scheid, M. K. Hoffmann, K. Komuro, U. Hammerling, J. Abbott, E. A. Boyse, G. H. Cohen, J. A. Hopper, R. S. Schulof and A. L. Goldstein, *J. Expt. Med.* *138*, 1027 (1973).
17. V. Daniels, G. Litwack, and G. M. Tomkins, *Proc. Nat. Acad. Sci., U.S.* *70*, 76 (1973).
18. J. Watson, R. Epstein and M. Cohn, *Nature* *246*, 405 (1973).

19. J. W. Hadden, E. M. Hadden, M. K. Haddox and N. D. Goldberg, *Proc. Nat. Acad. Sci. U.S. 69*, 3024 (1972).
20. R. W. Dutton, M. M. McCarthy, R. I. Mishell, and D. J. Raidt, *Cellular Immunol. 1*, 196 (1970).
21. R. I. Mishell and R. W. Dutton, *J. Expt. Med.* (1967).
22. J. Watson, *J. Expt. Med.* submitted (1974).
23. J. Andersson, O. Sjoberg and G. Moller, *Transplantation Reviews 11*, 131 (1972).
24. J. Watson, *J. Immunol. 111*, 1301 (1973).
25. A. L. Steiner, C. W. Parker and D. M. Kipnis, *J. Biol. Chem. 247*, 1106 (1972).
26. D. H. Katz, J. M. Davie, W. E. Paul and B. Benacerraf, *J. Expt. Med. 134*, 201 (1971).
27. D. H. Katz and D. P. Osborne, *J. Expt. Med. 136*, 455 (1972).
28. D. H. Katz, T. Hamoako and B. Benacerraf, *J. Expt. Med. 136*, 1404 (1972).
29. D. H. Katz, *Transplantation Rev. 12*, 141 (1972).
30. W. O. Weigle, J. M. Chiller, G. S. Habicht, in *Prog. Immunol. 1* (1971).
31. J. Chiller and W. O. Weigle, *J. Expt. Med. 137*, 740 (1973).
32. L. A. Smets, *Nature New Biol. 239*, 132 (1972).
33. J. R. Sheppard, *Nature New Biol. 236*, 14 (1972).
34. M. M. Burger, B. M. Bombik B. M. Breckenridge and J. R. Sheppard, *Nature New Biol. 239*, 161 (1972).
35. M. Feldman, *J. Expt. Med. 135*, 1049 (1972).
36. A. Coutinho and G. Moller, *Nature New Biol 245*, 12 (1973).
37. R. W. Dutton, R. Falkoff, J. A. Hirst, M. Hoffmann, J. W. Kappler, J. R. Kettmann, J. F. Lesley, D. Vann. *Prog. Immunol. 1*, 355 (1971).
38. P. S. Rudland, D. Gospodarowicz, W. Seifert, *Nature*, submitted (1974).

IDIOTYPIC RECEPTORS FOR ALLOANTIGEN ON T CELLS?

Hans Binz, Jean Lindenmann and Hans Wigzell*

Department of Medical Microbiology; University of
Zurich, Switzerland and *Department of Immunology
University of Uppsala, Sweden.

ABSTRACT: In rats injection of alloantibodies
(produced in one strain against transplantation
antigens of another strain) into F_1-hybrids between the two strains will induce the induction of
anti-alloantibodies. Radiolabelled anti-alloantibodies will bind to normal lymphocytes from rats
of the genotype that provided the alloantibody.
These lymphocytes are B cells and not T cells,
and their idiotypic surface marker has the same
antigen-binding specificity as the alloantibody
as shown by binding to allogeneic monolayers.
However, despite the negative findings in the
radioimmunoassay, anti-alloantibody serum can be
shown to react with immunocompetent T lymphocytes
of the correct parental strain. This was shown
both by the capacity of sera to selectively inhibit the binding of T cells to monolayers of
allogeneic cells and by the capacity to block the
induction of GvH-reactions of parental T cells if
inoculated into the F_1-hybrids. Adsorption experiments using F_1 or parental lymphocytes failed
to show that these effects on T cells were caused
by antigen-alloantibody complexes but emphasized
the antibody nature of these T cell inhibitory
factors.
    Thus, the present data are fully compatible
with the view that B and T lymphocytes reactive
against the same alloantigens may share idiotypic
determinants.

INTRODUCTION

Antibody molecules besides being able to bind
relevant antigenic determinants can also function
as immunogens. Anti-antibodies can thus be produced against various parts of an antibody molecule. Antibodies directed against the actual

533

antigen-binding sites or other unique parts of the
variable area of the antibody molecule are called
anti-idiotype antibodies (1). Such anti-idiotype
antibodies are commonly found to be produced in
F_1-hybrid animals, if they are injected with alloantibodies produced in one parental strain against
the other parent (2, 3). Proof that the F_1-hybrid
does indeed produce such anti-alloantibodies come
from an analysis of their allotype characteristics
(4), and the kinetics of synthesis (5).

Such anti-alloantibodies can be demonstrated
by actual binding tests using either radioimmune
assays (3) or gel precipitation (6). Also, the
anti-alloantibody containing sera have been found
to interfere in a specific way with in vitro or in
vivo recognition of immunocompetent parental cells
of the relevant alloantigen in some systems (7)
but not in others (8). Most striking with regard
to in vivo effects are the findings that such anti-
alloantibody serum if passively transferred can
suppress the in vivo graft-versus-host reactivity
of parental cells in F_1-hybrid recipients (6, 7).
This might imply the actual existence of idiotypic
determinants on the immunocompetent inoculated
parental T lymphocytes.

Using a combination of techniques involving
radiolabelled anti-alloantibodies, separation
procedures to produce "pure" B and T lymphocytes,
and allogeneic monolayers as specific immunosor-
bants we could find that isotype-labelled anti-
alloantibodies would only bind in significant
quantities to normal lymphocytes of B type (9).
Furthermore, from the relevant strain all idiotype-
positive B lymphocytes can be shown to express
similar antigen-binding specificity as evidenced
by their binding to the relevant, allogeneic fibroblast monolayer. If the cells are preincubated
with anti-alloantibody containing serum, specific
blocking of the binding of the relevant B lymphocytes to the monolayer did take place. These
results thus failed to demonstrate idiotypic receptors on T lymphocyte as measured by the direct
radioimmunoassay. However, we can demonstrate
that the anti-alloantibody containing sera will
display a selective inhibitory action on the binding of immunopotent T cells to the relevant monolayers as evidenced by subsequent tests in GvH

reactions.

In the present article, we have summarized our data on the capacity of anti-alloantibody containing sera to react with B and T lymphocytes. The results and their theoretical implications will be discussed.

MATERIALS AND METHODS

Detailed descriptions as to all technical details are to be found in ref. 7 and 9.

RESULTS

I. Significant uptake of ^{125}I-anti-alloantibody Ig by B but not T lymphocytes.- Normal lymphoid cells from DA or Lewis rats used were mixtures of lymph node and spleen cells. "Pure" T lymphocytes were obtained by filtration through columns and pure B cells were obtained by treatment with a rabbit-anti-T cell serum and complement. The starting population of cells contained approximately 40 - 45% B cells as judged by anti-T and complement cytotoxicity; the same test revealed between 0 - 3% of contaminating cells in purified suspensions of T and B cells. As seen in Table 1, uptake of the proper ^{125}I-labeled anti-alloantibody occurred to a significant degree only in populations containing B cells. In fact, uptake of the anti-alloantibody was proportional to the percentage of B cells of the relevant strain in the tested cellular population. In a further attempt to find idiotypic determinants on relevant T cells, parental thymocytes were inoculated into irradiated F1 hybrid animals for activation in vivo. These cells were subsequently recovered from the spleen, filtered through anti-Ig columns to remove possible contaminating B cells (10) leaving a T cell population known to be highly pure with regard to T cells, and with excellent specific immunocompetence of T cell type (11). However, even such immune T cells failed to express any selective binding of the relevant anti-alloantibody as shown in Table 2. Thus, as judged by uptake of radiolabeled anti-alloantibody, receptors with the idiotypes of alloantibodies

TABLE 1

Uptake of ^{125}I-Labled Anti-Alloantibody Ig by Purified B and

T Lymphocytes

Labeled anti-alloanti-body	Cells*	Uptake** of ^{125}I (cpm) by DA Cells		Lewis Cells	
anti-(DA anti-L)	B	2900	(1972)	946	
anti-(DA anti-L)	B+T	1470	(570)	738	
anti-(DA anti-L)	T	578	(68)	538	
anti-(L anti-DA)	B	928		3176	(2230)
anti-(L anti-DA)	B+T	900		1610	(872)
anti-(L anti-DA)	T	510		503	(-35)

*   B and T means more than 95% purity of each kind.
B+T = approximately 40% B cells.

**   Figures within brackets denote in cpm the actual specific cpm (uptake of relevant ^{125}I anti-alloantibody minus uptake of irrelevant ^{125}I Ig on the same cell population).

Figures denote the mean of 3-4 tubes/group.

TABLE 2

Uptake of ^{125}I-Labeled Anti-alloantibody by
Activated Thymocytes

Labeled Anti-alloantibody	Uptake of ^{125}I (cpm) by Thymocytes Activated for	
	Lewis Antigen*	DA Antigen*
anti-(L anti-DA)	992 ± 60	2638 ± 82
anti-(DA anti-L)	1160 ± 69	2525 ± 43

* DA or Lewis thymocytes were inoculated i.v. into
1000 r (DA x Lewis) Fl rats. Five days later
spleens were harvested and the cells filtered
through anti-Ig columns whereafter the ^{125}I-
uptake was measured. Results denote mean (±
S.E.)of triplicate measurements using 5 x 10^6
cells/tube.

were only to be found on B lymphocytes.

II. Cytotoxicity of anti-alloantibody Ig and complement on lymphocytes carrying idiotypic markers of the alloantibody. - To show that the idiotypic determinants present on B lymphocytes were produced by these cells, treatment with anti-alloantibody Ig and complement was carried out on normal parental strain lymphoid cells. Incubation with anti-alloantibody Ig in presence or absence of complement was carried out. Thereafter, the cells were treated with trypsin to remove antigen-antibody complexes from the cell surfaces and were subsequently allowed to recover overnight at 37° C, whereafter ^{125}I-anti-alloantibody was added to study the presence or absence of idiotype-containing cells in the population. The results, as shown in Table 3, clearly demonstrate that the anti-alloantibody in the presence of complement (but not in its absence) caused a specific elimination (most likely cytolytic) of cells with the relevant idiotypes.

Further evidence that idiotypic markers similar to those of alloantibodies were present on B lymphocytes in such a way as to make these cells sensitive to the cytolytic action of anti-alloantibodies and complement came from experiments in which rabbit antisera directed against either rat Ig or T cells were included in the cytolytic assays. Treatment with anti-Ig in the presence of complement caused an elimination of the idiotype-containing cells, whereas this was not the case when the anti-T serum was used.

III. The uptake of ^{125}I-anti-alloantibody Ig on normal B lymphocytes is due to the presence of idiotypic receptors with specificity for alloantigens. - We applied immunosorbent techniques with monolayers (12) to demonstrate that the cells with idiotypic receptors expressed the expected antigen-binding capacity. Normal lymphoid cells of DA or Lewis origin were incubated at 37°C for 90 min on DA or Lewis fibroblast monolayers in the presence of normal Fl serum, of the relevant anti-alloantibody serum or of rabbit anti-T or rabbit anti-Ig serum.

TABLE 3

Cytotoxicity of Anti-alloantibodies for Lymphoid Cells.
Comparison of uptake of ^{125}I anti-alloantibody Ig by cells after treatment
with anti-alloantibody plus complement and anti-alloantibody alone.

Cells	Treatment	Labeled Anti-alloantibody	Uptake of ^{125}I (cpm $\pm$ SE*)
L	anti-(L anti-DA)	anti-(L anti-DA)	5239 $\pm$ 363
L	anti-(L anti-DA)	anti-(DA anti-L)	2328 $\pm$ 52
L	anti-(L anti-DA) + C'	anti-(L anti-DA)	1825 $\pm$ 97
L	anti-(L anti-DA) + C'	anti-(DA anti-L)	2086 $\pm$ 108
DA	anti-(DA anti-L)	anti-(DA anti-L)	6992 $\pm$ 289
DA	anti-(DA anti-L)	anti-(L anti-DA)	2159 $\pm$ 42
DA	anti-(DA anti-L) + C'	anti-(DA anti-L)	3757 $\pm$ 129
DA	anti-(DA anti-L) + C'	anti-(L anti-DA)	3865 $\pm$ 296

* Underlined values indicate groups where specific uptake occurred.
  If only specific uptake minus non-specific uptake is compared,
  none of the anti-alloantibody and complement treated cells displayed any surviving idiotype-positive cells (-261 cpm for Lewis
  cells and -108 cpm for DA cells, respectively).

The lymphocytes in the supernatant and the bound,
EDTA-eluted cells were subsequently trypsin-treated,
left overnight to recover and then assayed for
presence of idiotype-containing cells using ^{125}I-
anti-alloantibody Ig.

As shown in Table 4, normal Fl serum did not
inhibit adsorption of idiotype-carrying cells to
the monolayers, as evidenced by the fact that the
unadsorbed cells fixed little radioactive anti-
alloantibody, whereas the eluted cells, representing a population enriched in the specific receptor,
fixed much more. Anti-alloantibody of the proper
specificity, however, prevented adsorption, yielding higher radioactivity in the unadsorbed fraction
and lower radioactivity in the eluted fraction.
The same effect could be induced with rabbit anti-
rat Ig serum, but not with rabbit anti-T serum.
This suggests that the bulk of radioactivity must
have been taken up by B cells, and that these cells
when carrying idiotypic determinants present in
alloantibodies of a given specificity, also expressed the same antigen-binding specificity at the
cellular level.

IV.   The capacity of anti-alloantibody-containing
      serum to inhibit GvH reactivity. Anti-allo-
antibody-containing serum produced in F_1-hybrid
animals by the injection of alloantibodies from one
parental strain induced against the other parental
strain can be shown to allow specific suppression
of the GvH reactivity of lymphocytes from that
parental strain (8, 6). That the factor causing
this inhibition was an antibody reactive against
the GvH-reactive cells and not an alloantibody-
antigen complex caused by the immunization procedure was strongly suggested by the following facts:
The inhibitory capacity of such anti-alloantibody
containing sera was not removed by incubation with
either F_1-hybrid cells or with lymphocytes from
the other parental strain but only by lymphocytes
provided for by animals of the genotype that provided the original alloantibodies. The possibility, however, that the anti-alloantibodies could
have as their primary target the B lymphocytes
creating antigen-antibody complexes when reacting
with the idiotype-containing cells and this in a
secondary manner causing an inhibitory effect on

TABLE 4

Idiotypic Determinants on Surface Receptors for Alloantigens Present on Normal B Cells.

Binding to Allogeneic Monolayers and its Interference with Anti-alloantibody IgG.

Lymphoid Cells	Fibroblast Monolayers from Strain	Inhibitors	Labeled Anti-alloantibody	Uptake* of ^{125}I (cpm) by Cells	
				Remaining in the Supernatant	Eluted from the Monolayers and Allowed to Recover
L	DA	normal F1 serum	anti-(L anti-DA)	997	3893
		F1 anti-(L anti-DA)		<u>4020</u>	<u>1386</u>
		rabbit-anti-rat Ig		<u>5146</u>	<u>1221</u>
		rabbit-anti-T		1182	3908
DA	L	normal F1 serum	anti-(DA anti-L)	1923	3350
		F1 anti-(DA anti-L)		<u>6832</u>	<u>1910</u>
		rabbit-anti-rat Ig		<u>7974</u>	<u>1590</u>
		rabbit-anti-T		2687	6323

* Underlined values indicate experiments where specific interference of binding to allogeneic monolayers occurred. Uptake of a non-specific kind on supernatant cells was 1813 for anti-(DA anti-L)-^{125}I on L cells and 1994 for anti-(L-anti-DA)-^{125}I on DA cells. Each value in the Table represents the mean of triplicates.

541

the GvH reaction could not be excluded. Thus, we
now tested highly purified T lymphocytes from either
parental strain for their capacity to inflict a GvH
reaction in the presence of anti-alloantibody containing serum of the two parental specificities.
As seen in Table 5, even when using "pure" T lymphocytes there was a selective, significant inhibition
of the GvH reaction caused by the presence of the
relevant anti-alloantibody-containing serum. We
would thus conclude that the inhibitory activity of
anti-alloantibody serum as measured in the local
popliteal lymph node assay is a measure of direct
inhibition of T lymphocyte activities.

V. Capacity of anti-alloantibody-containing sera
    to block the binding of specific T lymphocytes
    to the relevant monolayers. In a series of
tests we analyzed the impact of anti-Ig, anti-T or
normal F_1 or anti-alloantibody sera on the capacity
of GvH-reactive cells to bind to syngeneic or allogeneic monolayers. In previous experiments (see
Table 4) we have already described that with regard
to B cell binding to monolayers, both anti-Ig and
anti-alloantibody sera are effective blockers. As
seen in Table 6 when potential GvH-reactive cells
were incubated in the presence of the various sera
on syngeneic monolayers, there was no differential
distribution of GvH-reactive cells in the supernatants as compared to cells binding to monolayers
and thereafter eluted. However, in all 6 experiments where either anti-Ig, anti-T or normal F_1
serum was used together with the GvH-reactive cells
on allogeneic monolayers there was a significant
shift in the ratio, in so far that more specific
GvH-reactive cells were now found in the bound and
eluted portions. Thus, again we could show that
indeed in this system we have binding of relevant
GvH-reactive cells to allogeneic monolayers. If
now specific anti-alloantibody containing serum was
included in the experiments with the allogenic mono
layers we observed a blocking of the binding of
GvH-reactive cells to the monolayers (see underlined combinations) as evidenced by a change in the
ratios of GvH-reactive cells in supernatant versus
eluate. From the data in Tables 4 and 6 we would
conclude that a) GvH-reactive cells can be removed
by preincubation in vitro with relevant monolayers

TABLE 5

The Effect of Injection of Parental Alloantibodies in $(DA \times Lewis)F_1^+$ Rats. Specific Inhibition of GvH by Injected T lymphocytes

	DA T cells/Lewis T cells	
	DA anti-Lewis antibodies	Lewis anti-DA antibodies
Mean of ratio $\pm$ S.E.	-0.240 ± 0.044	0.314 ± 0.028
(log_{10} units)	(12)	(10)

Difference between two groups significant at 0.001 level.

Popliteal lymph node assays 5×10^6 DA or Lewis T cells injected into each hind foot pad, assayed 7 days later. F_1-rats immunized by two injections of 1 ml alloantibody-serum 2 weeks before cell injection.

543

TABLE 6

Binding and Elution of GvH Reactive Cells to Cellular Monolayers.
Interference by Anti-Ig, Anti-T and Anti-Alloantibody sera

Cells	Monolayers	Inhibition	Ratio[x]
L	DA	R → Ig	-0.192 ± 0.019
L	DA	R → T	-0.111 ± 0.043
L	DA	(DA x L)F₁ normal	-0.175 ± 0.077
L	DA	(DA x L)F₁ anti-(L anti-DA)	0.297 ± 0.018
L	L	R → Ig	0.035 ± 0.010
L	L	R → T	0.033 ± 0.014
L	L	(DA x L)F₁	0.000 ± 0.046
L	L	(DA x L)F₁ anti-(L anti-DA)	0.007 ± 0.030
DA	DA	R → Ig	-0.006 ± 0.039
DA	DA	R → T	-0.020 ± 0.060
DA	DA	(DA x L)F₁	0.008 ± 0.032
DA	DA	(DA x L)F₁ anti-(DA anti-L)	-0.056 ± 0.016
DA	L	R → Ig	-0.151 ± 0.024
DA	L	R → T	-0.148 ± 0.044
DA	L	(DA x L)F₁	-0.304 ± 0.018
DA	L	(DA x L)F₁ anti-(DA anti-L)	0.425 ± 0.060

x Log 10 means ± S.E. of the individual ratios of the lymph nodes.
Underlined values denote blocking of specific adsorption. GvH
reactivity evoked by supernatant versus eluted cells.

544

and b) of the sera tested for blocking of this binding relevant anti-alloantibody-containing sera would cause blocking of both GvH-reactive cells and B lymphocytes, whereas c) anti-Ig serum would only block the binding of B lymphocytes.

VI. Cytotoxic effects of anti-alloantibody serum on GvH-reactive cells. We have previously found that anti-alloantibody sera contain antibodies which in the presence of complement are cytotoxic for the relevant, idiotype-positive B lymphocytes as shown in Table 3. We now tested whether anti-alloantibody-containing serum in the presence of complement would be cytotoxic in vitro for GvH-reactive lymphocytes. Cells to be tested were incubated with anti-alloantibody serum in the presence or absence of complement or with complement alone, washed and then tested for capacity to induce GvH-reactions as measured in the local popliteal lymph node assay. As controls anti-Ig or anti-T sera were tested for cytotoxic activity in the same assay. As seen in Table 7, anti-T or anti-alloantibody-containing sera were all active as cytotoxic antisera in this assay whereas, as expected from the previous findings, anti-Ig and complement had no inhibitory activity on the GvH potential. It should be realized that cytotoxicity induced by anti-alloantibody serum was not apparent by trypan blue uptake, indicating a low frequency of antiserum-sensitive cells. The finding that anti-alloantibody-containing sera were cytotoxic for relevant GvH-reactive cells was not true for all sera tested; in fact, out of 8 sera tested in the rat system only 4 sera were found positive despite the fact that by other criteria they behaved like anti-alloantibody-containing sera.

We would thus conclude that several of our anti-alloantibody-containing sera behaved like they contained antibodies potentially cytotoxic for the relevant GvH-reactive T lymphocytes.

VII. Miscellaneous Preliminary Observations. Instead of using alloantibodies for the induction of anti-alloantisera we have also used parental lymphocytes. Here both mixtures of B and T lymphocytes as well as purified T lymphocytes

545

TABLE 7

GvH Reaction of Parental Lymphoid Cells Treated with Anti-alloantibodies plus Complement in Comparison to the GvH-Reaction of Parental Lymphoid Cells Treated with Anti-alloantibodies or Complement Alone

Cells Injected	Host	Treatment of the Injected cells with	Mean of Lymph node weights[x] ± S.E. (mg)	Mean of log ratio[xx] ± S.E.
DA	$(DAxBN)F_1$	anti-(DA anti-BN)+C'	17.7 ± 1.0	-0.327 ± 0.038
DA	$(DAxBN)F_1$	anti-(DA anti-BN)	37.8 ± 2.4	
DA	$(DAxBN)F_1$	anti-(DA anti-BN)+C'	18.3 ± 1.1	-0.209 ± 0.031
DA	$(DAxBN)F_1$	Complement	30.5 ± 3.2	
Lewis	$(LxBN)F_1$	anti-(L anti-BN)+C'	15.7 ± 0.8	-0.208 ± 0.027
Lewis	$(LxBN)F_1$	anti-(L anti-BN)	25.3 ± 1.2	
Lewis	$(LxBN)F_1$	anti-(L anti-BN)+C'	13.6 ± 0.9	-0.238 ± 0.024
Lewis	$(LxBN)F_1$	Complement	23.5 ± 1.0	

[x] Mean of between 16 and 22 lymph nodes

[xx] All values different from 0.000 at a p-value less than 0.005

have been shown to function in this respect; now
measuring the assumed production of anti-alloantibodies by specific inhibition of GvH-reactions.
Furthermore, such immunized F_1-hybrid animals inoculated with purified parental T lymphocytes can
be shown to frequently have in their sera cytotoxic
antibodies against the relevant parental T lymphocytes as measured by inhibition of GvH reactions.
The production of these anti-T antibodies is both
time and dose dependent. We have not tested such
positive sera as yet whether they also contain anti-
alloantibodies reactive with B lymphocytes as measured by the radioimmunoassay. The idiotypic nature of the T factors is suggested by preliminary
third party experiments where either in GvH inhibitions or by killer cell inhibition in vitro using
Cr^{51} assay selective inhibition in the "correct"
target combination did take place.

DISCUSSION

In the present article we have presented data
supporting the view that antisera produced in F_1-
hybrids via the inoculation of alloantibodies produced in one parental strain against alloantigens
of the other parental strain contain antibodies
reactive with antigen-binding receptors on T lymphocytes. Such receptors would be present on T
lymphocytes from the donor strain that produced the
alloantibodies used for inoculation into the F_1-
hybrid animals, and would carry specificity for
the alloantigens of the other parental strain. The
evidence for this comes from the findings that
"pure" T lymphocytes are selectively inhibited in
their GvH-reactivity when inoculated into F_1-hybrids
containing such supposed anti-alloantibodies.
Furthermore, binding of GvH-reactive cells to relevant allogeneic monolayers is inhibited by anti-
alloantibody-containing sera. And finally, in
several experiments we could demonstrate a cytotoxic activity against relevant T lymphocytes by in
vitro incubation in the presence of anti-alloantibody serum and complement. Our data thus confirm
and extend earlier preliminary reports on the
specific inhibitory activity of anti-alloantibody
serum on the GvH-reactivity (7), and demonstrate

that the effect is actually occurring at the level
of the T lymphocyte.

There exist, however, several seemingly contradictory findings in this field. Anti-alloantibody IgG radiolabelled with I^{125} could be shown to
bind in a significant manner to the relevant parental lymphocytes but only in a detectable manner to
B lymphocytes. Yet, the same serum (pure IgG has
not been tested) would inhibit the binding of T
lymphocytes to relevant allogeneic monolayers or
inhibit the GvH-reactivity of inoculated T lymphocytes in vivo (present article and 7). This could
then mean several different things. Firstly, the
anti-alloantibodies directed against the idiotype-
positive B cells might not react with T cells because the latter cells would not express the same
idiotype-containing receptors on their outer cell
surface. This would mean that either T lymphocytes do not use the same spectrum of idiotype-
positive antigen-binding receptors as do the B
lymphocytes. Alternatively, they have the same
receptors as B lymphocytes as the B cells but do
not express them in a way allowing binding assays
to be made at the cell surface of T cells. Alternatively, the specific factor in the anti-alloantibody-containing sera that reacts with T lymphocytes
might be a complex consisting of alloantibody and
antigen of the other parental strain type, produced
in the F_1-hybrid as a consequence of the injection
of alloantibody. The strongest argument against
this latter possibility would seem to be the results in the present article where anti-alloantibody sera were shown, in the presence of complement,
to exert a cytotoxic activity on the T lymphocytes
as measured by inhibition of GvH-reactivity. Although it would seem theoretically possible that
antigen-antibody complexes in antigen excess might
bind to the relevant antigen-binding T cells,
whereafter the attached antibody could fix complement and kill the T lymphocyte in an indirect
manner we would not favour this interpretation as
the most likely one.

However, we consider it possible that in the
alloantibody serum injected into the F_1-hybrids to
produce the anti-alloantibodies there might have
been some soluble T cell "antibodies", leading to

production of anti-antibodies of specific T type.

We already know that "pure" T lymphocytes can be used for the induction of antibodies reactive with the antigen-binding receptors on T lymphocytes as assessed by the GvH assay (13), and it has previously been found that in a system that presumably measured T lymphocytes reacting against foreign alloantigens (2) the same is true (14). Using inhibition of cytolytic killer cell activity in vitro as assay system, production of anti-T idiotype receptor serum was reported using specific mouse "killer" cells across an H-2 barrier as the immunogen in rabbits (15). Here, after proper adsorptions only inhibition of killer cells against the relevant target cells was obtained supporting the concept of true anti-idiotype antibodies for T cell receptors.

In conclusion, the present article shows that in F_1-hybrids inoculated with alloantibodies produced in one parental strain against alloantigens of the other parent, antibodies will appear in the serum capable of reacting with B and T lymphocytes of the alloantibody-donor genotype. Similar specific factors can also be induced by the inoculation of parental lymphoid cells. It is unknown whether the specific antibodies reactive with B and T lymphocytes from the same donor are the very same factor (s). In order to analyze whether the antibodies reactive with T and B lymphocytes are directed against the same determinants, we will do absorptions with purified B or T lymphocytes or alternatively use purified Fab-fragments of alloantibodies as immunogen looking for specific anti-T cell induction. Until now, however, the present data are fully compatible with the view that B and T lymphocytes directed against the same alloantigens might have shared or identical idiotypes; the B lymphocytes expressing them on the outer surface in a way accessible for radioimmunoassays using anti-receptor antibodies whereas such direct binding could not be demonstrated on the T cells.

ACKNOWLEDGEMENTS

This work was supported by the Swedish Cancer Society, by the Roche Foundation and by contract NIH-NCI-NOI-CB-33859.

References

1. Hopper, J.E., and A. Nisonoff. 1971. Individual antigenic specificity of immunoglobulins. Adv. Immunol. 13: 58.
2. Ramseier, H., and J. Lindenmann. 1971. Cellular receptors. Effect of anti-alloantibodies on the recognition of transplantation antigens. J. Exp. Med. 134: 1083.
3. Binz, H., and J. Lindenmann. 1972. Cellular receptors. Binding of radioactively labeled anti-alloantiserum. J. Exp. Med. 136: 872.
4. Binz, H., and J. Lindenmann. 1973. Allotypes of anti-alloantibodies. Cell. Immunol. (in press).
5. Binz, H., H. Ramseier, and J. Lindenmann. 1973. Anti-alloantibodies: A de novo product. J. Immunol. 111: 1108.
6. McKearn, T.T. 1974. Antireceptor antiserum causes specific inhibition of reactivity to rat histocompatibility antigens. Science 183: 94.
7. Binz, H., J. Lindenmann, and H. Wigzell. 1973. Inhibition of local graft-versus-host reaction by anti-alloantibodies. Nature 246: 146.
8. Fischer-Lindahl, K. 1972. Antisera against recognition sites. Lack of effect on the mixed leucocyte culture interation. Eur. J. Immunol. 2: 501.
9. Binz, H., J. Lindenmann, and H. Wigzell. 1974. J. Exp. Med. (in press).
10. Wigzell, H. K.G. Sundqvist, and T.O. Yoshida. 1972. Separation of cells according to surface antigens by the use of antibody-coated columns. Fractionation of cells carrying immunoglobulins and blood group antigen. Scand. J. Immunol. 1: 75.
11. Wigzell, H., P. Golstein, E.A.J. Svedmyr, and M. Jondal. 1972. Impact of fractionation procedures on lymphocyte activities in vitro and in vivo. Separation of cells with high concentrations of surface immunoglobulin. Transplant. Proc. 4: 311.
12. Golstein, P.E., A.J. Svedmyr, and H. Wigzell. 1971. Cell mediating specific in vitro cytotoxicity. I. Detection of receptor bearing lymphocytes. J. Exp. Med. 134: 1385.

13. Binz, H., and H. Wigzell, unpublished.

14. Ramseier, H. 1973. Activation of T and B thymus cells to recognize histocompatibility antigens. Cell. Immunol. 8: 177.
15. Kimura, A. J. Exp. Med., in press.

MANIPULATION OF A TOLERANT STATE: CELLS AND SIGNALS

Jacques M. Chiller, Jacques A. Louis, Barry J. Skidmore
and William O. Weigle

Department of Experimental Pathology
Scripps Clinic and Research Foundation
La Jolla, California 92037

ABSTRACT. The state of immunological unresponsiveness induced in mice with a tolerogenic form of the antigen human IgG can be cellularly characterized into phases of either T and B cell tolerance or T cell tolerance. In those circumstances when specific T cells appear tolerant while B cells are not, bacterial lipopolysaccharide (LPS) was able to modulate the biological effect of tolerogen from its capacity to induce tolerance to a capacity to induce specific immunity. This property of LPS was demonstrated under conditions where it could also act as a B cell mitogen. In two experimental situations in which LPS could be shown to be non-mitogenic, namely in the C3H/HeJ mouse strain or after chemical modification as a result of base hydrolysis, it could not affect the normal induction process of tolerance.

INTRODUCTION

There exists a body of experimental evidence which details that heterologous serum proteins can induce a state of immunological tolerance not only in neonates but also in adult animals (see reviews of Dresser and Mitchison (1) and of Weigle (2)). In particular, γ-globulins treated in a way so as to render them monomeric in solution are highly tolerogenic (3). The state of tolerance which can be induced in mice with such monomeric (ultracentrifuged) preparations of purified human IgG (HGG) has been well delineated insofar as the cellular parameters which are involved (4). For example, it was initially demonstrated that the antibody response obtained following the injection of an immunogenic preparation of aggregated HGG (AHGG) was T dependent and that the lack of the response to AHGG observed in mice initially treated with a tolerogenic preparation of deaggregated HGG (DHGG) could be explained cellularly by tolerance in both specific B and specific T cells (5). Furthermore, each specific cell population displayed unique temporal kinetic patterns of tolerance induction, maintenance and spontaneous termination (6) in that T cells not only became unresponsive faster than B cells but also remained tolerant for a much longer period of time than B cells. The fact that the persistence of tolerance in the animal followed a pattern which was kinetically superimposable on that determined for unresponsiveness in T cells suggested that a cellular lesion restricted to specific T cells was sufficient to maintain a state of immunological unresponsiveness.

The "phenotype" of tolerance demonstrable after a single injection of DHGG may be viewed cellularly as the sequential expression of three temporary phases: early and late phases each of which could be characterized as having the "cellular genotype" of tolerant T and non-tolerant B cells and an intermediate phase which could be characterized as having the "cellular genotype" of tolerant T and tolerant B cells. Predictably, only within the early or late phase could it be possible to affect the tolerant state to HGG by those experimental manipulations which would circumvent the immunological block created by tolerant T cells.

In the present paper it will be shown that it is in fact possible to affect both the induction and the maintenance of tolerance at certain times and that this effect can be mediated by using bacterial lipopolysaccharide (LPS). Furthermore, experimental evidence will be presented which suggests that there exists a correlation between the ability of LPS to modulate the tolerant state and its capacity to induce B cell mitogenesis. Finally, these data will be considered in view of possible cellular manifestations which they may reflect.

METHODS

Methods used within the context of the experiments which follow have been described in previous publications (4, 6, 7). Cohn fraction II from human sera was obtained through the courtesy of the American Red Cross National Fractionation Center. E. coli K235 LPS was generously provided by Dr. Floyd McIntire from the Laboratory of Microbiology and Immunology, National Institute for Dental Research, Bethesda, Md. Dr. David C. Morrison at Scripps Clinic and Research Foundation kindly supplied LPS from various rough bacterial mutants as well as Lipid A (8).

RESULTS

Manipulation of tolerance to HGG: Effect on the maintenance of unresponsiveness. Adoptive transfer studies have shown previously that normal thymocytes can restore the immunocompetency of tolerant spleen cells obtained from unresponsive animals early or late after tolerance induction but not at times in between (9). Alternative to cellular reconstitution as a means of modulating a tolerant state to HGG, LPS given at appropriate times in conjunction with immunogen has also been shown to result in the specific termination of tolerance (10). In this case, the form of antigen does not appear to be germane to the subsequent biological effects. That is, termination of tolerance is observed not only when LPS is given with an immunogenic challenge of AHGG (10) but also when it is administered following an injection of the otherwise tolerogenic form of DHGG. The latter is shown in Table I. Mice initially given an intraperitoneal injection of 2.5 mg of DHGG do not respond to a subsequent (day 98) injection of either AHGG or DHGG but do form specific antibody if at that time they are injected with DHGG and also with LPS. In contrast, none of the same treatments affect a tolerant state which had been induced in mice some 49 days earlier. In view of the kinetic curves for T and B cell tolerance (6), these data may be interpreted as the ability of LPS to modulate the maintenance of a tolerant state only at a time when unresponsiveness is maintained solely by T cells. However, tolerance in B cells cannot be similarly modified by LPS.

Manipulation of tolerance to HGG: Effect on the induction of unresponsiveness. Since LPS is capable of inducing an immune response in T cell tolerant mice when given in conjunction with a tolerogenic form of HGG and since a parallel transient state of tolerant T cell, non-tolerant B cell exists in the induction phase of tolerance to HGG, LPS should predictably mediate a similar effect when given early in the induction process. In fact, Claman (11) originally observed that mice given LPS after a normally tolerogenic dose of bovine gamma globulin did not become tolerant. A quantitative extension of these studies demonstrated that animals so treated became primed to the antigen (12). Table 2 reveals the details of such an experiment. Mice injected with 2.5 mg DHGG and with saline 3 hours later are completely tolerant to a subsequent challenge of the immunogenic form of AHGG. On the other hand, mice treated with tolerogen and then with LPS respond vigorously to the challenge of AHGG, exhibiting an immune response some 30 times greater than that seen in mice initially treated with saline and with LPS.

A more direct demonstration that LPS modulates the immunological action of DHGG from its normal ability to induce tolerance to a capacity to induce immunity is seen from the data presented in Figure 1. Mice injected with 1.0 mg DHGG and with 50 µg LPS three hours later make a primary immune response to HGG. In

TABLE 1

Termination of tolerance to HGG in mice given tolerogen (DHGG) and bacterial lipopolysaccharide (LPS).

Mice	Challenge	Indirect PFC per spleen
Day 98 Tolerant	DHGG + LPS	5625
" "	DHGG	25
" "	AHGG	177
Day 49 Tolerant	DHGG + LPS	181
" "	DHGG	154
" "	AHGG	158

A/J male mice were injected on day 0 with 2.5 mg deaggregated HGG (DHGG) given ip. At a time, either 49 or 98 days following this treatment, groups of 5 mice were injected with either 1.0 mg DHGG ip and 3 hours later with 50 µg E. coli 0111:B4 LPS iv or 1.0 mg DHGG ip or 0.4 mg aggregated HGG (AHGG) given iv. Twelve days after this challenge, spleen cells from individual mice were quantitated for direct or indirect plaque forming cells (PFC) specific to HGG. The data presented show only numbers of indirect PFC since no direct PFC were observed at that time.

TABLE 2

Effect of LPS on the induction of immunological unresponsiveness to HGG.

Initial Treatment	Challenge	Response Indirect PFC/Spleen ($\pm$ SE)
DHGG	AHGG	63 ($\pm$ 49)
DHGG + LPS	AHGG	103,317 ($\pm$ 29,080)
LPS	AHGG	3,876 ($\pm$ 1,691)

A/J male mice were injected on day 0 with either 2.5 mg of deaggregated HGG (DHGG) given ip or 2.5 mg DHGG given ip followed 3 hours later with 50 µg E. coli 0111:B4 LPS given iv or 50 µg LPS given iv. 25 days after this initial treatment all mice were challenged with 100 µg aggregated HGG (AHGG) given iv. 5 days after challenge, spleens from individual mice were quantitated for indirect plaque forming cells (PFC) specific to HGG. The response of each group represents the arithmetic mean of 5 mice per group. The numbers in parentheses represent the standard error (SE) of the mean for the response of each group.

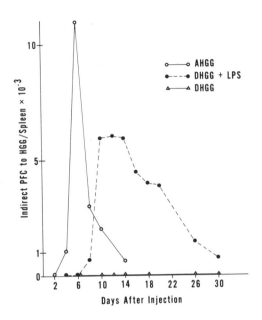

Fig. 1. Kinetic profile of the response to HGG of mice injected with either tolerogen, tolerogen and LPS, or immunogen. Normal A/J male mice were injected on day 0 with either 1.0 mg deaggregated HGG (DHGG) or 1.0 mg DHGG followed 3 hrs later with 50 µg E. coli 0111:B4 LPS or 0.4 mg aggregated HGG (AHGG). At various time points thereafter, spleens from such mice were assayed individually for direct and indirect plaque forming cells (PFC) specific to HGG. The results show only the indirect PFC responses since little or no direct PFC were detected throughout the kinetic profile. Each point represents the arithmetic mean of the response of 5 mice.

comparison with the kinetics of a response obtained following the injection of AHGG, animals which receive the dual treatment of tolerogen and LPS display a shifted kinetic pattern in that the maximal response occurs between days 8 and 14 rather than on day 6. Additionally, LPS seems to prolong the appearance of detectable antibody forming cells in that some 25 to 30 days are required to bring the level of the response down to that obtained within 12-15 days in those mice challenged with AHGG alone.

Relationship between the capacity of LPS to modify the tolerant state and its ability to act as a B cell mitogen. The property of LPS to induce B cell mitogenesis (see review of Andersson et al. (13)) has been shown to be mediated by the lipid A moiety of the molecule (8, 14, 15, 16). Lipid A also possesses the capacity to affect the induction of tolerance. Table 3 reveals that lipid A or any LPS preparation which contains lipid A including those from mutant bacterial strains whose LPS do not have the O polysaccharide (J5 and Re 595) can convert a tolerogenic effect into an immunogenic stimulus. The data also show that although this effect can be seen when tolerogen and LPS injections are separated by an interval of 3 hours, the injection of LPS 10 days after tolerogen does not lead to an immune response. As before, these temporal limitations are interpreted as reflecting the ability of LPS to function in spite of T cell tolerance but not in a state of B cell tolerance to HGG.

What is the effect of LPS on tolerance induction under conditions where LPS is not mitogenic? This can be determined by using a mouse strain whose spleen cells are refractive to the induction of mitogenesis by LPS. Table 4 shows that, as originally described by Sultzer and Nilsson, C3H/HeJ mice do not show ^{3}H thymidine incorporation following exposure to a wide range of LPS concentrations. This appears to be an effect specifically restricted to C3H/HeJ mice in that other C3H strains (exemplified by the C3H/St) respond in a normal fashion. Moreover, although the present data show results obtained from 2 day cultures, the absence of LPS induced mitogenesis in C3H/HeJ spleen cells is evident at each day of a four day culture period (18). In this strain of mice, LPS is incapable of altering the normal induction process of tolerance. This is shown in Table 5. A dose of LPS which in conjunction with tolerogen produces immunity in the A/J strain has no effect in influencing the induction of tolerance in C3H/HeJ mice. This observation is not due to a difference in the ability of the two strains to respond to the antigen HGG since the data demonstrate that both strains respond equally well to AHGG.

TABLE 3

Capacity of various LPS preparations and of Lipid A to modulate the induction of tolerance to HGG.

Injections Deaggregated HGG and	Time Injected	Response Indirect PFC per Spleen
Saline	3 hours	70
LPS	"	7,730
J5-LPS	"	10,470
Re 595-LPS	"	11,740
Lipid A	"	12,270
Saline	10 days	60
LPS	"	100
Re 595-LPS	"	110
Lipid A	"	70

A/J male mice were injected ip at time 0 with 1.0 mg deaggregated HGG. Either 3 hours or 10 days later, groups of 5 mice each were injected iv with saline or 50 µg of one of the following preparations: E. coli 0111:B4 LPS, E. coli 0111:B4 LPS obtained from the epimeraseless mutant J-5, S. minnesota LPS obtained from the mutant strain Re 595, or Lipid A obtained by mild acid hydrolysis of E. coli 0111:B4 LPS. 12 days after the second injection, spleen cells from individual mice were assayed for indirect plaque forming cells (PFC) specific to HGG. Preparation of the various LPS fractions was performed as previously described (10).

TABLE 4

Strain differences in responsiveness of spleen cells to LPS-induced mitogenesis.

Mitogen (µg/ml)	CPM/Culture		
	A/J	C3H/St	C3H/HeJ
None (Saline)	675	994	181
LPS (0.1)	—	7,270	156
" (1)	5,271	15,942	144
" (10)	5,271	16,807	174
" (100)	3,245	13,484	112
Con A (5)	47,997	29,468	26,746

The culture methods used are based on those developed by Mishell and Dutton (33). Spleen cell cultures were prepared containing 2×10^6 viable cells in 1 ml of medium supplemented with 5% FCS. Duplicate cultures were incubated for 2 days in the presence of either saline, LPS, or Con A, after which time the stimulation of DNA synthesis was assessed by a 4 hr pulse with ^{3}H-TdR (1 µCi/ml, 5 Ci/mmole). Cells were then harvested, washed, precipitated with 5% TCA, and the precipitates collected onto Millipore filters. Radioactive measurements were made after overnight accommodation of samples in Aquasol scintillation fluid. A/J and C3H/HeJ mice were purchased from Jackson Laboratories, Bar Harbor, Maine and C3H/St mice were purchased from L. Strong Laboratories, Del Mar, Calif.

TABLE 5

Effect of LPS on the induction of tolerance to HGG in A/J and C3H/HeJ strains.

Initial Treatment	Challenge	Response (Indirect PFC/Spleen)	
		A/J	C3H/HeJ
DHGG + Saline	AHGG	291	632
DHGG + LPS	AHGG	21,308	15
Saline	AHGG	8,958	8,075

Male mice of either the A/J or C3H/HeJ strains were injected ip on day 0 with 2.5 mg of deaggregated HGG (DHGG) and 3 hours later with either saline or 50 μg of E. coli K235 LPS given iv. 15 days after this initial treatment, all mice were challenged with 100 μg aggregated HGG (AHGG) given iv, and 4 days after this injection, plaque forming cells (PFC) specific to HGG were quantitated in individual spleens. To measure the primary response to AHGG in both strains, mice initially treated with saline were injected iv with 100 μg AHGG and plaqued 6 days later, at the peak of the response. The response represents the arithmetic mean of that obtained in 5 mice.

Base hydrolysis of LPS is a treatment which removes ester-linked fatty acids from the lipid A moiety of the molecule without altering the polysaccharide portion (19). This chemical modification also greatly reduces the mitogenic activity of LPS (14, 15, 16, 18). In addition, Table 6 reveals that base hydrolyzed LPS has no effect on the induction process of tolerance in A/J mice. That is, those mice given tolerogen and base hydrolyzed LPS are as unresponsive to a challenge of AHGG as are those animals treated with tolerogen alone. Thus, under two conditions in which LPS is non-mitogenic, namely in the C3H/HeJ mouse and after chemical modification with base hydrolysis, LPS cannot alter the normal induction process of tolerance to HGG.

DISCUSSION

The ability of LPS to interfere with the maintenance or the induction of a tolerant state to HGG in mice is a phenomenon whose in situ mechanism is extremely difficult to dissect. For one thing, a hypothetical treatise on the observation that LPS modulates the induction of tolerance to stimulation of specific antibody demands some details of the in vivo biological basis of cellular cooperation which leads to antibody formation. Thus far however none of the competing theories (20, 21, 22) has been either ruled in or ruled out. An added burden to a rational interpretation of this phenomenon is the fact that LPS has a myriad of biological activities which can affect a broad spectrum of physiological systems and their controls (23). Finally, the nature of immunological tolerance has itself been the object of divergent interpretation. The more classical view of functional clonal elimination (24) has been challenged by a concept of regulatory homeostatic balance perhaps mediated by a population of T cells with a specialized suppressive capacity (see individual papers by Baker, Droege and Gershon in this volume).

If one assumes that 3 cell types, T and B lymphocytes and macrophages, integrate their efforts in the eventual formation of specific antibody, then it is necessary to consider which of these cells can be functionally affected by LPS. There is evidence that LPS can act directly on B cells to stimulate both cellular replication and IgM synthesis (13), although more recent data would suggest that LPS induced mitogenesis requires both T cells and macrophages (25). The adjuvant effect of LPS on antibody formation has been regarded as potentiating specific T cell helper function possibly due to an increase in the interaction between macrophages and T cells resulting in

TABLE 6

Inability of base hydrolyzed LPS (BH-LPS) to interfere with the induction of tolerance to HGG in A/J mice.

Initial Treatment	Challenge	Response Indirect PFC/Spleen
DHGG + Saline	AHGG	36
DHGG + LPS	AHGG	7,785
DHGG + BH-LPS	AHGG	0

A/J male mice were injected ip with 2.5 mg deaggregated HGG (DHGG) and 3 hours later with an iv injection of either saline, 50 μg of E. coli 0111:B4 LPS or 50 μg of E. coli 0111:B4 LPS which had been base hydrolyzed. 24 days after the initial treatment, all groups were challenged with 100 μg aggregated HGG (AHGG) given iv. 4 days following this injection, plaque forming cells (PFC) specific to HGG were quantitated in individual spleens. The response represents the arithmetic mean of that obtained in 5 mice.

specific T cell proliferation (26, 27, 28). Macrophage activation by LPS (29, 30) is another biological effect which merits the utmost consideration inasmuch as both inductive (31) and suppressive (32) roles have been implicated for this cell type in immunological reactions.

Critical to the question of how LPS affects a state of tolerance is whether the phenomenon can occur in spite of absolute T cell tolerance. Although it has been previously reported that mice making specific antibody to HGG following the injection of DHGG and LPS had tolerant thymocytes (12), the scope of peripheral T cell unresponsiveness has not yet been critically evaluated. More recent experiments which utilize a set of antigens that demonstrate T cell cross-reactivity but little B cell cross-reactivity (HGG and equine gamma globulin (EGG)) indicate that the dual treatment of LPS and DHGG allows the expression of a state of immunity to HGG although the animals show a marked suppression in their ability to respond to a challenge with EGG. Although admittedly indirect, these observations suggest that a normal complement of specific T cell helper function may not be necessary to obtain the effect seen with LPS. They do not however eliminate the possibility that LPS and antigen may amplify a residual population of non-tolerant specific T cells. An alternative to the requirement of antigen specific T cell help may be a T cell activity non-specifically stimulated (? via LPS activated macrophages) or even T cell activity specifically recognizing LPS bound on B cells. What is clearly apparent from the previous discussion is that consideration of the precise mechanism by which LPS modulates a tolerant state requires more defined parameters than those presently on hand and that esoteric cellular interpretations of this phenomenon at the present are premature.

ACKNOWLEDGMENTS

This is publication number 827 from the Department of Experimental Pathology, Scripps Clinic and Research Foundation, La Jolla, Ca. We thank Ms. Emma Lum, Lee Cunningham and Linda Lewis for their excellent technical assistance.

This work was supported by U. S. Public Health Service Grant AI-07007, American Cancer Grant #IM-42D and AEC Contract AT (04-3)410. J.M.C. and J.A.L. are each supported by Dernham Fellowships of the California Division of the American Cancer Society (No. J-209 and D-202 respectively), B.J.S. by USPHS Training Grant AI-00453 and W.O.W. by USPHS Career Development Award 5-K6-GM-06936-13.

REFERENCES

1. Dresser, D.W. and Mitchison, N.A., Advances in Immunol. 8, 129 (1968).
2. Weigle, W.O., Advances in Immunol. 16, 61 (1973).
3. Dresser, D. W., Immunology 5, 378 (1962).
4. Chiller, J. M. and Weigle, W. O., Contemporary Topics in Immunology I, M. Hanna (Ed.), Plenum Pub. Corp., New York, 1971, p. 119.
5. Chiller, J. M., Habicht, G. S. and Weigle, W. O., Proc. Nat. Acad. Sci. U.S., 65, 551 (1970).
6. Chiller, J. M., Habicht, G. S. and Weigle, W. O., Science 171, 813 (1971).
7. Habicht, G. S., Chiller, J. M. and Weigle, W. O., Immune Response at the Cellular Level, T. P. Zacharia (Ed.), Marcel Dekker Inc., New York, 1973, p. 141.
8. Chiller, J. M., Skidmore, B. J., Morrison, D. C. and Weigle, W. O., Proc. Nat. Acad. Sci. U.S., 70, 2129 (1973).
9. Chiller, J. M. and Weigle, W. O., J. Immunol. 110, 1051 (1973).
10. Chiller, J. M. and Weigle, W. O., J. Exp. Med. 137, 740 (1973).
11. Claman, H. N., J. Immunol. 91, 833 (1963).
12. Louis, J. A., Chiller, J. M. and Weigle, W. O., J. Exp. Med. 138, 1481 (1973).
13. Andersson, J., Sjöberg, O. and Möller, G., Transpl. Reviews 11, 131 (1972).
14. Andersson, J., Melchers, F., Galanos, C. and Lüderitz, O., J. Exp. Med. 137, 943 (1973).
15. Peavy, D. L., Shands, J. W., Adler, W. H. and Smith, R. T., J. Immunol. 111, 352 (1973).
16. Rosenstreich, D. L., Nowotny, A., Chused, T. and Mergenbagen, S. E., Inf. and Imm. 8, 406 (1973).
17. Sultzer, B.M. and Nilsson, B. S., Nature New Biol., 240, 198 (1972).
18. Skidmore, B. J., Chiller, J. M., Morrison, D. C. and Weigle, W. O., Fed. Proc. 33, 600 (1974).
19. Rietschel, E. T., Gottert, H., Lüderitz, O., and Westphal, O., Eur. J. Biochem. 28, 166 (1972).
20. Bretscher, P. and Cohn, M., Science, 169, 1042 (1970).
21. Feldman, M. and Nossal, G. J. V., Transpl. Rev. 12, 3 (1972).

22. Coutinho, A., Gronowicz, E., Bullock, W. W. and Möller, G., J. Exp. Med. 139, 74 (1974).

23. Neter, E., Current Topics in Microbiology and Immunology, W. Braun (Ed.), Spinger-Verlag, Berlin, 1969, Vol. 47, p. 92.

24. Burnet, F. M., The Clonal Selection Theory of Acquired Immunity, Cambridge Univ. Press, Cambridge, 1959.

25. Kagnoff, M. F., Billings, P. and Cohn, M., J. Exp. Med. 139, 407 (1974).

26. Allison, A. C. and Davies, A. J. S., Nature 223,330 (1971).

27. Hamaoka, T. and Katz, D. H., J. Immunol. 111, 1554 (1973).

28. Armerding, D. and Katz, D. H., J. Exp. Med. 139, 24 (1974).

29. Alexander, P. and Evans, R., Nature, New Biol. 232, 76 (1971).

30. Gery, I. and Waksman, B. H., J. Exp. Med. 136, 143 (1972).

31. Schrader, J. W., J. Exp. Med. 138, 1466 (1973).

32. Yoshinaga, M., Yoshinaga, A. and Waksman, B. H., J. Exp. Med. 136, 956 (1972).

33. Mishell, R. I. and Dutton, R. W., J. Exp. Med. 126, 423 (1967).

THE ROLE OF HISTOCOMPATIBILITY GENE PRODUCTS IN COOPERATIVE CELL INTERACTIONS BETWEEN T AND B LYMPHOCYTES

David H. Katz and Baruj Benacerraf

Department of Pathology
Harvard Medical School
Boston, Massachusetts 02115

ABSTRACT. Three different experimental systems are described which support the hypothesis that active regulation of B cell responses is mediated through either direct membrane interaction with T cells or by the interaction with soluble mediators produced and released by T cells. The collective evidence presented here has led us to formulate an hypothesis that histocompatibility gene products may serve as the molecules largely responsible for regulating cell interactions required for development of most humoral immune responses.

INTRODUCTION

Delineation of the complex events involved in requisite cooperative interactions between thymus-derived (T) and bone marrow-derived (B) lymphocytes in the development of antibody responses to all but a selected class of antigens has been the subject of intensive analysis in many laboratories (reviewed in Ref. 1). Several hypotheses have been developed over the past years to explain the mechanism of T-B cell cooperation. These have included direct or indirect antigen presentation by T cells, and the active regulation of B cell responses by either direct membrane interaction with T cells or by the interaction with soluble mediators produced and released by T cells (1). The latter hypothesis stems largely from the demonstration that T cells activated by means other than the constituent determinants of the antigen employed, such as by allogeneic cell interactions, were highly effective in providing helper function for antigen-specific B cells (1).

In this paper, we will discuss three different experimental systems currently under active investigation in our laboratory which support the latter hypothesis mentioned above. These different approaches include: 1) the identification of genes and gene products in the major histocompatibility gene complex and of their products in governing optimal T-B cell cooperative interactions: 2) the biological and biochemical properties of a non-specific mediator produced by populations of activated T cells and its activi-

ty on the in vitro antibody responses of mouse lymphocytes:
and 3) the elicitation of hapten-specific antibody responses
in vivo by stimulation of carrier-specific T cells and hapten-specific B cells by their relevant determinants administered independently and on separate molecules. Based on
these collective observations, we will develop a model to
explain the possible role of histocompatibility gene products
in regulating humoral immune responses.

GENETIC RESTRICTIONS OF T-B CELL INTERACTIONS

In order to minimize possible confusion of terminology,
the phenomenon of the allogeneic effect has been distinguished from interactions between normally isologous antigen-specific T and B lymphocytes by referring to the latter, for
the purposes of brevity, as "physiologic" T-B cell cooperation. The "allogeneic effect" is that pheonomenon in which
specific B lymphocytes become readily activated by antigen
in the absence of antigen-specific helper T cells by virtue
of a direct interaction with histoincompatible T lymphocytes
recognizing surface antigen differences on such cells (1, 2).
In our studies, several approaches have been employed to answer the question of physiologic cooperative interactions between histoincompatible T and B lymphocytes in humoral immune responses. The experimental schemes were designed specifically to circumvent the possible contribution to the results of a complicating allogeneic effect (2) based on our
unexpected earlier observations that a heavily irradiated
mouse (600 R) possesses sufficient numbers of active residual T cells to exert this effect on a small population of
adoptively transferred histoincompatible primed B lymphocytes (3). This was accomplished for in vivo cell transfer
studies by using an F1 hybrid host as the recipient of limited number of carrier-primed T lymphocytes from one parent
(irradiated in situ after transfer) and DNP-keyhole limpet
hemocyanin (KLH)-primed B lymphocytes from the opposite parental strain. The latter cells are depleted of T lymphocytes
by treatment with anti-θ serum and complement prior to transfer to eliminate development of a fatal graft-vs.-host reaction in the irradiated F1 recipient (4, 5).
This protocol takes advantage of the fact that: 1)
primed mature mouse T lymphocytes are relatively radioresis-
tant when they are subjected to x-irradiation in situ after
adoptive transfer and a suitable period for migration to the
recipient lymphoid organs has elapsed (6); and 2) semi-
allogeneic recipients are genetically incapable of reacting
against histocompatibility specificities of either parental

strain lymphocytes. Since the F_1 host is genetically incapable of reacting against either parental donor cell population, and since the irradiated carrier-primed parental cells are present in restricted numbers, the allogeneic effect has been avoided. Furthermore, the fact that the transferred parental DNP-specific B cells in the F_1 recipient, which would be the potential target for the allogeneic effect, constitutes but a small proportion of the cells against which the T cells from the second parent can react in the F_1 environment is an additional argument for the absence of allogeneic effects in our experiments.

The protocol and results of one series of combinations of T and B cells in which the DNP-primed B cells were derived from A/J ($H-2^a$) donor mice are shown in Fig. 1 (5). For convenience, the relevant genetic similarities and/or differences are listed for each combination. Groups I and II demonstrate the intact cooperative functional capacities of the irradiated (in situ) bovine gamma globulin (BGG)-primed and the anti-θ-treated DNP-primed cells of syngeneic A/J origin within the environs of (AxB10)F_1 irradiated recipients (Group II) as compared to control recipients of normal cells (Group I). Similarly, BGG-primed T cells derived from congenic-resistant B10.A donors, which are identical with A/J at the major $H-2^a$ locus but dissimilar with respect to background genotypes, are capable of exerting a clear helper effect in cooperating with A/J B cells (Groups III and IV). In sharp contrast, T cells from A.By or B10 donors, which are both $H-2^b$, fail to cooperatively interact with A/J B lymphocytes (Groups V-VIII). This is true irrespective of whether or not the genetic background other than H-2 is identical such as in the case of A.By donor cells (Group VI).

Comparable results using reciprocal strains combinations are summarized in Table 1 and provide definitive proof that the gene or genes restricting physiologic T and B cell cooperation do indeed belong to the major H-2 gene complex (5).

There are several possible explanations for the failure of physiologic T-B cell cooperation to occur across the major histocompatibility barrier. Certain of these possibilities which appear to be quite unlikely include the following:

1) Failure of transferred T and B cells to migrate to appropriate sites in the lymphoid organs in vivo, and/or rejection of one or the other cell type. These possibilities have been eliminated by using the F_1 host as a neutral environment in which very good cooperative interactions could be obtained between H-2 identical cell mixtures and, moreover, by the corroboration of these data in a fully in vitro system (4, and see below).

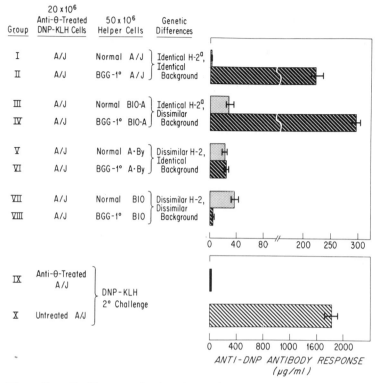

Fig. 1. Failure of physiologic cooperative interactions to occur between T and B lymphocytes differing at the major histocompatibility locus. The scheme followed is described in text. Recipients for all cell combinations were (AxB10)F₁ hybrids. Combinations and strain origins of T and B cells and the relevant genetic differences are indicated. Recipients in groups I-VIII were secondarily challenged with 50 μg of DNP-BGG; groups IX and X received 20 μg of DNP-KLH. Mean serum anti-DNP antibody levels of groups of 5 mice on day 7 after secondary challenge are illustrated. Horizontal bars represent ranges of the standard errors. (5)

TABLE 1

CAPACITY OF T AND B LYMPHOCYTES OF VARIOUS STRAIN ORIGINS
TO PHYSIOLOGICALLY INTERACT

B Cells	T Cells	Genetic Differences	Cooperative Response
A (H-2^a)	A (H-2^a)	None	Yes
A (H-2^a)	B10.A (H-2^a)	Background	Yes
B10.A (H-2^a)	B10.A (H-2^a)	None	Yes
B10.A (H-2^a)	A (H-2^a)	Background	Yes
A.By (H-2^b)	A.By (H-2^b)	None	Yes
A (H-2^a)	A.By (H-2^b)	H-2 alone	No
A (H-2^a)	B10 (H-2^b)	H-2 and Background	No
B10.A (H-2^a)	B10 (H-2^b)	H-2 alone	No
B10.A (H-2^a)	A.By (H-2^b)	H-2 and Background	No
A.By (H-2^b)	A (H-2^a)	H-2 alone	No
A.By (H-2^b)	B10.A (H-2^a)	H-2 and Background	No

(Ref. 5)

2) A "block" of some sort to cell-cell interaction by
the presence of a foreign major histocompatibility specificity on the cell surface of one or the other of the lymphocyte
classes. This has been ruled out in our initial studies by
experiments demonstrating highly effective cooperation between reciprocal combinations of parental and F_1 hybrid T
and B lymphocytes and provided that the carrier antigen employed is one to which both parental strains involved are
genetic responders (4). An example of this (in one direction) is illustrated in Fig. 2. These findings demonstrate,
moreover, that the existence of one common major H-2 haplotype is sufficient for effective interaction to occur between
two cell populations even though the F_1 cells also possess a
set of foreign H-2 specificities.

3) Ineffective or inefficient macrophage-lymphocyte interaction due to major histocompatibility differences. This
possibility plays little, if any, significant role in these
data since the major macrophage component is most likely provided by the irradiated F_1 host. The latter not only share
a common haplotype with both parental H-2 specificities but
also support good cooperative responses between adoptively
transferred isogeneic T and B cells. Furthermore, other
studies from our laboratory have provided evidence that, in
in vitro mouse spleen cell cultures, antigen-bearing macrophages from allogeneic donors are as effective as those from
syngeneic donors in presenting DNP-KLH to T and B cells in
the elicitation of secondary anti-DNP responses (7).

4) Non-specific suppressive influences exerted by the
adoptively transferred allogeneic T cells on the DNP-specific
B cells. This seems remote since nonspecific enhancement,
rather than suppression, due to allogeneic effects was the
major difficulty to overcome in developing the system (3).
Moreover, primed parental T cells were shown to serve as effective helper cells for F_1 B cells under circumstances where
comparable suppressive effects, had they existed, might be
expected to manifest themselves (4). Finally, in an experiment designed to test this possibility directly, proof has
been obtained that no appreciable nonspecific suppressive influence exists to explain the absence of cooperative responses between histoincompatible T and B cells (8). Thus,
as shown in Table 2, concomitant transfer of histoincompatible carrier-primed T cells does not appreciably diminish the
cooperative response between isogeneic T and B cells (Group
VII).

This reasoning has led us to conclude, therefore, that
the genetic restrictions for physiologic cooperation between
T and B cells in the immune response concern the actual co-

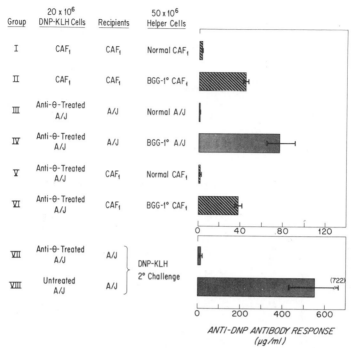

Fig. 2. Demonstration of physiologic cooperative interactions between T and B lymphocytes sharing one major histocompatibility specificity in common and differing by another:
Using F₁ hybrid helper T cells with parental B cells. The
donor cell-recipient strain combinations are indicated. Recipients in groups I - VI were secondarily challenged with
50 µg of DNP-BGG. Groups VII and VIII received 20 µg of DNP-
KLH. Mean serum anti-DNP antibody levels of groups of 6 mice
on day 7 after secondary challenge are illustrated. Horizontal bars represent ranges of the standard errors. (4)

TABLE 2

FAILURE OF HISTOINCOMPATIBLE T CELLS TO INTERFERE WITH PHYSIOLOGIC COOPERATION
BETWEEN SYNGENEIC T AND B LYMPHOCYTES

| | PROTOCOL* | | |
| | 20 x 10⁶ | 50 x 10⁶ Irradiated | |
Group	Anti-θ Treated DNP-KLH B Cells	Helper Cells	Antibody Responses**
			(µg/ml)
I	BALB/c	Normal BALB/c	1.2
II	BALB/c	BGG-1° BALB/c	152.7
III	A/J	Normal A/J	5.8
IV	A/J	BGG-1° A/J	173.4
V	BALB/c	Normal A/J	7.3
VI	BALB/c	BGG-1° A/J	4.9
VII	BALB/c	BGG-1° BALB/c + BGG-1° A/J	189.4

*50 x 10⁶ normal or BGG primed spleen cells were transferred intravenously to non-irradiated CAF₁ recipients; 24 hrs. later, the recipients were irradiated and then given a second transfer consisting of 20 x 10⁶ anti-θ-treated DNP-primed B lymphocytes from either syngeneic or allogeneic donors as indicated. Secondary challenge with 50 µg of DNP-BGG in saline was given intraperitoneally immediately thereafter.

**The data are expressed as geometric mean serum anti-DNP levels of groups of 5 mice on day 7 after secondary challenge. Statistical comparisons between the various groups yielded the following results: 1) groups I and II - 0.001>P; 2) groups III and IV - 0.001>P; 3) groups II and VII - 0.80>P>0.70. (Ref. 8)

576

operative interaction between these cells. The studies described above as well as similar observations of Kindred and Shreffler (9) thus far provide clear evidence that the relevant gene or genes involved belong to the major histocompatibility complex. It is now essential to identify more precisely the genetic region concerned with H-2 primarily involved. In our initial studies, no cooperation occurred with mixtures of T and B cells from BALB/c (H-2^d) and A/J (H-2^a) donors, respectively (4). These particular strains are identical at Ss and the entire D-end of the H-2 complex but possess major differences at the K-end. Many differences are known to exist in the I region as well. What this tells us is that gene identities only at Ss and D are insufficient to permit optimal cooperative interactions to occur under these conditions. It is important, therefore, to determine precisely what gene or combination of gene differences are sufficient to either permit or restrict physiologic T-B cell cooperation.

In view of these findings which indicate that differences at K and I gene regions prevent effective T-B cell cooperation, we next asked whether identities at only K and I are sufficient to allow effective cooperation. In the following experiment (10), we have utilized the micro-culture system developed in our laboratory for eliciting cooperative T-B cell responses to soluble DNP-carrier conjugates as described elsewhere (4, 11, 12). As shown in Fig. 3, DNP-primed B cells from A/J (H-2^a) donors effectively interact with irradiated KLH-primed T cells from isogeneic A/J and syngeneic B10.A donors. In addition, effective cooperative responses developed between A/J B cells and T cells from B10.BR donors which differ from A/J at genes in the Ss and D regions. In the reciprocal mixed cell cultures, DNP-primed B cells from B10.BR interacted with T cells from A/J and B10.A donors as well as isogeneic T cells to develop secondary in vitro anti-DNP antibody responses to DNP-KLH. Although not shown in this figure, these data do not reflect non-specific allogeneic effects as an explanation for successful cooperation between A and B10.BR lymphocytes since reciprocal controls using irradiated normal rather than KLH-primed cells failed to develop secondary responses to DNP-KLH. These results are, in essence, the reciprocal situation of our initial combination of BALB/c and A/J which failed to cooperate despite identities at Ss and D (4). The development of cooperative responses between A/J and B10.BR which differ for genes in Ss and D but are identical for K and I region genes indicate that the critical genes involved in T-B cell cooperation exist in the latter regions. It must be stated, however,

577

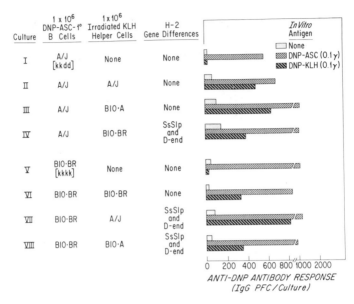

Fig. 3. In Vitro cooperative responses between cells differing at genes in the Ss and D-end of the H-2 complex. Spleen cells from DNP-ASC-primed A/J or B10.BR mice were cultured alone or together with irradiated KLH-primed spleen cells (as a source of helper T cells) from the strains indicated in the presence of either no antigen, 0.1 µg/ml DNP-ASC or 0.1 µg/ml DNP-KLH. The IgG anti-DNP antibody response after 4 days incubation in micro-cultures are shown. Letters in brackets symbolize the H-2 genotype of A/J and B10.BR strains. Relevant H-2 gene differences are listed in the column to the immediate left of the data.

that these results should be considered with some degree of caution until fully corroborated in an in vivo system. The data described above raise the intriguing possibility that identities at the I gene region either alone or together with K or D end identities are the critical determinants for T-B cell interaction. By taking advantage of our previous demonstration (Fig. 2) of highly effective cooperation between reciprocal combinations of parental and F1 hybrid T and B lymphocytes when the carrier molecule employed is one to which both parental strains are genetic responders (4), we next asked the question of whether F1 carrier-primed T cells can serve as helper cells for either or both parental B cells when: a) the carrier molecule employed is under genetic control such that one parental strain is a responder and the other is a non-responder, and b) the determinant specificity of the parental B cells being assessed is not under genetic control and bears no relationship to the specificity of the carrier molecule (13). The experimental system utilized an immune response gene controlling responses to the terpolymer L-glutamic acid-L-lysine-L-tyrosine (GLT) to which A strain mice (H-2^a) are non-responders whereas BALB/c (H-2^d) and (BALB/c x A)F1 hybrids, (CAF1) are responders. These studies demonstrated that GLT-primed T cells of CAF1 donors can provide for responder BALB/c, but not for non-responder A/J, the required stimulus for the anti-DNP responses of DNP-specific B cells of these respective parental strains to the DNP conjugate of GLT.

The protocol and results of this adoptive transfer experiment is shown in Fig. 4. As an extension of our previously published data (13), the experiment illustrated here includes secondary antigen challenge with macrophage-bound DNP-GLT in addition to the routinely employed intraperitoneal challenge with soluble DNP-carriers. As shown in Fig. 4, BALB/c (Group II) and A/J (Group VIII) DNP-specific B cells are effectively "helped" by KLH-specific T cells of CAF1 origin in developing secondary adoptive anti-DNP antibody responses to DNP-KLH. Similarly, GLT-primed CAF1 T cells cooperate very well with B cells from BALB/c donors in response to either soluble or macrophage-bound DNP-GLT (Groups IV and VI). In marked contrast, however, is the failure of these same GLT-specific F1 T cells to serve as helper cells for DNP-specific B cells from A/J donor mice irrespective of whether soluble or macrophage-bound DNP-GLT is employed for secondary challenge (Group X and XII). There is no possibility that the different results obtained with BALB/c and A/J B cells reflect marked functional disparities between them since the same pool of cells of respective origins were used

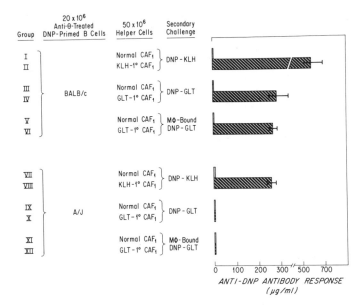

Fig. 4. Involvement of I gene in control of T and B lymphocyte interactions. Recipients for all cell combinations were CAF₁ hybrids. The transfer scheme is described in the text. Combinations, strain origins and specificities of T and B cells are indicated. Secondary challenge was performed intraperitoneally with either 20 μg of soluble DNP-KLH or 100 μg of soluble DNP-GLT or intravenously with 10^7 F₁ macrophages (Mφ) containing 2.4 μg DNP-GLT per mouse as indicated. Mean serum anti-DNP antibody levels of groups of 5 mice on day 7 after secondary challenge are illustrated. Horizontal bars represent ranges of the standard errors.

in the cooperating mixtures in recipients of CAF₁ KLH-primed cells in which intact function was manifested in both cases (Groups II and VIII). The same reasoning applies in the case of the GLT-primed CAF₁ cells which functioned very well as helpers for BALB/c B cells (Groups IV and VI), although failing to do so for A/J cells (Groups X and XII). It is not possible to conclude, as yet, whether identity at the I region alone is sufficient for successful and efficient physiologic cooperation. Experiments currently underway with appropriate recombinant strains should resolve this issue. The possibility clearly exists that: 1) identity at the entire H-2 complex is required or 2) identity at the I region together with genes coded for at either the K or D-end of H-2 are sufficient. However, if this is the case, the present experiments establish that insofar as the CAF₁ T cell is concerned, the I gene cannot function efficiently with the possibly required K or D-end genes when in the -trans position.

It is essential to emphasize the point that what these experiments demonstrate is that certain identities of H-2 genes are required for the most effective T-B cell interactions; such identities may not constitute an absolute requirement for T-B interactions to occur under certain circumstances. Thus, Bechtal, et al (14) have observed that tetraparental mice derived from responder and non-responder strains may produce antibodies of non-responder allotype under conditions of hyperimmunization. More recent studies from our own laboratories by Benacerraf, et al (15) demonstrated that in a totally in vitro system, (responder x non-responder)F₁ T cells primed to the terpolymer L-glutamic acid, L-alanine, L-tyrosine (GAT), which fail to provide helper function for non-responder B cells in response to GAT added to cultures in free soluble form, will "help" such B cells when the GAT is added to cultures in small quantities attached to macrophages. However, as shown above DNP-GLT on macrophages failed to elicit a cooperative DNP response between F₁ responder T cells and parental non-responder B cells in vivo. Finally, it should be reiterated that as seen in the allogeneic effect, activated allogeneic T cells provide the necessary stimulus for triggering antigen-activated B cells if the specificity of the T cell is directed against surface alloantigen differences.

BIOLOGICAL AND BIOCHEMICAL PROPERTIES OF A T CELL PRODUCT ACTIVE IN TRIGGERING B LYMPHOCYTES

A major effort in studies on the mechanism of T-B cell interactions has been focused on the identification of various biologically active substances capable of influencing lymphocyte function in antibody responses to different antigens elicited in in vitro systems. The demonstration by Dutton, Kettman and their colleagues (16) that supernatants obtained from short-term cultures of histoincompatible mouse spleen cells contained a non-antigen-specific biologically active mediator capable of markedly affecting in vitro antibody responses to thymus-dependent antigens provided evidence for the existence of such a possible mediator. In this section, we will briefly review some very recent data of Armerding and Katz (12) on the biological and certain biochemical properties of an active moiety produced in supernatants of short-term (24 hours) in vitro reactions between T cells specifically activated to foreign alloantigens and the corresponding target cell population.

The basic points to which we have addressed these studies can be summarized as follows: 1) Can an active material be generated during in vitro reactions between histoincompatible lymphocyte populations that operates in a virtually identical biological fashion on in vitro antibody responses as the phenomenon we termed the "allogeneic effect" (17) operates in in vivo antibody responses? 2) What are the biochemical properties of such material(s)? and 3) Are there identifiable similarities in the genetic restrictions governing the biological action of such material on lymphocytes in vitro as has been documented to exist in T-B cell interactions in vivo and in vitro (4, 5, 8, 13)?

1) Can allogeneic effect factors (AEF) be generated in vitro? One of the reasons of great concern in asking this question is the fact that, heretofore, studies with allogeneic cell culture supernatants have been largely performed on in vitro responses to particulate antigens, such as heterologous erythrocytes of haptenated erythrocytes, in which circumstances positive results have been rather reproducibly obtained (2, 16, 18-27). On the other hand, in the one previously published study in which the activity of allogeneic cell supernatants on in vitro responses to soluble DNP-carriers was examined, the enhancing effect could only be observed on responses to a thymus-independent DNP-carrier (20).

This apparent distinction between the capacity of allogeneic factors to stimulate B cell responses to particulate but not soluble antigens has been clarified by the following observations in our studies (12). AEF can reconstitute helper cell function in responses of T cell-depleted primed spleen cells to soluble DNP-proteins, but the extent to which AEF will either exhibit a reconstituting effect or permit the

development of secondary in vitro anti-DNP responses to heterologous DNP-carriers is clearly determined by the form in
which the specific DNP determinants are presented to the B
cell. Thus, as shown in Fig. 5, cultures of DNP-KLH-primed
lymphocytes in which the presence of AEF failed to stimulate
responses to the heterologous conjugate, DNP-fowl gamma globulin (FγG), added to the culture in free soluble form could
develop very good secondary responses to the same conjugate
bound to macrophage surface membranes. Moreover, the response to macrophage-bound DNP-FγG in the presence of AEF
was totally abolished by addition of free soluble DNP-FγG to
the same culture. It appears, therefore, that the presence
of a sufficient quantity of free DNP-carrier molecules might
render all or some of the DNP-specific B cells refractory to
the action of AEF or, for that matter, the product(s) of
carrier-stimulated T cells if the latter are in any way different from AEF.

The strongest evidence that our active AEF acts directly on B cells stems from the capacity of AEF to stimulate B
cells exposed to DNP conjugated to the D-glutamic acid, D-
lysine (D-GL) copolymer. This compound has been demonstrated to be highly tolerogenic for DNP-specific B cells
both in vivo and in vitro under normal circumstances (28-30).
However, when administered to appropriately-primed animals
during a critical time period after induction of an in vivo
allogeneic effect, DNP-D-GL can provide a definite inductive
stimulus for primary or secondary anti-DNP antibody responses (1, 2, 28). Since no demonstrable T cell function
specific for the D-GL carrier has been demonstrated, these
observations provided the strongest indirect proof that the
allogeneic effect is mediated by a direct interaction on the
responding B cells. The capacity of AEF to permit in vitro
responses to DNP-D-GL (not shown) constitutes conclusive
evidence, therefore, that the active moiety involved is acting directly on B lymphocytes (12).

2. What are the biochemical properties of AEF? The experiments performed thus far have demonstrated the following
salient physicochemical features of the active enhancing
molecule in AEF (12): a) it is a trypsin-sensitive protein;
b) it is labile to heating (56°C, 1 hour), thereby indicating the importance of tertiary structure to activity; and
c) it has a molecular weight in the range of 30,000-40,000.
Thus, as shown in Fig. 6, the active moeity in AEF capable
of triggering B lymphocyte responses to SRBC elutes from
Sephadex G-100 in a fraction corresponding to that of an insulin marker which has a m.w. of around 36,000.

583

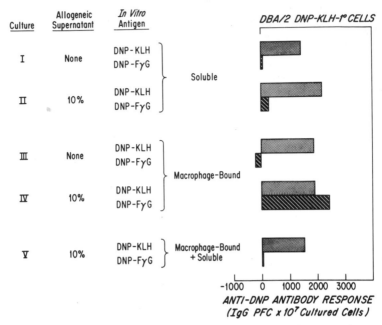

Fig. 5. The capacity of AEF to bypass the requirement for carrier-specific helper T cells in secondary in vitro anti-DNP antibody responses. Spleen cells from DNP-KLH-primed (4 months) DBA/2 were cultured at a cell density of 1.67 x 10⁶ cells/ml with or without antigen in the presence or absence of 10% allogeneic supernatant as indicated. Soluble DNP-KLH or DNP-FγG were added at a concentration of 1 µg/ml (cultures I, II and V). Macrophage-bound antigen was added on 2.5 x 10⁴ macrophages per well (cultures III, IV and V). The IgG anti-DNP responses after 4 days are shown. Background values for non-antigen stimulated control cultures have been subtracted from each corresponding experimental value for purposes of clarity. (10)

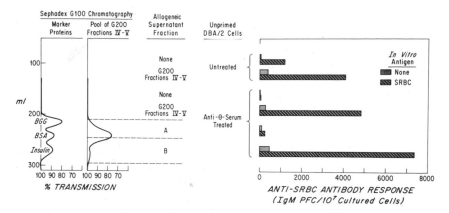

Fig. 6. Comparison of activities of unseparated and Sephadex G-100-fractionated AEF on primary anti-SRBC responses of untreated and anti-θ serum-treated DBA/2 spleen cells. Fractions IV and V from G-200 were pooled and subjected to further chromatography on G-100. The elution patterns of this supernatant and the corresponding markers BGG (m.w. 150,000), BSA (m.w. 65,000) and insulin (m.w. 36,000 in hexameric form) are shown on the far left. The primary IgM anti-SRBC responses of untreated and anti-θ serum-treated DBA/2 cells in the presence of the various fractions indicated (50% concentration in reference to the original unseparated supernatant) are shown. (10)

3. Are there genetic restrictions governing the biological
activity of AEF? This question is raised as a result of the
observations discussed in the preceding section which demonstrate that most effective cooperative T-B cell interactions
occur when the respective cell populations possess identical
genes located within the H-2 gene complex (4,5,8,13). It
occurred to us, therefore, that the active enhancing moiety
in AEF might indeed represent one such molecule and, if so,
should manifest some relationship to histocompatibility
specificities. One might predict, for example, that the
active enhancing molecule should act best or preferentially
on B cells derived from the same histocompatibility type as
the effector T lymphocytes producing the molecules.

The studies carried out thus far are not definitive in
this regard. However, there is a clear suggestion of the
possible preferential activity of AEF on syngeneic B lymphocytes (12). Thus, as shown in Table 3, AEF from supernatants of mixed cultures containing DBA/2 activated T cells
and irradiated C3D2F₁ target cells clearly exhibit the
greatest enhancing and reconstituting effects on B lymphocytes from DBA/2 and C3D2F₁ mice, both of which possess the
DBA/2 (H-2^d) histocompatibility molecules. The purified
AEF, although fully reconstituting C3H (H-2^k) and BALB/c
(H-2^d) B cell responses, only partially reconstituted
responses to sheep erythrocytes (SRBC) of B cells from
C57Bl/6 mice (Table 4). Of course, it is not surprising to
observe activity on the cells bearing the C3H haplotype
since the target cells bearing such surface antigens might
also release active molecules with preferential activity on
C3H cells. Moreover, preliminary absorption studies with
various spleen cell populations have demonstrated that
spleen cells from normal DBA/2 mice are considerably more
effective than cells of other strains in absorbing the biological enhancing activity from AEF derived from DBA/2 T
cells (31).

ELICITATION OF ANTI-HAPTEN ANTIBODY RESPONSES BY
NON-LINKED HAPTEN AND CARRIER DETERMINANTS

In earlier studies from our laboratory on T cell
regulation of IgE antibody responses in mice, we found that
adoptively transferred DNP-KLH-primed cells could be stimulated to develop secondary anti-DNP responses in vivo by
administration of the relevant haptenic and carrier determinants (i.e. DNP and KLH) on distinctly separate molecules
(32). This demonstration was indeed surprising in view of
our own, as well as that of others (33-37), failure to

TABLE 3

RECONSTITUTION OF HELPER CELL FUNCTION IN SECONDARY IN VITRO ANTI-DNP ANTIBODY RESPONSES OF VARIOUS MOUSE STRAINS WITH ALLOGENEIC EFFECT FACTORS. *

Exp.	Strain	Cells	In Vitro Antigen	IgG ANTI-DNP RESPONSE	
				No AEF	AEF (20%)
1	DBA/2	Untreated	None	26	1,440
			DNP-KLH	3,400	3,780
		anti-θ-serum treated	None	146	68
			DNP-KLH	440	3,000
2	C3H	Untreated	None	203	317
			DNP-KLH	1,000	1,680
		anti-θ-serum treated	None	160	239
			DNP-KLH	234	510
3	(C3D2)F1	Untreated	None	200	1,202
			DNP-KLH	2,760	4,500
		anti-θ-serum treated	None	26	1,320
			DNP-KLH	360	1,920
4	BALB/c	Untreated	None	66	168
			DNP-KLH	5,400	2,400
		anti-θ-serum treated	None	80	360
			DNP-KLH	360	840

*DNP-KLH-primed, untreated or anti-θ-serum treated, spleen cells (cell-density = 1.67 x 10[6] cells/ml) from various mouse strains were cultured with or without DNP-KLH (1 µg/ml) in the absence or presence of AEF for 4 days. Figures presented are PFC per 10[7] cultured cells. Donors were primed 3 months (Exp. 1), 5 months (Exp. 2) and 3-1/2 months (Exp. 3 & 4). (Ref. 10)

TABLE 4

RECONSTITUTION OF HELPER CELL FUNCTION IN PRIMARY IN VITRO ANTI-SRBC ANTIBODY RESPONSES OF VARIOUS MOUSE STRAINS WITH UNPURIFIED AND SEPHADEX G-200-PURIFIED ALLOGENEIC EFFECT FACTORS.*

Culture	Strain	Cells	In Vitro Antigen	IgM ANTI-SRBC RESPONSE		
				No AEF	Unpurified AEF (10%)	Purified AEF (2%)
1	DBA/2	Untreated	None	50	184	200
			SRBC	450	1,710	3,420
		anti-θ-serum treated	None	50	167	351
			SRBC	60	3,930	6,180
2	C3H	Untreated	None	67	67	412
			SRBC	300	340	1,200
		anti-θ-serum treated	None	40	93	665
			SRBC	40	700	2,060
3	BALB/c	Untreated	None	267	251	251
			SRBC	1,050	570	1,920
		anti-θ-serum treated	None	13	186	519
			SRBC	60	300	2,730
4	C57BL/6	Untreated	None	468	134	268
			SRBC	1,200	300	2,400
		anti-θ-serum treated	None	0	106	240
			SRBC	40	60	720

*Normal, untreated or anti-θ-serum treated spleen cells from various mouse strains (cell density = 1.67 x 10^6 cells/ml for C57BL, 3.33 x 10^6 cells/ml for DBA/2 and BALB/c, and 5 x 10^6 cells/ml for C3H) were cultured with or without SRBC (1%) in the absence or presence of AEF for 4 days. Figures presented are PFC per 10^7 cultured cells. (Ref. 10)

588

elicit responses in a similar manner in earlier studies. Initially, the responses we observed to non-linked determinants occurred only in the IgE antibody class, but when additional carrier-primed cells were added to the transferred DNP-primed population, thus increasing the frequency of specific helper T cells, responses in the IgG class could be stimulated as well (32).

More recently, we have performed a series of experiments to extend these observations by investigating whether the antigens bearing the two determinants would be effective if administered at different times and, if so, the length of time over which respective stimulation of the T and B cells involved in the response would be effective (38).

The protocol and data from one such experiment is summarized in Fig. 7. Irradiated (550 R) CAF$_1$ recipients were injected intravenously on day 0 with 30 x 10^6 cells from syngeneic DNP-Ascaris (ASC)-primed donors. On various days after cell transfer groups of recipients were secondarily challenged intraperitoneally with alum-adsorbed DNP-ASC, DNP-KLH, ASC alone or a mixture of DNP-KLH plus ASC. All recipients were bled 7 days after challenge with one or the other DNP-proteins. As shown in Fig. 7, recipients challenged with DNP-ASC 4 days after the cell transfer developed high titers of anti-DNP antibodies in both IgE and IgG classes (Group I). Recipients challenged at the same time with DNP-KLH alone (Group II) manifested only weak responses in both classes. However, when a mixture of ASC and DNP-KLH was employed for challenge, recipients developed substantially better responses in both IgE and IgG classes (Group III). The magnitude of the secondary IgE and IgG anti-DNP response was even higher when ASC was administered 1 or 2 days prior to DNP-KLH (Groups IV and V). When ASC was administered 3 days before DNP-KLH (Group VI), the IgE response fell to the level obtained with simultaneous challenge (Group III) whereas the IgG response diminished to background titers (Group II).

These data demonstrate, therefore, that not only can anti-hapten antibody responses be effectively generated by stimulation of the respective T and B cells with their specific determinants on distinct molecules, but, moreover, that the stimulation of the two lymphocyte classes can be temporally dissociated within finite limits. The possibility that administration of a very strong antigen, such as ASC or KLH, may stimulate T cells specific for these molecules, respectively, and result in an adjuvant-like milieu that in turn promotes very rapid development of helper T cells specific for the carrier moiety on which the DNP determinant

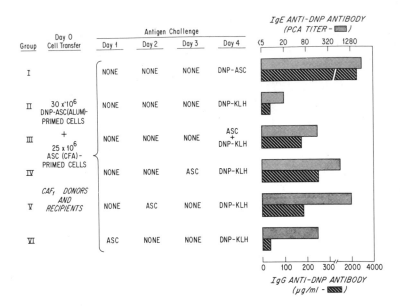

Fig. 7. Temporal requirements for administering hapten and carrier determinanats in eliciting secondary IgE and IgG anti-DNP responses by non-linked molecules. Irradiated (550 R) CAF₁ recipients were injected intravenously on day 0 with 30 x 10⁶ cells from syngeneic donors primed 2 months earlier with DNP-ASC in alum plus 25 x 10⁶ cells from donors primed 4 months earlier with ASC in CFA. On various days after cell transfer, groups of recipients were secondarily challenged intraperitoneally with alum-adsorbed DNP-ASC (10 µg), DNP-KLH (2 µg), ASC (10 µg) or a mixture of DNP-KLH (2 µg) plus ASC (10 µg) as indicated. The IgE and IgG anti-DNP responses of groups of 4 mice on day 7 after DNP-carrier challenge are shown. The differences in IgG responses were statistically significant (0.01>P) in groups II or VI vs. III, IV and V). (36)

is administered, has been tested in our recent studies (36). The capacity to elicit such responses with DNP coupled to a carrier, L-GL, for which no T cell function apparently exists in the mouse, essentially rules out this possibility at least in conditions where the T and B cell determinants are administered together (38).

HYPOTHETICAL SCHEME OF T-B CELL INTERACTIONS

In this last section we will attempt to develop a hypothetical model for T-B cell cooperative interactions based on the collective data presented in the preceding sections. Clearly, much additional work is needed to define precisely which gene(s) in the major histocompatibility complex are most critically involved in T-B cell interactions. However, we do not need to identify the gene or the gene product concerned with physiologic T-B interaction to be able to evaluate the significance of the need for a common gene product on T and B cells for physiologic cooperation to be effective in the immune response to hapten-protein conjugates. The requirement for a common gene product on T and B cells for physiologic cooperation to occur clearly suggests something of critical importance relevant to the mechanism by which such interactions occur.

We have recently proposed that these genetic considerations provide evidence for the existence on the B lymphocyte surface membrane of a site closely related to the histocompatibility specificity that is critically involved in physiologic T-B cell interaction (4,5,13). We envisage this relevant site as an "acceptor" molecule either for the active T cell product or the T cell itself. The necessity for the T and B cells to possess the same gene or genes for physiologic cooperation requires that the same gene product is expressed on both cells or, alternatively, if two gene products are expressed in the respective cell types, the genes concerned have remained closely linked.

The number of specific H-linked Ir genes that have been identified and the specific manner in which they permit immune responses to distinct antigens to take place, particularly at the T cell level, has suggested that they are involved in the specificity of the T cell antigen receptors and may, therefore, be clonally expressed in this class of lymphocytes. Our experiments on the F_1-parent cooperative responses to DNP-GLT indicate, but do not establish, that Ir genes may also be expressed in B cells and demonstrate that their activity is concerned with successful T-B cell interactions in specific immune responses involving carrier recognition. These results clearly indicate that as far as B cells are concerned, if the Ir gene required for T-B cell interactions is indeed expressed in such cells, their products and functional roles are not clonally restricted.

However, an alternative explanation for our results is that GLT-activated F_1 T cells, under control of the relevant I gene on one of its H-2 alleles is limited to effective cooperation only with the B lymphocytes of the parent expressing the histocompatibility specificities coded for by the allele possessing the GLT Ir gene. According to this alternative, there would be no requirement for the functional expression of the Ir gene product in the B cell, but only a requirement for the Ir gene product from the T cell to govern the interaction with the B cell at the histocompatibility site on the B cell surface. This alternative would, however, require that identity at either K alone or K and D end of the H-2 complex exist for successful cooperation to occur. A choice between the two alternatives discussed above would require, as stated earlier, a determination of whether the entire H-2 complex or restricted regions are involved in T-B cell cooperation.

The studies of Armerding and Katz (12) summarized above indicate that a soluble T cell product derived from allo-antigen-activated T cells, and which clearly interacts directly with B lymphocytes to mediate successful triggering, may be related to products of genes in the histocompatibility complex. The observations on temporal dissociation of challenge with relevant carrier and hapten determinants which nonetheless results in good cooperative responses (38) suggest that following activation by antigen, T lymphocytes exist for a finite period of time in a state capable of exerting their influence on B cells and possibly other T cells. If B cells become similarly triggered to a state of receptivity for the T cell signal, then effective cooperation will occur. The intriguing possibility exists that the event of antigen interaction with surface receptors on lymphocytes may induce a critical steric or structural alteration in other cell surface molecules, namely those involved in T-B cell interactions. These data suggest that within a finite period of time this molecular alteration on the T cell surface allows that cell to effectively interact with the similarly altered "acceptor" molecule on the B cell surface.

To elaborate further, we envisage the following sequence involved in effective T-B cell interactions: The antigen-activated T lymphocyte, in close proximity to the appropriate B cell, either engages direct contact at the specific "acceptor" site(s) on the B cell surface and/or releases the active products (AEF) that have specific complementarity for, and bind to, the specific "acceptor" sites on the B lymphocyte. The relevant surface molecules involved are conceivably histocompatibility gene products. It is likely that the antigen-binding event on the specific B cell surface Ig receptors has already taken place before the relevant interaction with the T cell or its product occurs. Perhaps one of the important consequences of the antigen-binding event followed by subsequent movement, capping and endocytosis of the B cell surface immunoglobulin receptors (39) is to either appropriately expose greater numbers of "acceptor" sites or even induce steric conformational changes in the acceptor molecule. Likewise, as suggested above, it is conceivable that the process of activation of the T cell results in a critical steric or structural alteration in the active moiety which allows it then to interact with the B cell acceptor. This mechanism would explain the discriminant regulation involved in normal immune responses since only those T and B lymphocytes whose surface sites have been either appropriately exposed or structurally altered by activation events would be capable of successful interaction. The salient features of this scheme are depicted in Fig. 8.

ACKNOWLEDGMENTS

We are deeply indebted to our colleagues and assistants who have worked so diligently on the studies herein: Drs. Dieter Armerding, Martin Dorf, Toshiyuki Hamaoka and David Osborne, Jr., and Mr. Peter Newburger, Miss Mary Graves, Mr. Henry Dimuzio and Mr. Peter McKenna. We also appreciate the excellent secretarial assistence of Ms. Candace Maher in the preparation of the manuscript.

This work supported by Grants AI-10630 and AI-09920 from the National Institutes of Health, U. S. Public Health Service.

REFERENCES

1. D. H. Katz and B. Benacerraf, Adv. Immunol. 15:1 (1972).
2. D. H. Katz, Transpl. Rev. 12:141 (1972).
3. T. Hamaoka, D. P. Osborne, Jr. and D. H. Katz, J. Exp. Med. 137:1393 (1973).
4. D. H. Katz, T. Hamaoka and B. Benacerraf. J. Exp. Med. 137:1405 (1973).
5. D. H. Katz, T. Hamaoka, M. E. Dorf and B. Benacerraf, Proc. Nat. Acad. Sci. 70:2624 (1973).

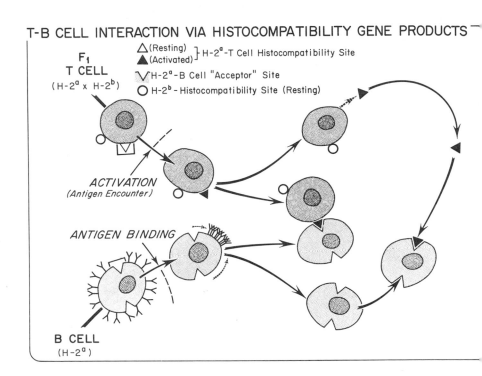

T-B CELL INTERACTION VIA HISTOCOMPATIBILITY GENE PRODUCTS

F_1
T CELL
($H-2^a$ x $H-2^b$)

△(Resting)
▲(Activated) } $H-2^a$-T Cell Histocompatibility Site

∨$H-2^a$-B Cell "Acceptor" Site

○ $H-2^b$- Histocompatibility Site (Resting)

ACTIVATION
(Antigen Encounter)

ANTIGEN BINDING

B CELL
($H-2^a$)

Fig. 8. T-B cell interaction via histocompatibility gene products. The T cell depicted here is an F_1 bearing both parental H-2 alleles. In the case of activation by an antigen, the response to which is under Ir gene control, the scheme depicts alteration of only the parental allele associated with positive Ir status (H-2^a in the figure). The acceptor site on the B cell becomes appropriately exposed after antigen binding and is then reacted upon by the active T cell product either via direct membrane contact or via free molecules released from the T cells.

6. T. Hamaoka, D. H. Katz and B. Benacerraf. Proc. Nat. Acad. Sci. 69:3453 (1972).
7. D. H. Katz and E. R. Unanue, J. Exp. Med. 137:967, (1973).
8. D. H. Katz, T. Hamaoka, M. E. Dorf and B. Benacerraf, J. Immunol. 112:855 (1974).
9. B. Kindred and D. C. Shreffler, J. Immunol. 109:940, (1972).
10. D. H. Katz, M. E. Dorf and B. Benacerraf. Manuscript submitted.
11. D. Armerding and D. H. Katz, J. Exp. Med. 139:24,(1974).
12. D. Armerding and D. H. Katz, J. Exp. Med. In press, (1974).
13. D. H. Katz, T. Hamaoka, M. E. Dorf, P. H. Maurer, B. Benacerraf, J. Exp. Med. 138:734 (1973).
14. K. B. Bechtal, L. A. Herzenberg and H. O. McDevitt, Fed. Proc. 31:777 (1972), Abstract.
15. B. Benacerraf, J. Kapp, C. W. Pierce and D. H. Katz, Manuscript submitted.
16. R. W. Dutton, R. Falkoff, J. A. Hirst, M. Hoffmann, J.W. Kappler, Progress in Immunol. p.355 (1971).
17. D. H. Katz, W. E. Paul, E. A. Goidl and B. Benacerraf, J. Exp. Med. 133:169 (1971).
18. A. Ekpaha-Mensah and J. C. Kennedy, Nature New Biol. 233:174 (1971).
19. A. Schimpl and E. Wecker, Nature New Biol. 237:15 (1972).
20. M. Feldmann and A. Basten, J. Exp. Med. 136:722 (1972).
21. S. Britton, Scand. J. Immunol. 1:89 (1972).
22. O. Sjöberg, J. Andersson and G. Möller, J. Immunol. 109:1379 (1972).
23. A. Schimpl and E. Wecker, J. Exp. Med. 137:547 (1972).
24. R. M. Gorczynski, R. G. Miller and R. A. Phillips, J. Immunol. 110:968 (1972).
25. D. C. Vann and P. C. Galloway, J. Immunol. 110:1542 (1972).
26. R. M. Gorczynski, R. G. Miller and R. A. Phillips, J. Immunol. 111:900 (1973).
27. J. Watson, J. Immunol. 111:1301 (1973).
28. D. H. Katz, J. M. Davie, W.E. Paul and B. Benacerraf, J. Exp. Med. 134:201 (1971).
29. D. H. Katz, T. Hamaoka and B. Benacerraf, J. Exp. Med. 136:1404 (1972).
30. G. J. V. Nossal, B. L. Pike and D. H. Katz, J. Exp. Med. 138:312 (1973).
31. D. Armerding and D. H. Katz, Manuscript in preparation.

32. T. Hamaoka, D. H. Katz and B. Benacerraf, J. Exp. Med. 138:538 (1973).
33. N. A. Mitchison, Eur. J. Immunol. 1:18 (1971).
34. K. Rajewsky, V. Schirrmacher, S. Nase and N. K. Jerne, J. Exp. Med. 129:1131 (1969).
35. T. Hamaoka, K. Takatsu and M. Kitagawa, Immunol. 21:259 (1971).
36. J. Kettman and R. W. Dutton, Proc. Nat. Acad. Sci. 68:699 (1971).
37. E. R. Unanue and D. H. Katz, Eur. J. Immunol. 3:559 (1973).
38. D. H. Katz, T. Hamaoka, P. E. Newburger and B.Benacerraf, Manuscript submitted.
39. E. R. Unanue and M. J. Karnovsky, Transp. Rev. 14:184 (1973).

Ir GENES AND ANTIGEN RECOGNITION[1]

Hugh O. McDevitt, Kathleen B. Bechtol[2],
Günter J. Hämmerling[3], Peter Lonai[4],
Terry L. Delovitch[5]

Division of Immunology, Department of Medicine
Stanford University School of Medicine
Stanford, California 94305

INTRODUCTION

During the past several years, it has become apparent that the specific immune response to a wide variety of synthetic polypeptide, protein, and isoantigens is under histocompatibility-linked genetic control. Almost all of these genetic controls of specific immune responses affect carrier recognition functions, and similar types of genetic controls have now been identified in the mouse, the rat, the guinea pig and man. The initial findings, the general characteristics of this type of genetic control, and the extensive studies carried out in a number of laboratories to attempt to analyze the mechanism by which these genes work have been extensively reviewed elsewhere [1,2,3].

The Ir gene puzzle now focuses on three primary problems: 1) The type of immunocompetent cell in which Ir genes are expressed -- in particular whether they are expressed in T cells alone or in T cells and B cells; 2) The relationship between Ir genes and the many other functions which are now known to be a property of the I region of the H-2 major histocompatibility complex; and 3) The nature of the Ir gene product itself. Figure 1 shows the map of the H-2 major histocompatibility complex with the newly designated Ir-1A and Ir-1B regions which control specific immune response to different antigens. In the bottom part of the figure are shown the suggested map positions for a series of antigenic specificities which are

[1]This research supported by USPHS research grant AI 07757
[2]Recipient of Dernham Fellowship J-197
[3]Recipient of Dernham Fellowship J-195
[4]Recipient of Senior Dernham Fellowship D-195
[5]Recipient of Senior Dernham Fellowship D-207
All from the American Cancer Society, California Division

expressed on almost all B lymphocytes, on some T lymphocytes, and which appear to be distributed throughout the I region of the H-2 complex so that the I region comprises Ir-1A, Ir-1B and Ir-C(?) at a minimum. No immune response gene functions have been yet ascribed to the region tentatively designated as Ir-C(?), which appears to code primarily for lymphocyte cell surface antigens of the type described above and now designated as Ir-associated or Ia antigens.

These three major subdivisions of the I region control a number of biological functions which are listed in Table 1. These major properties include the Ir genes themselves, the antigens which stimulate in the mixed lymphocyte culture reaction (MLR) in vitro and which elicit the graft versus host (GvH) reaction in vivo, the Ia antigens which have been described above and a number of effects on cellular inter-action which appear to be properties of the major histo-compatibility complex [4], but which have not yet been assigned a definite map position. From the map shown in Figure 1, and the properties listed in Table 1, it is now becoming apparent that the I region subdivision of the H-2 complex is a complex region controlling a variety of cellu-lar recognition phenomena as well as recognition of anti-genic foreignness. Adequate understanding of the function of Ir genes and the possible nature of the Ir gene products will require a complete understanding of the interrelationship between the various functions controlled by the I region as well as a clear determination of which particular immunocom-petent cell types express the various properties controlled by the I region.

The subsequent sections of this paper will deal with a series of experiments designed to determine the cellular site of expression of the Ir genes, to characterize the expression of the Ia antigens and their relationship to the Ir genes, and to the MLC reaction and to begin preliminary characterization of these Ia antigens. Although no attempt has been made to include a comprehensive review of the literature, pertinent experiments from other laboratories which bear on the points at issue will be referred to in the course of each sub-section.

THE ANALYSIS OF THE RESPONDING CELL TYPE
IN TETRAPARENTAL CHIMERIC MICE

The I region controls specific immune responses and cell surface antigens which are a function of or expressed

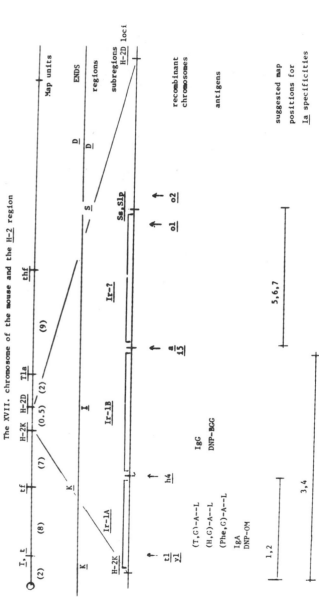

Figure 1   A schematic representation of the XVII mouse chromosome. The first line is an approximate linkage map of the entire chromosome but does not include all the mapped loci. The second line is a subdivision of the H-2 complex into its four major regions, K, I, S, D. The third line is subdivision of the I region into its major subregions. The small letters followed by numbers (e.g., tl, yl) designate the recombinant H-2 chromosomes which define a particular subregion and separate it from the regions to the right and to the left. The bottom series of lines are tentative map locations for the genes controlling the various Ia antigenic specificities. These specificities have been defined and designated primarily by D.C. Shreffler and C.S. David and this tentative designation is reproduced here with their kind permission.

599

Table 1

Properties of the I region

1) Ir genes   − affect T and possibly (?) B cell carrier recognition

2) MLC   − responding cell = T cell

                 − stimulating cell = B and T cell

3) GvH   − ? in vivo correlate of MLC

4) Ia antigens − B cells +++

                 − T cells $\pm$

5) Effect on cellular interaction − not yet mapped

preferentially on B cells or T cells [3,5,Lonai unpublished data]. These functions and cell surface antigens may be the consequence of several genes or several clusters of genes, each of which is involved in a different step of the complex sequence of interactions which leads to production of an antibody response.

In order to elucidate the cellular expression of Ir-1A, the I region gene which controls the specific immune response to (T,G)-A--L, we have performed an inductive cell interaction experiment in tetraparental mice [6]. In these mice, T and B cells of high responder and low responder origin are present in an operationally histocompatible environment and are free to interact during both primary and secondary immunization. The input strains used for construction of the tetraparental mice are coisogenic on the C3H genetic background. The high and low responder embryos which are aggregated to form each tetraparental mouse (Fig. 2) differ at their H-2 region, including Ir-1A, and also differ for immunoglobulin allotype. It is this allotype difference which allows the monitoring of the activity of high and low responder B cells in the specific response to immunization with (T,G)-A--L. Thus, if only the high responder genotype B cells produce high titers of anti-(T,G)-A--L response, then there should be only b (high responder strain) allotype anti-(T,G)-A--L antibody detected. If, on the other hand, both high and low responder B cells produce a high titered response under the influence of cells in the tetraparental mouse, then both a (low responder strain) and b (high responder) allotype anti-(T,G)-A--L antibodies should be produced in proportions approximating their ratio in the total serum immunoglobulin.

We have found, in a genetic situation where there can be no allogeneic effect against the low responder B cells, that the low responder and high responder B cells respond with equal titers of anti-(T,G)-A--L antibodies [7]. That is, in tetraparental mice constructed from C3H ($H-2^{k/k}$, $Ir-1A^{low/low}$, $Ig-1^{a/a}$) low responders to (T,G)-A--L and (CKB x CWB)F$_1$ ($H-2^{k/b}$, $Ir-1A^{low/high}$, $Ig-1^{b/b}$) high responders to (T,G)-A--L, many of the mice produced approximately equal titers of a (low responder strain) and b (high responder) allotype anti-(T,G)-A--L antibody. Thus, in these animals, the B cells of low responder origin appear to be activated to specific antibody secretion and production of memory cells with the same efficiency as are high responder B cells. This is not the case in intact low responder

(a)

high responder
embryo

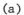 zona pellucida

→ pronase →

low responder
embryo

→

→

24 hrs.

→

chimeric
blastocyst

(b)	Input Strain Genotype		
Gene Complex	low responder	high responder	Tetraparental
Ir-1A for (T,G)-A--L	low/low	(high/low)F_1	low/low + high/low
H-2	k/k	(b/k)F_1 ⟹	k/k + b/k
Ig-1	a/a	b/b	a/a + b/b

Figure 2

(a) Method of production of tetraparental mice.

(b) Genotype of coisogenic strains on the C3H genetic background used for production of C3H↔(CKBxCWB)F_1 tetraparental mice.

parental strain mice or in tetraparental mice produced between two histoincompatible low responder strains (CKB↔C3H/Q; CKB = $H-2^{k/k}$, $Ir-1^{low/low}$, $Ig-1^{b/b}$; C3H/Q = $H-2^{q/q}$, $Ir-1^{low/low}$, $Ig-1^{a/a}$). In these genetically low responder mice there is little or no increased response following the secondary immunization with (T,G)-A--L [7].

Thus, the direct expression of the Ir-1A gene appears to be at a level other than B cell potential for activation. Several lines of evidence suggest that the Ir-1A gene affects T cell reactivity [3]. Other evidence suggests that Ir-1A may be expressed in B cells [8] or in both B cells and T cells [9,2,Session I]. The present results tend to argue against expression of the Ir-1A gene in the B cell. In tetraparental mice, at least, the low responder B cell has the potential to react to the specific antigen and the capacity to interact with specific stimulating T cells to produce antibody and memory cells.

We have shown that, under certain conditions, H-2 disparate lymphoid cells can interact to produce a high titered specific immune response. Other investigators [4,10, 11], using different experimental conditions, have found that lymphoid cells which differ at the major H locus are restricted in their ability to interact in specific immune responses.

It is apparent that the interaction of lymphoid cells can utilize many pathways. It remains to be determined whether one major pathway, or an interplay of several pathways is integral to specific immune responsiveness in the normal animal.

ANTIGEN BINDING B AND T CELLS IN HIGH
AND LOW RESPONDER MICE

In the preceding paragraphs, evidence has been presented suggesting the exclusive expression of the Ir-1 gene(s) in T cells. The molecular nature of the Ir-1 gene product(s) is still a matter of speculation but, due to the antigen specificity of Ir-1, it appears justified to assume that Ir-1 is involved in antigen recognition by T cells. If this hypothesis is correct, then two predictions could be made: (a) one would expect to find differences in the interaction of antigen with B and T cells, and (b) the frequency of antigen specific T cells should be higher in high responder than in low responder mice.

^{125}I-(T,G)-A--L binding lymphocytes were studied by autoradiographic methods [12 & 13]. Short exposure times (4 days) of autoradiographs permitted selective detection of antigen binding B cells (B-ABC) in unfractionated lymph node cell populations, whereas antigen binding T cells were found after 14 day exposure time in purified T-cell populations which were obtained by elimination of B cells utilizing column fractionation [14 & 15].

Comparative analysis of B-ABC and T-ABC demonstrated clearcut differences in the interaction of antigen with T and B cells. It was observed that temperature and metabolic state had a marked effect on T-ABC, but not on B-ABC. When antigen was allowed to react with cells at 37°C, approximately 2-3 times more T-ABC were found as compared to 4°C [12]. This T-cell phenomenon could be blocked by nonlethal concentrations of sodium azide, suggesting a partial dependence on cellular metabolism of antigen binding to T cells.

When the specificity of T-ABC and B-ABC was investigated, striking differences were again found. The synthetic polypeptides, (T,G)-A--L, (H,G)-A--L and (Phe,G)-A--L are strongly crossreactive at the serum antibody level. Therefore, it was not unexpected to find inhibition of ^{125}I-(T,G)-A--L binding B cells by a tenfold excess of all three unlabeled chemical analogues. In contrast, as can be seen from Table 2, ^{125}I-(T,G)-A--L binding T cells from unimmunized mice or immunized mice could only be blocked by preincubation with non-radioactive (T,G)-A--L, but not by (H,G)-A--L or (Phe,G)-A--L, demonstrating dramatic differences in the specificity of T and B cells, which in this case appears to be extraordinarily restricted and precise for T cells.

This difference is in agreement with the lack of cross-immunogenicity of (T,G)-A--L and (H,G)-A--L in in vivo [16] and in vitro systems [17]. In these experiments, successful secondary responses could only be achieved when the same polypeptide was used for primary and secondary immunization.

Because of the close relationship between Ir-1 and H-2 complex, and because of the evidence that Ir-1 is involved in antigen recognition by T cells, anti-H-2 sera and anti-immunoglobulin sera were employed in inhibition studies [13]. It was observed that specific anti-μ heavy chain sera partially blocked T-ABC from normal and immunized mice. When anti-H-2 sera were employed, complete blocking of T-ABC was

Table 2

Inhibition by chemical analogs of ^{125}I-(T,G)-A--L
binding to B and T cells from CWB mice

Immuni-zation	Inhibitor	B cells		T cells	
		ABC/10^4	% Inhi-bition	ABC/10^4	% Inhi-bition
Unimmu-nized	−	12	−	27	−
	(T,G)-A--L	1	92	2	92
	(H,G)-A--L	3	75	24	11
	(Phe,G)-A--L	2	83	25	7
Immu-nized	−	44	−	53	−
	(T,G)-A--L	2	95	5	90
	(H,G)-A--L	6	86	52	2
	(Phe,G)-A--L	8	82	49	8

For inhibition, cells were incubated with 3 μg of nonradioactive inhibitor. Then 0.3 μg radiolabeled (T,G)-A--L were
added without performing an intermediate washing step.
B-ABC were selectively detected in the total cell population
by 4 day exposure time of autoradiographs. T-ABC were
studied in column purified T-cell populations by 11 day
exposure times.

found, whereas no inhibitory effect on B-ABC was detected. One possible explanation is that due to the close linkage of Ir-1 and H-2, anti-H-2 sera contain activity against the Ir-1 gene product and thus specifically block binding of antigen to T cells.

However, blocking of T-ABC by anti-Ig and anti-H-2 sera should be regarded with reservations because (a) any membrane perturbation may interfere with antigen binding to T cells, and (b) anti-Ig does not inhibit in vitro antigen induced DNA synthesis by T cells [17]. Blocking of T-ABC by anti-Ig has also been described by other investigators [18 & 19]. This appears to support the idea that the T-cell receptor is an immunoglobulin, but could also be explained by reaction of anti-Ig with cytophilic B-cell derived IgM bound to T-cell surfaces (which does not act as receptor for antigen, as indicated by our demonstration of different specificity of T and B-ABC) and subsequent steric interference with the actual T receptor. Thus, these blocking studies do not permit final conclusions concerning the possible role of histocompatibility antigens and immunoglobulins in the function of the T-cell antigen receptor.

In summary, studies of antigen binding cells demonstrate striking differences in antigenic specificity and in dependence on metabolic activity of antigen binding to T and B cells. Together with the differential inhibition of T-ABC and B-ABC by anti-H-2 sera, marked differences concerning the nature of T and B-cell receptors for antigen are strongly suggested. These differences are a prerequisite for the hypothesis of selective expression of the Ir-1 gene in only one cell line, namely in thymus derived cells, where it controls antigen recognition.

When the effect of immunization on the frequency of T-ABC was determined, it was found that only high responder T-ABC, but not low responder T-ABC, proliferate after antigenic stimulation (see Fig. 3) again suggesting a defect in low responder T-cell function [Hämmerling, G.J. unpublished] However, to date, no significant differences in the frequency of T-ABC in unimmunized high and low responder mice could be found. This could reflect the fact that these studies have been performed in large excess of antigen, which may obscure potential affinity differences in high and low responder T-cell receptors. Therefore, T-ABC were prepared with increasing amounts of ^{125}I-(T,G)-A--L in the incubation mixture. It can be seen from Fig. 4 that the dose

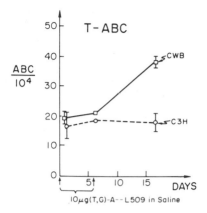

Figure 3   Influence of immunization into hind footpads on
frequency of T-ABC.   T cells were obtained from popliteal
and inguinal lymph nodes by nylon fiber fractionation [15].
CWB = high responder for (T,G)-A--L, C3H = low responder.

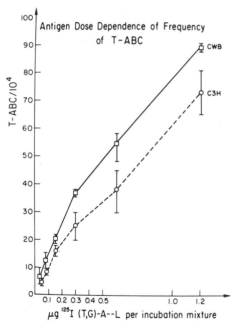

Figure 4   Antigen dose dependence of frequency of T-ABC.
Aliquots containing equal numbers of high responder (CWB) or
low responder (C3H) T cells from unimmunized mice were incubated with increasing concentrations of radiolabeled
(T,G)-A--L and then processed for autoradiography.

607

dependence curves for T-ABC in unimmunized high responder
(CWB) and low responder (C3H) are very similar [Hämmerling,
G.J. unpublished data]. One explanation could be that the
method used is inadequate for detecting differences in the
affinity of T-cell receptors. The other conclusion would
be that Ir genes do not interfere with antigen binding T-
cells, but they control some step(s) in the process of T-cell
stimulation taking place after the original antigen binding
event. Thus, these studies fail to support the previously-
mentioned hypothesis that the Ir-1 gene is involved in antigen binding by T lymphocytes. However, it should be remem-
bered that any theory concerning the mechanism of action of
Ir genes has to be in agreement with the basic observations
demonstrating the antigen-specific effect of Ir genes on
T-cell function.

THE USE OF IN VITRO LYMPHOCYTE TRANSFORMATION
FOR THE STUDY OF Ir-1 REGULATED IMMUNE REACTIONS

The simplest, if not necessarily the best, way to study
the identity and function of cell surface structures is to
react the cells with reagents thought to be specific for
given surface components in a system where the cells are
performing the function assumed to depend on the structures
under investigation, and to measure the ensuing changes in
the cellular activity as a function of the reagents added.
We have established such a system for the study of Ir-1A.
Mouse lymphocytes from the draining nodes or from the
peritoneal cavity of animals immunized with the synthetic
antigens (T,G)-A--L, (H,G)-A--L, or (Phe,G)-A--L, were cultured in the presence of the homologous antigen, and the
antigen-induced cell transformation was measured by determining ^{3}H-thymidine uptake. Using this system, we have
studied the cellular, physiological, and genetic conditions
required, and the effect of anti-H-2 and anti-immunoglobulin
sera on specific antigen-induced lymphocyte transformation.

The stimulation of sensitized lymphocytes with antigen
in culture is largely dependent on T cells, since the effect
can be prevented by anti-θ serum and C' treatment. We have
shown that T-cell fractions purified on nylon wool columns,
from in vivo sensitized lymph node cell suspensions, can be
stimulated by the homologous antigen in the same manner as
the whole lymph node cell population, suggesting that T
cells alone, or in the presence of minimal numbers of B
cells and macrophages, are sufficient for the reaction.
Therefore, it appears that the experimental system for

practical purposes can be regarded as measuring a T-cell dependent function.

It was of interest to determine whether genetic regulation by the Ir-1 gene(s), as measured by humoral antibody formation, correlates with this in vitro T-cell reaction. It was found that the H-2^b haplotype was a responder to (T,G)-A--L and (Phe,G)-A--L, but a nonresponder to (H,G)-A--L; haplotype k was a nonresponder to (T,G)-A--L, but a responder to (H,G)-A--L and (Phe,G)-A--L; haplotype q responded only to (Phe,G)-A--L, while haplotype s behaved as a nonresponder to all three of the antigens (see Table 3 and 17, 20, 21). This pattern of the in vitro regulation is identical to that observed at the level of antibody formation. The effect in the in vitro system did not appear as a quantitative, but rather as a qualitative trait. This finding is compatible with the hypothesis of expression of the Ir-1 gene product on T cells [16,20].

The antibodies produced against the three synthetic antigens used here are broadly crossreactive [16]. The in vitro reaction offered the possibility of testing whether antigen recognition by T cells in this system is similar to that of humoral antibodies. Lymphocytes of mice immunized with one of the three synthetic antigens were cultured in the presence of each of the other two antigens. If there were an antibody-like crossreactivity in the T cell recognition, a certain degree of "cross-stimulation" would have been expected. This was not the case. The sensitized lymphocytes responded only to the homologous immunizing antigen, suggesting that T cell recognition in the in vitro system has a different specificity than humoral antibody specificity (see Table 4 and reference 21). These results were in good agreement with studies on antigen binding T cells [12], which also demonstrated the same difference in specificity of T and B cells.

The binding of antigen to antibody or to B lymphocytes is not temperature dependent. In contrast, the in vitro stimulation of T cells by these synthetic antigens was found to be temperature dependent. If the antigen was added for only a few hours to the cultures and later washed away, the cultures responded with stimulation if the antigen was present at 37°C, but not if it was present at an incubation temperature of 4°C (see Table 5 and references 17,20,21). Insufficient antigen binding at low temperatures seems to be a characteristic of T cells, since similar differences were

Table 3

H-2 linked immune responsiveness to synthetic polypeptides as measured by in vitro stimulation.

Strain	H-2	Stimulation Index in the Presence of:		
		(T,G)-A--L	(H,G)-A--L	(Phe,G)-A--L
CWB	b	12.03	0.98	5.31
C3H	k	0.99	12.06	2.55
C3H.Q	q	n.d.	1.15	4.47
B10.S	s	1.12	n.d.	0.56

Footnote: n.d. = not done

Table 4

The absence of cross-stimulation by the synthetic antigens in vitro

Strain	Immunizing Antigens	Antigen in Culture	cpm ^{3}H-T
C3H.Q	(Phe,G)-A--L	-	5120
C3H.Q	(Phe,G)-A--L	(Phe,G)-A--L	37680
C3H.Q	(Phe,G)-A--L	(H,G)-A--L	4980
C3H	(H,G)-A--L	-	2860
C3H	(H,G)-A--L	(H,G)-A--L	12480
C3H	(H,G)-A--L	(Phe,G)-A--L	2980

Table 5

The effect of low temperature on the in vitro stimulation
of primed C3H.Q lymphocytes by (Phe,G)-A--L

Conditions for Antigen Stimulation			
Time	Temperature	Antigen	cpm ^{3}H-T
3 hours	37°C	–	3260
3 hours	37°C	(Phe,G)-A--L	16280
3 hours	4°C	–	1872
3 hours	4°C	(Phe,G)-A--L	3064
5 days	37°C	–	1912
5 days	37°C	(Phe,G)-A--L	20130
3 hours 3 hours	4°C & 37°C	–	5120
3 hours 3 hours	4°C & 37°C	(Phe,G)-A--L	27631

shown in antigen binding T cells [12].

The effect of anti-H-2 and anti-immunoglobulin sera on the in vitro stimulation of lymphocytes by (T,G)-A--L, (H,G)-A--L, or (Phe,G)-A--L, was studied by adding the sera (in appropriate dilution) to the cells together with the antigen for three hours. Both reagents were then removed by washing and the cultures were incubated until the end of the reaction period (5 days). Anti-H-2 antibodies directed against the H-2 type of the lymphocytes had a strong inhibitory effect, while the addition of polyvalent anti-mouse immunoglobulin antisera had no measurable effect (Table 6). To investigate whether the inhibitory effect of the anti-H-2 sera was due to the perturbation of the cell membrane by the adherence of antibody molecules, the cells were also reacted with anti-θ serum. This treatment had no effect, suggesting that, for blocking the lymphocyte transformation reaction, it is not sufficient if any antibody reacts with the cell membrane (Table 6). Anti-immunoglobulin serum inhibited E. coli lipopolysaccharide and pokeweed mitogen stimulation, showing that the antiserum is able to block B-cell stimulation.

These experiments demonstrate that histocompatibility-linked regulation of immune responsiveness is expressed in reactions in which the main or possibly the only lymphocyte component is the T cell; that the physiology and specificity of recognition by these cells is different in certain respects from that of B cells; and that early steps in antigen recognition by these cells are blocked by antisera to H-2 antigens but not by anti-immunoglobulin sera.

ANTIGENS CONTROLLED BY THE I REGION OF THE MOUSE H-2 COMPLEX

If Ir genes code for lymphocyte determinants, then their detection and biochemical analysis with appropriate antisera should be possible. However, alloantigenic differences in the I region would normally be extremely difficult to recognize, because I-region differences will usually be associated with differences in H-2K and H-2D regions. Therefore, detection of antibodies against determinants coded for by the I region became possible only when congenic mice were available which had identical H-2K and H-2D region specificities but different I regions. Reciprocal immunization with lymphocytes of such an I-region congenic pair, A.TL and A.TH, yielded an A.TH anti-A.TL serum [5]. Extensive serological investigation of this antiserum permitted

Table 6

The effect of alloantisera on in vitro antigen stimulation

Mouse Strain	Antigens	Alloantiserum (50λ)	cpm ^{3}H-T
Exp. 1.			
C3H.Q	–	–	3420
C3H.Q	(Phe,G)-A--L	normal mouse	22300
C3H.Q	(Phe,G)-A--L	anti-H-2^q	7820
C3H.Q	(Phe,G)-A--L	anti-IgG+IgM+IgA	18200
C3H.Q	PHA	–	64300
C3H.Q	PHA	anti-H-2^q	65220
C3H.Q	PHA	anti-IgG+IgM+IgA	72300
C3H.Q	PWM	–	61820
C3H.Q	PWM	anti-H-2^q	45600
C3H.Q	PWM	anti-IgG+IgM+IgA	8970
Exp. 2			
CSW	–	–	1970
CSW	(Phe,G)-A--L	–	5260
CSW	(Phe,G)-A--L	anti-H-2^b	1328
CSW	(Phe,G)-A--L	anti-Thy 1.2	7340

PHA – phytohemagglutinin; PWM – pokeweed mitogen

613

the identification of cellular antigens which were designated
Ia antigens (I-region-associated antigens) [22]. Analysis of
anti-Ia sera revealed the existence of several different Ia
specificities which may be controlled by different genes,
some of which are common to strains with different H-2 haplotypes [5,23]. Table 7 shows the tissue distribution of Ia
antigens as identified with the anti-A.TL serum. To date,
Ia antigens can be detected on lymphocytes [5], spermatocytes, and probably on epidermal cells and macrophages
(Hämmerling, G.J., and Goldberg, E., unpublished data). It
is not clear yet whether Ia is present only on a subpopulation of spermatocytes and macrophages, or whether the weak
reaction is due to a low density of Ia on the respective
cell types.

Of particular importance is the observation that Ia
antigens are predominantly expressed on mature B lymphocytes
[5]. Similar conclusions have been drawn by Sachs and Cone
[24] who detected B-cell specific anti-Ia antibody in anti-
H-2 sera, by Shreffler and colleagues [25] and by Hauptfeld
and colleagues [26], who investigated several anti-Ia sera,
and by Delovitch (unpublished data; see this article,
Section 5), who could demonstrate biosynthesis of Ia antigens only in B cells, but not in T cells. However, a negative reaction with T cells does not mean absence of Ia
antigens in T cells. The failure to detect Ia on T lymphocytes could be due to the insensitivity of the methods
applied. In fact, other investigators have recently described anti-Ia sera containing anti-T-cell activity [23,27,
28]. Moreover, P. Lonai [29] obtained mixed lymphocytes
reactions in I-region congenic combinations when highly
purified T cells were used, suggesting the expression on
T-cell surfaces of structures controlled by the I region.
Thus, it appears that the I region codes for determinants
on both B and T cells, some of which are more readily detectable by serological techniques, and others by MLC reactions.

ISOLATION AND CHARACTERIZATION OF Ia ANTIGENS

The Ia antigens represent a group of cell surface proteins whose expression is regulated by genes mapping in the
I region [23]. This region contains genes that control
several immunological reactions involving cellular and/or
antigen recognition, e.g., specific immune responses (Ir),
MLC, GVH and graft rejection [30,31,32]. In order to understand the possible mechanisms of these recognitive processes,
it is of prime importance to localize, isolate and charac-

Table 7

Tissue distribution of Ia antigens

Tissue	Cytotoxic Index [%]	Absorption of Serum with Tissue
Spleen	40 - 55	+++
Lymph Node	25 - 35	++
Thymus	0	-
Bone Marrow	5 - 15	nd [a]
'B' Cells [b]	70 - 95	+++
'T' Cells [c]	0 - 5	-
Erythrocytes	0 [d]	nd
Epidermal Cells	nd	+
Sperm Cells	20 - 50	+
Macrophages	10 - 30	+
Kidney	nd	-
Liver	nd	-
Brain	nd	-

(a) nd = not tested

(b) B cells were prepared by treatment of spleen or lymph node cells with anti-Thy-1.2 serum and complement

(c) T cells were isolated by column fractionation of lymph node cells [4]

(d) Tested by hemagglutination

terize the related functional membrane components [3,33,34].

Several attempts to identify the presently known Ia alloantigenic specificities on different lymphoid cells, using cytotoxic and adsorption tests performed with anti-Ia antisera raised in Ir congenic recombinant strains, have been reported [5,23,24,27,28]. These assays unexpectedly revealed that Ia antigens can be identified primarily on lymph node and splenic B cells. However, they may be present, but in much lower amount on peripheral T cells. An initial biochemical characterization of these cellular antigens examined by SDS-polyacrylamide gel electrophoresis of radiolabeled, NP-40 solubilized and anti-Ia precipitated membrane-associated proteins demonstrated them to have a M.W. of approximately 30,000 daltons, under reducing conditions, thus differing in size from H-2 antigens [33,34]. This type of analysis has been extended by determining whether these proteins could be isolated from membranes of T and B cells, as well as other cell types.

Polyacrylamide gel electrophoretic patterns of reduced immune precipitates formed between an (A.TH x B10.S) anti-(A.TL x B10.S) antiserum and NP-40 extracts [33,34] of ^{3}H-leucine labeled splenic B cells and lymph node T cells prepared [5] from mice of several H-2 haplotypes are shown in Fig. 5. These profiles indicate that membrane proteins of approximately 30,000 M.W. are isolatable by this method from B cells and not from T cells. No such peaks of radioactivity were obtained in the control precipitates of either cell type using normal mouse serum. Thus, the cellular and strain distributions of these Ia antigens as well as their size heterogeneity correlate closely with the pattern of reactivity reflected by the cytotoxic assays previously described (see Table 7). This antiserum reacts predominantly with B cells of Ir^k, cross-reacts with B cells which are Ir^d and Ir^b, but shows no reactivity with B cells of Ir^s (Fig. 5 and Table 8). It should be noted that while the anti-Ia serum does not react with purified T cells, anti-K^k and anti-K^s antisera do react with the appropriate T cells (Table 8). In other experiments (Delovitch, unpublished data), a congenic anti-Thy 1.2 antiserum precipitates about 1-2 percent of the label in the T cell lysates. These results suggest that B cells definitely possess Ia antigens. While these antigens are not detectable on T cells under the conditions employed, it is possible that they are present in reduced quantities on T cells.

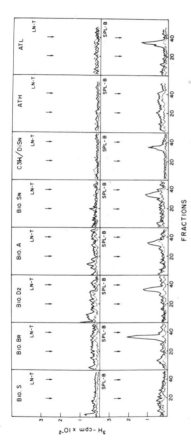

Figure 5   Strain distribution of Ia antigens on mouse T and B cells. Patterns of electrophoresis on 12.5 percent acrylamide gels run according to Laemmli [35] of NP-40 solubilized, anti-Ia precipitated extracts of T and B cells labelled with ^{3}H-leucine (25 µCi/ml) for 3 hr at 37°C are shown. Extracts were isolated from approximately 25 x 10^6 T or B cells prepared as described in Table 8. Cells were incubated in Eagle's minimal essential medium minus leucine (GIBCO) at a concentration of 5 x 10^6 cells/ml. Immunoprecipitation with the anti-Ia antiserum of the labeled proteins was performed as previously described following removal of ^{3}H-labeled H and L chains from the extracts [33,34]. Extracts were precipitated with an excess of anti-Ia (–) or normal mouse serum (---) and an equivalent amount of goat anti-mouse γ-globulin. The positions of migration of ^{14}C-labeled myeloma H and L chains are indicated by arrows. LN-T, lymph node nylon wool column purified T cells. SPL-B, anti-Thy 1.2 and C' treated spleen cells.

617

Table 8

Immunoprecipitation of Lysates of ^{3}H-leu Labelled Mouse Lymphocytes*

Strain	H-2 Haplotype	Cells**	% Radioactivity Immunoprecipitated***				
			α-Ir^k	α-K^k	α-K^s	NMS	α-BSA
ATL	tl	T	0.9	1.1	5.3	0.9	1.0
		B	6.2	1.4	5.4	0.8	0.8
ATH	th	T	0.9	0.6	5.1	0.7	0.9
		B	1.2	0.9	5.3	0.8	0.8
C3H/DiSn	k	T	1.0	5.1	---	0.7	1.0
		B	5.8	5.5	---	0.5	1.0
		LN(Con A)	5.2	---	---	0.4	0.9
B10.A	a	T	1.1	6.1	1.3	1.5	1.1
		B	5.9	6.2	1.4	1.6	1.3
B10.Sn	b	T	1.2	---	---	1.9	1.2
		B	5.9	---	---	1.7	1.1
B10.D2	d	T	1.8	2.8	1.0	2.6	2.8
		B	8.8	3.3	1.0	3.1	1.8
B10.BR	k	T	1.8	6.4	1.5	1.2	0.9
		B	6.3	6.7	1.4	1.2	1.8
		Thy	0.9	---	---	0.8	0.2
		BM	2.2	---	---	0.9	0.3
B10.S	s	T	1.7	2.1	7.9	1.6	1.4
		B	3.2	2.6	9.6	3.2	1.7

*   Cell suspensions contained 20–40 x 10^6 cells, with the following exceptions:

      B10.BR Thy 175 x 10^6 cells
               BM   150 x 10^6 cells

** T: Lymph node cells twice fractionated on nylon wool columns
      (3–5% B cells)
    B: Spleen cells treated with anti-Thy 1.2 + C' and fractionated
      on 35% BSA (3–5% T cells)
    LN(Con A): Lymph node cells stimulated for 50 hr by 0.1 µg/ml Con A
    Thy: Thymocytes
    BM: Bone marrow cells

***Total acid precipitable CPM incorporated by the cell suspensions varied
between 1–20 x 10^5. Aliquots containing 25,000 CPM were used except for
B10.BR Thy and BM where 100,000 CPM aliquots were tested. An optimum
amount of BSA was added to Rabbit anti-BSA treated samples, while an
optimum amount of Goat anti-mouse IgG was added to the other antisera,
each used at a 1:16 dilution.

A quantitative difference in the amount of Ia antigens on B and T cells was also apparent from absorption experiments presented in Fig. 6. A 30,000 M.W. peak was isolated from anti-Ia precipitated extracts of C3H/HeJ lymph node and spleen cells labeled for 3 hr with ^{3}H-leucine. The lymph node cell peak could be removed by prior absorption of the anti-Ia serum with an equal number of lymph node cells or half as many spleen or spleen B cells. No absorption was effected with lymph node T cells. Similarly, the spleen cell peak could be absorbed with as many spleen cells or half as many spleen B cells. However, this peak was reduced by half after absorption with lymph node cells, but remained in equal amount following absorption with lymph node T cells. These results seem to restrict the presence of Ia antigens to B cells and suggest that the C3H/HeJ antigens detected with this antiserum are identical on lymph node and splenic B cells.

The Ia antigens isolated seem to constitute only a small proportion of the total labeled protein in the B cell NP-40 lysates. Approximately 5 percent of the acid precipitable radioactivity in these preparations is specifically immunoprecipitable with the anti-Ia antiserum (Table 8). However, only about 30-40 percent of the radioactivity on the gels (Fig. 5) is present in the 30,000 M.W. region; no other distinct peaks are evident. Thus, the Ia antigens comprise only 1-2 percent of the ^{3}H-leucine labeled intracellular and membrane-bound proteins.

Tissue distribution studies indicate that Ia antigens may be present on other cell types in addition to B cells. A 30,000 M.W. peak was apparent in the gel patterns depicting the anti-Ia precipitates of extracts derived from C3H/HeJ macrophages [36], 14 day old fetal liver cells, epidermal cells [37] and B10.BR bone marrow cells (Fig. 7). The peaks in the latter two preparations are rather heterodisperse. These peaks are absent in B10.BR thymus cells. These results coincide with the cytotoxic data previously described.

In conclusion, the data presented here corroborates previous findings on the isolation and characterization of Ia antigens [33,34]. These antigens may be isolated with anti-Ia antisera from the membrane of murine lymph node and splenic lymphocytes and have an apparent M.W. of 30,000 as estimated by gel electrophoresis under reducing conditions. They seem to differ from H-2 antigens with respect to size, composition and serological reactivity [33]. The large

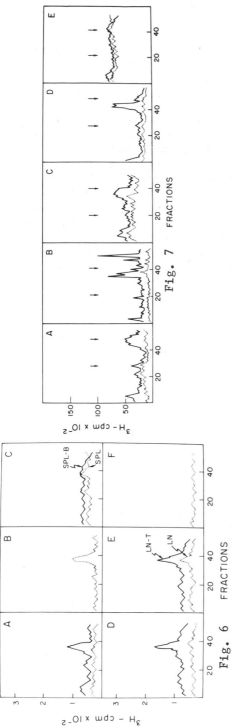

Fig. 7

Fig. 6 FRACTIONS

Figure 6 Distribution of Ia antigens on C3H/HeJ T and B cells following absorption of the anti-Ia antiserum with T or B cells. Ia antigens were isolated from 50 x 10⁶ lymph node (A-C) or spleen cells (D-F) using the anti-Ia antiserum that was unabsorbed (-) or absorbed with 25-50 x 10⁶ cells (---). The serum was absorbed for 30 min at 4°C with 50 x 10⁶ lymph node cells (A), 25 x 10⁶ lymph node T cells (B), 25 x 10⁶ spleen or spleen B cells (C), 50 x 10⁶ spleen cells (D), 25 x 10⁶ lymph node T cells (E) and 25 x 10⁶ spleen B cells (F).

Figure 7 Tissue distribution studies of Ia antigens. ³H-leucine labeled proteins were isolated, immunoprecipitated and electrophoresed as described in Fig. 5. The patterns shown represent equal aliquots taken from extracts prepared from approximately 50-100 x 10⁶ cells of each tissue. Samples were prepared from C3H/HeJ (A,B,D) or B10.BR (C,E) mice: (A), epidermal cells; (B), macrophages; (C), bone marrow cells; (D), fetal liver cells and (E), thymocytes. They were treated with anti-Ia (-) or normal mouse serum (---). No 30,000 M.W. peak of radioactivity was observed when extracts prepared from 25 x 10⁶ cells or normal mouse serum controls shown here (Delovitch, unpublished data) were examined. The patterns of extracts isolated from the same tissues of B10.S mice were were similar to the normal mouse serum controls shown here (Delovitch, unpublished data).

degree of cross-reactivity of anti-Ia sera with cells of
varying H-2 haplotypes and the heterodisperse pattern of the
Ia peaks demonstrated here supports the concept of possible
heterogeneity of Ia antigens previously reported [23,33,34].

Cellular and tissue distribution studies of Ia antigens
on lymphoid as well as non-lymphoid cells reveal several
interesting points. There seems to be a quantitative difference in the amount of Ia antigens on T and B cells. While
detectable quantities of radiolabeled Ia can be isolated
from B cells, the 30,000 M.W. peak is absent from extracts
of equivalent numbers of T cells. However, different methods
of preparation of T cells as well as extracts of increased
numbers of T cells must be employed before the presence of
Ia antigens on these cells can be ruled out. Of particular
interest are the findings that these antigens may appear on
other cell types such as macrophages, bone marrow and epidermal cells, but are not found on all cells, as are H-2
antigens. In addition, they seem to appear early in differentiation since they can be detected on fetal liver cells,
which provide a source of lymphoid stem cells [38].

Further characterization of Ia antigens on fetal, neonatal and adult lymphocytes should assist the elucidation
of the possible role of these cell surface antigens in
cellular interactions involved in the immune response.

MIXED LYMPHOCYTE REACTION STUDIES ON THE DISTRIBUTION
OF ANTIGENS ON T AND B LYMPHOCYTES CONTROLLED
BY THE I REGION OF THE H-2 COMPLEX

Three immunological traits have been shown to be associated with the I-region of the H-2 complex: 1) The Ir
genes regulating immune responsiveness to certain antigens
[39]; 2) the Lad genes controlling structures responsible
for lymphocyte stimulation in allogeneic mixed lymphocyte
(MLR) [30] or graft versus host reaction (GVHR) [31];   •
and 3) the Ia genes controlling lymphocyte cell surface
antigens as detected by alloantisera in serological reactions [23]. It is assumed that all these structures are
expressed on the lymphocyte cell membrane. Whether the
three traits known to be controlled by the I region are
in fact three independent genetic units controlling different functions, or are different experimental manifestations
of the same genetic region, is not known. It seems reasonable to assume that the Ia and Lad antigens are in fact cell
surface structures recognized as antigens by humoral immune

reactions and lymphocyte proliferation respectively.

In the present study, the MLR reaction was used to detect the cellular distribution of antigens coded by the I region. The strategy of the experiments was the following: purified T or B cells were used as stimulator cells in MLR reactions across I-region different combinations. The degree of stimulation by the two lymphocyte subpopulations was compared, and inferences were drawn as to whether the I region controls antigens which are expressed on both lymphocyte subpopulations, or only on one of them.

First we have shown that thymocytes do stimulate in the MLR across differences incorporating the whole H-2 complex [40]. Seven H-2 haplotypes have been studied. In one of these H-2 different combinations, we have shown that purified peripheral B and T cells both stimulate in the MLR. Peripheral T cells or thymocytes gave about 2 - 5 times less stimulation than B cells or whole lymph node cell suspensions. Dose response experiments demonstrated that the minimal stimulating dose in this system for B cells is about 15-25% of the total number of stimulator cells used, suggesting that it is unlikely that the stimulation observed by thymocytes or isolated lymph node T-cells would have been solely due to B-cell contamination [40].

For critical interpretation of our data, it was important to ascertain that the stimulation observed for T or B cells was indeed caused by the irradiated stimulator cells. It is known that irradiated T cells can recognize allogeneic lymphocytes and stimulate them, presumably by humoral factors [41]. Since, in most of our experiments lymph node cell suspensions were used as responder cells, the possibility existed that the stimulation observed was not due to the recognition of the stimulator T cells, but was due to the recognition of the B-cells in the responder fraction by the irradiated stimulator T-cells. To clarify this problem, a number of our experiments were repeated using nylon wool column purified stimulator and responder T cells. The results were identical with the experiments in which lymph node cell suspensions were used as responder cells, demonstrating that the recognition event in the experiments using purified T-cells as stimulator cells, was indeed the effect of the recognition of T-cell surface products. (Compare Tables 9 and 10).

Table 9

MLR ACROSS I-SUBREGION DIFFERENCES: ISOLATED T AND B CELLS AS STIMULATOR CELLS

Exp.	Responder	Stimulator	c.p.m.	± S.E.	Stimulation index	H-2 map					
						H-2K	Ir-1A	Ir-1B	I-C	Ss,Slp	H-2D
1.	B10.AQR-L	B10.AQR-T	2017	464		q	k	k	d	d	d
	B10.AQR-L	B10.T(6R)-T	5134	480	2.55	q	q	q	q	q	d
	B10.AQR-L	B10.T(6R)-B	5932	287	2.94						
2.	A.TL-L	A.TL-T	24719	2097		s	k	k	k	k	d
	A.TL-L	A.TH-T	122205	23933	4.95	s	s	s	s	s	d
	A.TL-L	A.TL-B	13200	3251							
	A.TL-L	A.TH-B	44308	6544	3.86						
3.	$(A.TL \times B10/Sn)F_1$-L	$(A.TL \times B10/Sn)F_1$-T	3850	346		s/b	k/b	k/b	k/b	k/b	d/b
	$(A.TL \times B10/Sn)F_1$-L	B10.HTT-T	11510	335	3.00	s	s	s	k	k	d
	$(A.TL \times B10/Sn)F_1$-L	$(A.TL \times B10/Sn)F_1$-B	668	97							
	$(A.TL \times B10/Sn)F_1$-L	B10.HTT-B	1066	268	1.60						
4.	$(B10.HTT \times A/J)F_1$-L	$(B10.HTT \times A/J)F_1$-T	2924	503		s/k	s/k	s/k	k/d	k/d	d/d
	$(B10.HTT \times A/J)F_1$-L	A.TH-T	13563	978	4.64	s	s	s	s	s	d
	$(B10.HTT \times A/J)F_1$-L	$(B10.HTT \times A/J)F_1$-B	1808	754							
	$(B10.HTT \times A/J)F_1$-L	A.TH-B	2161	43	1.20						
5.	B10.S(7R)-L	B10.S(7R)-T	5416	1747		s	s	s	s	s	d
	B10.S(7R)-L	B10.HTT-T	12051	1034	2.23	s	s	s	k	k	d
	B10.S(7R)-L	B10.S(7R)-B	18334	4476							
	B10.S(7R)-L	B10.HTT-B	17844	2833	0.97						

Table 10

MLR reaction across I region differences.
T-responder cells against T or B stimulator cells

Exp.	Responder	Stimulator	c.p.m.	± S.E.	Stimulation index	H-2K	Ir-1A	Ir-1B	I-C	Ss,Slp	H-2D
1.	A.TL–T	A.TL–T	1892	663		s	k	k	k	k	d
	A.TL–T	A.TH–T	8701	748	4.60	s	s	s	s	s	d
	A.TL–T	A.TL–B	4009	1382							
	A.TL–T	A.TH–B	10366	2013	2.59						
2.	A.TH–T	A.TH–T	28861	5972		s	s	s	s	s	d
	A.TH–T	A.TL–T	351259	50190	12.17	s	k	k	k	k	d
	A.TH–T	A.TH–B	27930	3953							
	A.TH–T	A.TL–B	245868	13301	8.80						

Experiments with combinations differing in the I and S regions, [A.TL versus A.TH;   B10.T(6R) versus B10.AQR]:   In these combinations, T and B cells stimulated to an equal extent or in some cases (A.TL versus A.TH) T cells stimulated slightly better than B cells, (Table 9, experiments 1 and 2, and Table 10).

Combinations differing in the Ir-1A and Ir-1B subregions [(A.TLxB10/Sn)F₁ versus B10.HTT]:   In this combination B cells gave a significantly weaker stimulation than T cells (Table 9, experiment 3).

Combinations differing in a region between Ir-1B and Ss, Slp (subregion I-C [42].)   [(B10.HTTxA/J)F₁ versus A.TH;   and B10.S(7R) versus B10.HTT]:   In these combinations, only T cells stimulated;   with B cells as stimulator cells, no significant degree of stimulation could be obtained (Table 9, experiments 4 and 5).

These findings suggest that antigens controlled by the I region are expressed on both T and B cells, as indicated by the MLR reaction. The fact that strain combinations exist which differ primarily in T-cell antigens, implies that at least some of the genes controlling the stimulatory structures are expressed exclusively on given lymphocyte subpopulations. A similar observation has been made by Fathman et al. [43], who found stimulation exclusively by B cells in the B10.A(4R) versus B10.A(2R) and the B10.A versus B10.D2 combination. The genetic difference between these combinations, however, comprises a larger chromosome segment than that tested in our last combination above. We have compared our data with the genetic localization of Ia antigens, as described by Shreffler's group [23,42], and found good agreement. Specifically, the combinations differing in specificities assigned to the third I subregion (I-C) separate this subregion and describe only T cell antigens as recognized in the MLR. The MLR combinations also correspond well with the Ia specificities assigned to the subregions according to their H-2 genotype. If these correlations can be continued in following experiments, then there will be a good possibility of investigating the specificity of the MLR and the possible identity of the Lad and Ia loci. To investigate the relationship between Lad loci and Ir genes, other studies will be needed. The comparison of the map position of Ir genes and Lad loci and their cellular distribution might give useful information provided that narrow enough genetic regions can be studied by the use of appropriate

recombinant strains. Another approach would be the use of
well-defined Ia antisera for inhibition of in vitro lymphocyte stimulation by antigen. In such systems, specific
inhibition of given reactions by sera controlled by Ia loci,
which map in the same position as the Ir gene regulating the
specific immune reaction studied, would suggest the identity
of some Ia and Ir genes. The existence of recombinant H-2
chromosomes which are identical at Ir-1A and Ir-1B but differ
for Ia antigens, and the MLR reactions observed in H-2^{t2}
versus H-2^{t3}, across subregion I-C which does not contain any
known Ir genes, already suggest that not all Ia or Lad antigens correlate with Ir gene function, and that these genes
may be separate and serve distinct functions.

DISCUSSION

It is clear that the available information on the properties of the I region and their relationship to specific Ir
gene function is not yet sufficient to permit a clear deci-
sion as to the major issues concerning Ir gene function and
its relation to antigen recognition. There is extensive circumstantial evidence to indicate that Ir genes are expressed
selectively in T cells and control foreign antigen recognition by T cells, perhaps because the Ir genes are structural
genes for the T cell antigen receptor [ref. 1,2,3]. However,
it must be emphasized that none of these experiments offers
definitive proof that Ir genes are expressed solely in T
cells. Indeed there are at least two lines of experimenta-
tion which question this hypothesis. The first is the demonstration of H-2 linked genetic control of specific immune
responses which has been shown by Mozes et al. [44] and by
Bluestein et al. [45]. The demonstration in these experiments that histocompatibility linked Ir genes affect not
only carrier antigenic recognition but the specificity of the
resultant antibody suggests that this type of gene might also
be expressed in B cells. The second type of experiment which
questions the hypothesis of Ir gene expression in T cells is
the limiting dilution studies of Shearer and Mozes [9,46].

In the absence of direct chemical information on the
nature of the Ir gene product, we are forced for the moment
to rely on a variety of biological experiments to attempt to
unravel the interrelationships between Ir genes, the antigens
responsible for the mixed lymphocyte culture reaction and
the graft vs. host reaction, the Ia antigens, and the cellular interaction effects of the major histocompatibility complex. The close relationship of all of these functions has

only recently been appreciated and experiments are now under way in a number of laboratories in an attempt to unravel the nature of these relationships. In the absence of definitive information, perhaps the best approach is the generation of a list of the most likely alternative in the relationships between these functions so that further experiments can be designed to test these alternate possibilities. Table 11 is a list of the possible relationships between Ir:MLC:GvH:Ia: and interaction functions of the I region.

The first alternative postulates that Ir genes are the structural genes for the T cell antigen receptor, and that the Ia genes are the genes that control cell surface structures which elicit the MLC and GvH reactions in allogeneic combinations and which are responsible for effective T-B cellular cooperation in syngeneic combinations. Thus Ir is postulated to be a separate function while Ia, MLC, GvH and cellular interaction are all functions of the same gene products. The major objection to this alternative is the experiments already referred to above which indicate genetic control of antibody specificity, and the limiting dilution cell transfer studies also referred to above. In any event, acceptance of this alternative would require isolation and characterization of the Ir gene product as well as isolation and characterization of the Ia antigens.

The second alternate suggests that Ia and Ir gene products are expressed in both T and B cells and in some manner, not specified, affect carrier antigenic recognition in both cell types. In this alternative, the cellular interaction function might be served by Ia gene products but could also be a function of some other gene in the I region of the major histocompatibility complex or even in the left hand half of the major histocompatibility complex. If one assumes that the Ia or Ir gene products expressed in both T and B cells are antigen specific and totally restricted in their expression, this model suffers from the problem of requiring coordinate recognition of both haptenic and carrier determinants on a particular antigenic molecule by the B cell population. If one assumes that there is approximately one cell per 10^4 specific for any given hapten [47] and approximately one cell per 10^4 specific for a particular carrier determinant, then the incidence of precursor cells for a particular hapten on a particular carrier would approach one in 10^8 or more cells. This is considerably below the lowest estimate for precursor cells. Therefore, clonally restricted Ir gene effects in B cells seems unlikely to be a viable model.

627

Table 11

Possible relationship between
Ir : MLC : GvH : Ia : interaction functions

---

1) Ir = T cell antigen receptor

    Ia = MLC and GvH antigens in allogeneic combinations

    = interaction signal in syngeneic combinations

2) Ia and Ir gene products are expressed in both T and
    B cells and affect and/or control carrier recognition
    in both cell types

    Ia or some other MHC product may affect cellular
    interaction

3) Ia = MLC antigen in allogeneic combinations

    = non-specifically "modulates" an Ig receptor on T
    and B cells, and facilitates cellular interaction

However, it is conceivable that a complex array of Ia gene products expressed on the surface of B cells might interact with immunoglobulin receptors to modify the interaction of antigen specific immunoglobulin receptors on the surface of B cells. The major argument against this possibility is the wide variety of specific antigens which are under H-2 linked Ir gene control and the precision in specificity of this type of genetic control. It seems highly unlikely that any small set of cell surface antigens could interact with immunoglobulin receptors in such a way as to have the antigenic specificity manifested by the H-2 linked Ir genes. However, this possibility cannot be ruled out on these grounds alone.

The third alternative is that Ia antigens are the antigens responsible for the mixed lymphocyte culture and graft vs. host reactions in allogeneic combinations and that, in syngeneic situations, they nonspecifically modulate any immunoglobulin receptor present on both T and B cells and also facilitate cellular interaction. This model is essentially a further extension of the second alternative and simply equates all the biological effects of the I region as being due to a single set of cell surface antigens -- the Ia antigens. In this version there would be no such thing as a specific Ir gene product. This model suffers from the same objection raised to the second model -- namely that the array in specificity of H linked Ir genes is both too large and too precise to envision them as the result of nonspecific interactions between two or three molecules on the cell surface and a particular immunoglobulin receptor.

It is clearly too early to chose between these alternative models and to limit the possible alternatives only to those already discussed. A step by step analysis of the relationship between the various functions of the I region in I-region congenic strains in mice should permit some discrimination between the alternatives already listed and the generation of new alternatives if this seems appropriate. Preliminary evidence already indicates that a definite genetic distinction can be made between the specific Ir genes and the Ia antigens. This statement is based on evidence from Meo and Shreffler [48] that they have found at least one strain combination in which the two partners in the combination differ for specific Ir gene functions but show no differences with respect to Ia antigens or mixed lymphocyte culture reaction. In addition, in the immediately preceeding section of this paper, evidence was presented that a strain combination has been identified which has the same <u>Ir</u> gene functions, but differs for Ia antigens and for mixed lymphocyte culture reactions. This is the combination comprised of H-2^{t2} and H-2^{t3} which differ in the <u>Ir-C</u>(?) region. This region does not contain any known <u>Ir</u> genes but does control differences in Ia antigens between these two <u>H-2</u> chromosomes and does exhibit a mixed lymphocyte reaction stimulated primarily by T cells. Such evidence is clearly preliminary and could be radically altered by the finding of specific <u>Ir</u> genes mapping in this region, but on present evidence it appears that <u>Ir</u> genes may be readily separable, through the use of <u>H-2</u> recombinant congenic strains, from Ia antigens and from the other major functions of the <u>I</u> region. This evidence thus constitutes a beginning analysis of the interrelationship between the various functions controlled by the <u>I</u> region, and should hopefully lead to an identification of the nature and cellular site of expression of the <u>Ir</u> gene products.

REFERENCES

1. McDevitt, H.O. and Benacerraf, B. Adv. Immunol. <u>11</u>, 31 (1969).
2. McDevitt, H.O. and Landy, M. (eds.) Genetic Control of Immune Responsiveness: Relationship to Disease Susceptibility. Academic Press, New York (1972).
3. Benacerraf, B. and McDevitt, H.O. Science <u>175</u>, 273 (1972).
4. Katz, D.H., Hamaoka, T., Dorf, M.E., Maurer, P.H., and Benacerraf, B. J. Exp. Med. <u>138</u>, 734 (1973).
5. Hämmerling, G.J., Deak, B.D., Mauve, G., Hämmerling, U., and McDevitt, H.O. Immunogenetics <u>1</u>, in press (1974).
6. Bechtol, K.B., Wegmann, T.G., Freed, J.H., Grumet, F.C., Chesebro, B.W., Herzenberg, L.A., and McDevitt, H.O. Cellular Immunol. (in press, 1974).
7. Bechtol, K.B. and McDevitt, H.O. Manuscript in preparation.
8. Mozes, E. and Shearer, G.M. J. Exp. Med. <u>134</u>, 141 (1971).
9. Shearer, G.M., Mozes, E., and Sela, M. J. Exp. Med. <u>135</u>, 1009 (1972).
10. Shevach, E.M. and Rosenthal, A.S. J. Exp. Med. <u>138</u>, 1213 (1973).
11. Shevach, E.M., Paul, W.E., and Green, I. J. Exp. Med. <u>136</u>, 1207 (1972).
12. Hämmerling, G.J. and McDevitt, H.O. J. Immunol. <u>112</u>, in press (1974).

13. Hämmerling, G.J. and McDevitt, H.O. J. Immunol. 112, in press (1974).
14. Basten, A., Sprent, J., and Miller, J.F.A.P. Nature, New Biol. 235, 178 (1971).
15. Julius, M.H., Simpson, E., and Herzenberg, L.A. Europ. J. Immunol. 3, 345 (1973).
16. McDevitt, H.O. and Sela, M. J. Exp. Med. 126, 969 (1967).
17. Lonai, P. Fed. Proc. 32, 993a (1973).
18. Roelants, G., Forni, L., and Pernis, B. J. Exp. Med. 137, 1060 (1973).
19. Warner, N.L. In: Contemporary Topics in Immunobiology, vol. 1 (ed. Hanna, M.G., Jr.) Plenum Press, New York and London, 1972, p. 87.
20. McDevitt, H.O., Bechtol, K.B., Freed, J.H., Hämmerling, G.J., and Lonai, P. Ann. Immunol. (Inst. Pasteur) 125 C, 175 (1974).
21. Lonai, P. and McDevitt, H.O. Manuscript in preparation.
22. Shreffler, D.C., David, C., Götze, D., Klein, J., McDevitt, H.O., and Sachs, D. Immunogenetics 1, in press (1974).
23. David, C.S., Shreffler, D.C., and Frelinger, J.A. Proc. Nat. Acad. Sci., USA 70, 2509 (1974).
24. Sachs, D.H. and Cone, J.L. J. Exp. Med. 138, 1289 (1973).
25. Shreffler, D.C., David, C.S., and Frelinger, J.A. Personal communication.
26. Hauptfeld, V., Hauptfeld, M. and Klein, J. J. Immunol. in press (1974).
27. Götze, D., Reisfeld, R.A., and Klein, J. J. Exp. Med. 138, 1003-1008 (1973).
28. Hauptfeld, V., Klein, D., and Klein, J. Science 181, 167-169 (1973).
29. Lonai, P. Manuscript in preparation.
30. Bach, F.H., Widmer, M.B., Bach, M.L., and Klein, J. J. Exp. Med. 136, 1430 (1972).
31. Klein, J. and Park, J.M. J. Exp. Med. 137, 1213 (1973).
32. Lozner, E.C., Sachs, D.H., Shearer, G.M., and Terry, W.D. Science 183, 757 (1974).
33. Cullen, S.E., David, C.S., Shreffler, D.C., and Nathenson, S.G. Proc. Nat. Acad. Sci. USA in press (1974).
34. Vitetta, E.S., Klein, J. and Uhr, J.W. Immunogenetics 1, in press (1974).
35. Laemmli, U.K. Nature 227, 680 (1970).

36. Gallily, R. and Feldmann, M. Immunology 12, 197 (1967).
37. Scheid, M., Boyse, E.A., Carswell, E.A., and Old, L.J. J. Exp. Med. 135, 938 (1972).
38. Tyan, M.L., Cole, L.J., and Herzenberg, L.A. Proc. Soc. Exp. Biol. Med. 124, 1161 (1967).
39. McDevitt, H.O. and Sela, M. J. Exp. Med. 122, 517 (1965).
40. Lonai, P. and McDevitt, H.O. Manuscript in preparation.
41. Harrison, M.R. and Paul, W.E. J. Exp. Med. 138, 1602 (1973).
42. Shreffler, D.C. Personal communication.
43. Fathman, C.G., Schwartz, R.H., Handwerger, B.S., Karpf, M., Paul, W.E., and Sachs, D. Manuscript in preparation.
44. Mozes, E., McDevitt, H.O., Jaton, J-C., and Sela, M. J. Exp. Med. 130, 1263 (1969).
45. Bluestein, H.G., Green, I., Maurer, P.H. and Benacerraf, B. J. Exp. Med. 135, 98 (1972).
46. Mozes, E. and Shearer, G.M. J. Exp. Med. 134, 141 (1971).
47. Klinman, N.R., Press, J.L., Pickard, A., Woodland, R., and Dewey, A.F. this volume (1974).
48. Meo, T. and Shreffler, D.C. Personal communication.